# TYPE A BEHAVIOR PATTERN

# TYPE A BEHAVIOR PATTERN

## RESEARCH, THEORY, AND INTERVENTION

Editors

B. KENT HOUSTON AND C. R. SNYDER
University of Kansas

WILEY

A Wiley-Interscience Publication

John Wiley & Sons

New York     Chichester     Brisbane     Toronto     Singapore

*Library of Congress Cataloging-in-Publication Data:*

Type A behavior pattern: research, theory, and intervention/ edited
  by B. Kent Houston and C. R. Snyder.
       p.     cm.—(Wiley series on health psychology/behavioral
  medicine)
     "A Wiley–Interscience publication."
     Updated and revised papers presented at a conference held in
  Lawrence, Kan., May 9–10, 1986.
     Includes bibliographies.
     ISBN 0-471-84591-4
     1. Coronary heart diseases—Psychosomatic aspects—Congresses.
  2. Type A behavior—Congresses.     I. Houston, B. Kent.     II. Snyder,
  C. R.     III. Series.
     [DNLM: 1. Coronary Disease—etiology—congresses.     2. Coronary
  Disease—prevention & control—congresses.     3. Type A Personality—
  congresses.     WG 300 T991]
  RC685.C6T97 1988
  616.1'2308—dc19

*To*
*Ray H. Rosenman, M.D., and Meyer Friedman, M.D.,*
*whose pioneering work provided the occasion for this book*

# Contributors

JOHN C. BAREFOOT, PH.D.   Medical Research Assistant Professor. Behavioral Medicine Research Center, Department of Psychiatry, Duke University Medical Center, Durham, North Carolina

GEORGE W. BLACK, M.P.H.   Senior Biostatistician, Department of Behavioral Medicine, SRI International, Menlo Park, California

JONATHAN D. CANICK, PH.D.   Research Associate, Biophysical Research Group, Langley Porter Psychiatric Institute, University of California, San Francisco, California

DORIT CARMELLI, PH.D.   Senior Biostatistician, Department of Behavioral Medicine, SRI International, Menlo Park, California

WILLIAM P. CASTELLI, M.D.   Director, Framingham Heart Study, National Heart, Lung, and Blood Institute, Bethesda, Maryland

MARGARET A. CHESNEY, PH.D.   Adjunct Associate Professor of Epidemiology and Behavioral Medicine, Department of Epidemiology and International Health, School of Medicine, University of California, San Francisco, California

RICHARD J. CONTRADA, PH.D.   Assistant Professor, Department of Psychology, Rutgers University, New Brunswick, New Jersey

ELAINE D. EAKER, Sc.D.    Behavioral Epidemiologist, Epidemiology and Biometry Program, National Heart, Lung, and Blood Institute, Bethesda, Maryland

JANEL K. HARRIS, PH.D.    Assistant Professor, Counseling Psychology Department, University of Southern Mississippi, Hattiesburg, Mississippi

SUZANNE G. HAYNES, PH.D.    Chief, Medical Statistics Branch, Division of Health Statistics, National Center for Health Statistics, Hyattsville, Maryland

MICHAEL H. L. HECKER, PH.D.    Senior Behavioral Scientist, Department of Behavioral Medicine, SRI International, Menlo Park, California

D. ROBIN HILL, M.A.    Doctoral Candidate, Department of Medical Psychology, Uniformed Services University of the Health Sciences, Bethesda, Maryland

B. KENT HOUSTON, PH.D.    Professor of Psychology, Department of Psychology, University of Kansas, Lawrence, Kansas

DAVID S. KRANTZ, PH.D.    Professor, Department of Medical Psychology, Uniformed Services University of the Health Sciences, Bethesda, Maryland

KAREN A. MATTHEWS, PH.D.    Associate Professor of Psychiatry, Epidemiology, and Psychology, Department of Psychiatry, Western Psychiatric Institute and Clinic, University of Pittsburgh, Pittsburgh, Pennsylvania

DIANE F. O'ROURKE, PH.D.    Assistant Professor of Psychiatry and Behavioral Science, Department of Psychiatry, University of Arkansas for Medical Sciences, Little Rock, Arkansas

JERRY R. PATTILLO, M.S.    Doctoral Candidate in Counseling and Health Psychology, Stanford University, Stanford, California

VIRGINIA A. PRICE, PH.D.    Private Practice, Palo Alto, California

RAY H. ROSENMAN, M.D.    Senior Research Physician, Department of Behavioral Medicine, SRI International, Menlo Park, California

LARRY SCHERWITZ, PH.D.    Assistant Professor, Department of Dental Public Health and Hygiene, School of Dentistry, University of California, San Francisco, California

C. R. SNYDER, PH.D.    Director, Graduate Training Program in Clinical Psychology, Professor of Psychology, Department of Psychology, University of Kansas, Lawrence, Kansas

GARY E. SWAN, PH.D.    Senior Health Psychologist, Department of Behavioral Medicine, SRI International, Menlo Park, California

CARL E. THORESEN, PH.D.   Professor of Education and Psychology, Stanford University, Stanford, California

REDFORD B. WILLIAMS, JR., M.D.   Professor of Psychiatry, Associate Professor of Medicine, Director, Behavioral Medicine Research Center, Duke University Medical Center, Durham, North Carolina

# Series Preface

This series is addressed to clinicians and scientists who are interested in human behavior relevant to the promotion and maintenance of health and the prevention and treatment of illness. *Health psychology* and *behavioral medicine* are terms that refer to both the scientific investigation and inter-disciplinary integration of behavioral and biomedical knowledge and technology to prevention, diagnosis, treatment, and rehabilitation.

The major and purposely somewhat general areas of both health psychology and behavioral medicine which will receive greatest emphasis in this series are: theoretical issues of bio-psycho-social function, diagnosis, treatment, and maintenance; issues of organizational impact on human performance and an individual's impact on organizational functioning; development and implementation of technology for understanding, enchancing, or remediating human behavior and its impact on health and function; and clinical considerations with children and adults, alone, in groups, or in families that contribute to the scientific and practical/clinical knowledge of those charged with the care of patients.

The series encompasses considerations as intellectually broad as psychology and as numerous as the multitude of areas of evaluation treatment and prevention and maintenance that make up the field of medicine. It is the aim of the series to provide a vehicle which will focus attention on both the breadth and the interrelated nature of the sciences and practices making up health psychology and behavioral medicine.

THOMAS J. BOLL

*The University of Alabama in Birmingham*
*Birmingham, Alabama*

# Preface

The Type A behavior pattern is probably the most widely known and extensively researched psychological variable that has been associated with cardiovascular disease. Research, theory, and clinical attention concerning the Type A behavior pattern span a period of almost 30 years. Several issues concerning Type A that have been addressed in the past continue to be discussed in the present. For example: How is the Type A behavior pattern defined? How is it assessed? What is the evidence that the Type A behavior pattern is associated with cardiovascular disease? What are the processes that are hypothesized to link the Type A behavior pattern and cardiovascular disease? What evidence is there for these processes? What are the origins of Type A behavior? Can Type A behavior be effectively altered? In addition, several issues concerning Type A have emerged in recent years. For example: Is the Type A behavior pattern a risk factor for women? What are the "toxic" components of Type A? Is Type A dead as a risk factor? Is hostility succeeding Type A as the major coronary-prone behavior? Thus Type A is at the crossroads, and the purpose of the present volume is to take stock of current knowledge concerning Type A and explore what the future directions may be in regard to this important topic.

This book grew out of a conference on Type A that was held in Lawrence, Kansas, May 9 and 10, 1986. The conference was the first in the Kansas University Series in Clinical Psychology. After the major issues regarding Type A were identified, scientists who were well known for their theoretical and/or empirical work concerning the issues were invited to make presentations at the conference. Each participant then prepared a chapter for this volume based on his or her presentation. This book, then, represents the collective wisdom of scientists of diverse training: health psychology, medicine, and epidemiology. Moreover, the volume should be of value to clinical, counseling, personality, social, and other psychologists who are interested in health psychology, and counselors, social workers, physicians, and other professionals who are interested in health psychology and behavioral medicine.

A number of individuals deserve our thanks for their assistance in preparing this volume. The faculty members, postdoctoral students, and predoctoral students of the Clinical Psychology Program at the University of Kansas played a key role in this project. Special thanks go to Nancy Hughes, who performed essential administrative work for the conference, and Janel Harris and Diane O'Rourke, who contributed significantly to the editing of the chapters. Finally, we would like to thank Herb Reich, our editor at Wiley, who gave helpful input at various stages in the preparation of this book.

B. Kent Houston
C. R. Snyder

*Lawrence, Kansas*
*March 1988*

# Contents

# TYPE A BEHAVIOR PATTERN

# 1

# Introduction

## B. KENT HOUSTON

Despite considerable advances in research and practice over the past three decades, cardiovascular disease remains the leading cause of death in the United States. Although there are other kinds of cardiovascular disease, including hypertension, stroke, and chronic diseases of the heart muscle or membranes, coronary heart disease (CHD) accounts for the vast majority of deaths from cardiovascular disease (American Heart Association, 1987). Moreover, approximately 45 percent of the deaths from CHD annually are premature, occurring in individuals under 65. Furthermore, CHD is a chronic disease with which approximately 4.8 million people in the United States must contend. Because of its great prevalence and the toll it takes on relatively young people, considerable attention has been given to investigating causes and interventions for CHD.

*Coronary heart disease* is the term given to cardiovascular diseases that are characterized by an inadequate supply of oxygen to the heart. The major symptomatic forms of CHD are angina pectoris, that is, severe chest pain, and myocardial infarction (MI), that is, heart attack. Coronary atherosclerosis (narrowing of coronary arteries) is considered the common substrate for the different forms of CHD.

1

There are a number of factors that traditionally have been regarded as conferring risk for CHD, among which are age, high blood pressure, diabetes, cigarette smoking, obesity, high serum cholesterol level, and low levels of physical activity (American Heart Association, 1987). It appears, however, that the traditional risk factors are unable to account for the majority of new cases of CHD (Jenkins, 1971). Recognition of this has spurred interest in considering the role that personality, behavioral, and social factors may play in the development of CHD.

Prior to the 1950s, several clinicians (Dunbar, 1943; Kemple, 1945; Menninger & Menninger, 1936; Osler, 1892) observed that certain personality or behavioral attributes, such as being hard driving, ambitious, aggressive, and so forth, seemed to characterize coronary-prone individuals. However, these observations had very limited effect on research and theory concerning risk for CHD.

It was not until work begun in the mid-1950s by cardiologists Friedman and Rosenman on the Type A behavior pattern (TABP) that serious, widespread consideration was given to the role that personality and/or behavioral factors may play in CHD. Individuals exhibiting the TABP are said to be characterized by impatience, chronic time urgency, enhanced competitiveness, aggressive drive, and hostility (Rosenman, 1978).

The TABP gained attention and some scientific credibility as investigators reported finding associations between the TABP and prevalence of CHD in retrospective studies (see Jenkins, 1971). The TABP gained more attention and substantially more scientific credibility when an association between the TABP and the incidence of CHD was found in a prospective study, namely, the Western Collaborative Group Study (WCGS) (Rosenman, et al., 1975), and investigators reported finding associations between the TABP and extent of coronary atherosclerosis (see Jenkins, 1976).

Enthusiasm regarding the Type A concept burgeoned in the 1970s. Widespread interest in Type A was stimulated by the publication in 1974 of a book for a general audience entitled *Type A Behavior and Your Heart* by Meyer Friedman and Ray Rosenman. In the scientific community, a growing number of investigators devoted attention to issues of the assessment of TABP, the physiological processes that might link Type A and CHD, the psychosocial correlates of Type A, the development of the TABP, and interventions for Type A. In this vein, an influential book entitled *Behavior Patterns, Stress, and Coronary Disease*, by David Glass, appeared in 1977; this book reviewed an extensive program of research concerning the psychosocial correlates of Type A.

Interest in the TABP and the evidence linking it to CHD was sufficient that the National Heart, Lung, and Blood Institute (NHLBI) sponsored a multidisciplinary conference, the Forum on Coronary-Prone Behavior, which was held in 1977 to review intensively the scientific status of the TABP. The conference addressed five major issues: (1) What evidence was there concerning the possible association between the TABP and CHD? (2) How is the TABP assessed? (3) What are the physiological processes that link the TABP with CHD? (4) How does Type A behavior develop? and (5) What interventions alter the TABP? The review of the literature regarding these issues that emanated from the conference was published in 1978 in another influential book entitled *Coronary-Prone Behavior* (Dembroski, Weiss, Shields, Haynes, & Feinleib, 1978).

Also in 1978, the NHLBI sponsored a conference of distinguished scientists who were "neutral" on the topic of Type A. The charge to this group was to carefully review and evaluate the proceedings of the previous year's Forum on Coronary-Prone Behavior, as well as all other data related to the TABP and CHD. The conclusion of this group was that Type A behavior was associated with an increased risk for CHD in employed, middle-aged U.S. citizens over and above that conferred by the traditional risk factors (Review Panel, 1981). Moreover, it was concluded that the risk conferred by Type A was comparable to the relative risk associated with the traditional risk factors. The review panel's findings were published in 1981 and stood as a landmark because, for the first time, a psychosocial factor had received authoritative recognition as a risk factor for CHD.

For many scientists and practitioners, however, the enthusiasm regarding Type A began to turn to ambivalence in the late 1970s and the early 1980s when reports appeared of failures to find associations between measures of Type A and coronary atherosclerosis. For some who were working in the area, the ambivalence changed to skepticism with the appearance in the 1980s of studies that reported failures to find associations between measures of Type A and incidence of CHD (see Matthews & Haynes, 1986). What had happened? Was global Type A no longer a risk factor? Were there assessment or other methodological problems with the more recent studies that obscured relations with Type A? Were there moderating variables that had been unaccounted for which were obscuring direct relations with Type A?

During the late 1970s and the early 1980s, certain other issues relevant to Type A also emerged or grew in prominence. One issue was whether Type A is a coronary-prone behavior in women. Another issue focused on the theoretical underpinnings of Type A. Yet another was whether only certain components of the TABP or characteristics associated with it confer risk of CHD.

This brief chronology of the history of the Type A concept brings us to the present. Where are we today in regard to this concept, and what will happen to the TABP in subsequent years? We find ourselves at a point where it is necessary to reevaluate the issues regarding Type A that have been of interest in this area for some time, to examine the issues that have emerged more recently, and to consider issues that may signal future directions. The chapters in this volume address these issues.

The first contributed chapter in this book is an overview of the TABP by one of its cooriginators, Ray Rosenman, and his colleagues. In this chapter, "Definition, Assessment, and Evolution of the Type A Behavior Pattern," Rosenman, Swan, and Carmelli elaborate on the definition of the TABP, review the measures of the TABP, survey the construct validation of Type A, and comment on some of the more recent issues regarding Type A, for example, which components may be coronary prone, the implications of research relating hostility to cardiovascular disease, and so on.

The next three chapters focus on studies that have examined the relations between Type A and coronary atherosclerosis and/or CHD. The first two of these chapters give special attention to the studies that have obtained null findings. Scherwitz, in Chapter 3, "Interviewer Behaviors in the Western Collaborative Group Study and the Multiple Risk Factor Intervention Trial Structured Interviews," discusses possible reasons for the null findings. In particular, Scherwitz focuses on differences in the style in which the Structured Interview (SI) method for assessing Type A has been given in recent years, and compares this interview style to that used in the WCGS in which a positive relation was found between the TABP and CHD.

In Chapter 4, "The Association of Type A Behavior with Cardiovascular Disease—Update and Critical Review," Haynes and Matthews critically review the studies relating Type A to CHD, coronary atherosclerosis, and other health outcomes. Further, as an outgrowth of their discussion of possible reasons for some of the recent null findings regarding Type A, they call for more consideration of how work and family milieu and other personality characteristics may influence the risk of Type A's for developing CHD.

Eaker and Castelli, in Chapter 5 "Type A Behavior and Coronary Heart Disease in Women: Fourteen-Year Incidence from the Framingham Study," give special attention to women in regard to the relation between Type A as measured by the Framingham Type A Scale and CHD.

Thoresen and Pattillo, in Chapter 6, "Exploring the Type A Behavior Pattern in Children and Adolescents," focus primarily on the issue of how Type A develops. First, they review procedures for measuring Type A in children and adolescents, the construct validity of these procedures, and research regarding the relative influence of nature and nurture on the development of Type A. Additionally, Thoresen and Pattillo include some thought-provoking theoretical considerations in their discussion of the research regarding parental influence on children's TABP.

In Chapter 7, "Self-Reference and Coronary Heart Disease Risk," Scherwitz and Canick review the intriguing research on self-referencing, cardiovascular reactivity, coronary atherosclerosis, and CHD. They also include some stimulating theoretical considerations concerning Type A, hostility, and social support in their discussion of this research.

The next three chapters address in one fashion or another the topic of Type A components. Chesney, Hecker, and Black devote the initial portion of Chapter 8, "Coronary-Prone Components of Type A Behavior in the

WCGS: A New Methodology," to a review of the previous attempts to identify the components of the TABP that predict coronary atherosclerosis, CHD, and cardiovascular reactivity. Then they describe their work, which involves examining the various components of the TABP that are predictive of CHD in the WCGS. In their presentation, they describe the components that were examined and the scoring criteria that were used. Hostility was one, but only one, of the components that was found to predict incidence of CHD in their analysis.

After reviewing some reasons for the recent null findings regarding relations between Type A and coronary atherosclerosis and CHD, the major portion of Williams and Barefoot's chapter, "Coronary-Prone Behavior: The Emerging Role of the Hostility Complex," is a review of the evidence that hostility is the crucial coronary-prone behavior. Because there is evidence that coronary atherosclerosis and CHD are predicted by somewhat different methods for measuring hostility, namely, the SI and the Cook-Medley Hostility scale from the MMPI, the term *hostility complex* is used to refer to the conceptual domain that encompasses these two measures. The chapter concludes with a discussion of the physiological responses that may mediate the relation between coronary-prone behavior and CHD.

Stimulated by the notion that exaggerated physiological responses may contribute to the relation between Type A and CHD, considerable research has been conducted on the relation between Type A and physiological responsivity to various stimulus situations. This research is reviewed in Chapter 10, "Cardiovascular and Neuroendocrine Reactivity, Global Type A, and Components of Type A Behavior," by Houston. Additionally, possible methods for improving the prediction of physiological responsivity are discussed. These include administering the SI in a facilitative style (as discussed in the chapter by Scherwitz) and using cluster analysis to identify people with different profiles of Type A components.

Rather than considering physiological reactivity as a consequence of Type A behavior and certain eliciting conditions, Contrada, Krantz, and Hill, in Chapter 11, "Type A Behavior, Emotion, and Psychophysiological Reactivity: Psychological and Biological Interactions," review evidence concerning the hypothesis that a predisposition for reactivity influences Type A behavior, or at least certain components of Type A behavior. Such an approach not only emphasizes the role of biology in the origins of Type A, but also delineates the process by which biology may enact this role.

The issue of intervention for Type A is addressed in Chapter 12, "Research and Clinical Issues in Treating Type A Behavior," by Virginia Price. After a brief review of previous intervention studies, Price describes a large-scale intervention study, the Recurrent Coronary Prevention Project (RCPP), that was conducted on individuals who had survived a heart attack. She then addresses a variety of issues regarding elements of intervention programs, measures of outcome, and populations to treat. Additionally, she focuses on an issue that should be part of any behavior change program, that is, emphasizing those behaviors to be encouraged (Type B behaviors) rather than attending solely to those behaviors (Type A behaviors) to be discouraged.

A wide array of interesting and sometimes controversial topics are covered by the contributors. In the final, summary chapter, an attempt is made by O'Rourke, Houston, Harris, and Snyder to underscore some of the topics regarding Type A that recurred across chapters, as well as to highlight some of the intriguing current trends and future directions in this fascinating area.

There is little doubt that the Type A construct has attracted popular interest and has captured the attention of a great number of scientists from different disciplines. Whether the concept is to continue as a viable one, however, will depend upon future work. The authors of this book provide current knowledge about the Type A behavior pattern, and they give us a glimpse of the key issues that need to be explored in the future.

At present, the Type A behavior pattern is undergoing a reevaluation with regard to its measurement and status as a coronary-prone behavior. Additionally, psychosocial variables associated in one way or another with the TABP, namely, hostility, self-referencing, and so on, are receiving considerable attention in regard to their measurement and status as coronary-prone behaviors. The future for research on coronary-prone behaviors promises to be lively.

## REFERENCES

American Heart Association. (1987). *1987 Heart facts*. Dallas, TX: American Heart Association.

Dembroski, T. M., Weiss, S. M., Shields, J. L., Haynes, S. G., & Feinleib, M. (Eds.). (1978). *Coronary-prone behavior*, New York: Springer-Verlag.

Dunbar, H. F. (1943). *Psychosomatic diagnosis*. New York: Paul B. Hoeber.

Friedman, M., & Rosenman, R. H. (1974). *Type A behavior and your heart*. New York: Knopf.

Glass, D. C. (1977). *Behavior patterns, stress, and coronary disease*. Hillsdale, NJ: Erlbaum.

Jenkins, C. D. (1971). Psychologic and social precursors of coronary disease. *New England Journal of Medicine, 284*, 244–255, 307–317.

Jenkins, C. D. (1976). Recent evidence supporting psychologic and social risk factors for coronary disease. *New England Journal of Medicine, 294*, 987–994, 1033–1038.

Kemple, C. (1945). Rorschach method and psychosomatic diagnosis: Personality traits of patients with rheumatic disease, hypertension, and cardiovascular disease, coronary occlusion and fracture. *Psychosomatic Medicine, 7*, 85–89.

Matthews, K. A., & Haynes, S. G. (1986). Type A behavior pattern and coronary disease risk: Update and critical evaluation. *American Journal of Epidemiology, 123*, 923–958.

Menninger, K. A., & Menninger, W. C. (1936). Psychoanalytic observations in cardiac disorders. *American Heart Journal, 11*, 10.

Osler, W. (1892). *Lectures on angina pectoris and allied states*. New York: Appleton.

The Review Panel on Coronary-Prone Behavior and Coronary Heart Disease. (1981). Coronary-prone behavior and coronary heart disease: A critical review. *Circulation, 63*, 1199–1215.

Rosenman, R. H. (1978). The interview method of assessment of the coronary-prone behavior pattern. In T. M. Dembroski, S. M. Weiss, J. L. Shields, S. G. Haynes, & M. Feinleib (Eds.), *Coronary-prone behavior*. New York: Springer-Verlag.

Rosenman, R. H., Brand, R. J., Jenkins, C. D., Friedman, M., Straus, R., & Wurm, M. (1975). Coronary heart disease in the Western Collaborative Group Study: Final follow-up experience of 8½ years. *Journal of the American Medical Association, 233*, 872–877.

# 2

# Definition, Assessment, and Evolution of the Type A Behavior Pattern

RAY H. ROSENMAN, GARY E. SWAN,
AND DORIT CARMELLI

## DEFINITION OF TYPE A BEHAVIOR PATTERN

The concept of the Type A behavior pattern (TABP) evolved in the mid-1950s after repeated observation of a relatively specific action–emotion complex particularly in younger and middle-aged patients with coronary heart disease (CHD). These patients, although they rarely despaired of losing, appeared to be in a chronic struggle to achieve poorly defined goals or to obtain an excessive number of things from their environment and to be in habitual conflict with others and with time. It was observed that these patients grappled aggressively with their perceived challenges and, in this regard, appeared to differ from individuals with anxiety or neuroses who tend to retreat from such challenges.

In the formulation of the TABP, Type A individuals of both sexes were considered to have the following characteristics: (1) an intense, sustained drive to achieve self-selected but often poorly defined goals; (2) a profound inclination and eagerness to compete; (3) a persistent desire for recognition and advancement; (4) a continuous involvement in multiple and diverse functions subject to time restrictions; (5) habitual propensity to accelerate the rate of execution of most physical and mental functions; (6) extraordinary mental and physical alertness; and (7) aggressive and hostile feelings (Friedman & Rosenman, 1959; Rosenman & Friedman, 1961; Rosenman et al., 1964).

The marked increase of CHD in most industrialized societies in the twentieth century (Rosenman & Chesney, 1982) may have resulted, in part, because these societies fostered the TABP by offering rewards to those who performed more quickly, aggressively, and competitively. The increased incidence of CHD has been associated with urbanization and population densification and the consequent increased need for finely synchronized, interdependent services. This new environment stimulated competitiveness and the hostility–anger dimensions that are associated with the unique new stresses not experienced either by earlier generations or by nonindustrialized contemporary populations. Therefore it was considered that the TABP may not stem solely from personality attributes, but rather that this cluster of specific behaviors and style of living emerges from the interaction of certain personality attributes with the environmental milieu (Rosenman, 1978). It is the enhanced competitiveness of Type A persons that leads to an aggressive and ambitious achievement orientation, increased mental and physical alertness, muscular tension, and explosive and rapid stylistics of speech. An associated chronic sense of time urgency leads to restlessness, impatience, and the habitual acceleration of most activities. This in turn may result in irritability and the enhanced potential for Type A hostility and anger, which is covert in many Type A individuals.

The TABP is thus defined as an action–emotion complex involving: (1) behavioral dispositions (e.g., ambitiousness, aggressiveness, competitiveness, and impatience); (2) specific behaviors (e.g., muscle tenseness, alertness, rapid and emphatic speech stylistics, and accelerated pace of most activities); and (3) emotional responses (e.g., irritation, hostility, and anger).

The TABP is considered to be neither a stressor situation nor a distressed response, and as such it is not synonymous with *stress*. It is based on an underlying set of values, thoughts, and approaches to interpersonal relationships; in turn these are manifested by characteristic gestures, facial expressions, respiratory pattern, motor activity and pace, and speech stylistics. It should be emphasized that the TABP stems from the interaction of an individual's personality attributes and predispositions, environmental milieu, and perception of milieu stressors as challenges. Because of these interactive processes, an aggressive, hostile, and time-urgent style of living emerges that is often associated with increased psychophysiological arousal.

In part, the TABP may be considered a response to maintain control over events that threaten the individual's sense of control over the environment (Glass, 1977, 1982). This attempt at control is reflected in the Type A drive and accelerated pace, and it often includes a vocational commitment in which other aspects of life are neglected.

In its conceptualization, the TABP was considered to be a relatively specific cluster of behaviors that were not equated with anxiety, worry, fear, depression, or neurosis. A converse, Type B, behavior pattern was conceived as being the relative absence of the TABP. Type B individuals were considered to be more relaxed, easygoing, and readily satisfied, and less concerned with achievement and acquisition needs. Over time it became apparent that the Type B behavior pattern was not merely the absence of most Type A behaviors; rather, Type B appeared to reflect a different coping style characterized by a lack of time urgency, impatience, and hostile responses (Rosenman & Chesney, 1982).

## ASSESSMENT OF THE TYPE A BEHAVIOR PATTERN BY THE STRUCTURED INTERVIEW

A Structured Interview (SI) was developed to assess TABP in the Western Collaborative Group Study (WCGS) (Rosenman, 1978; Rosenman et al., 1964). This was done to allow the senior author to assess the behavior patterns of all WCGS subjects from audiotaped SIs without knowledge of other risk factors.

The SI evolved over several years, during which time those items that were most capable of eliciting Type A were selected from a larger pool of questions. Specific questions originally were developed in order to assess the various component behaviors of the global TABP, and multiple questions were developed for each component behavior in order to provide a better basis for judgments. The assessment of the behaviors from the SI is based on the content of answers to the questions, speech stylistics, and overt nonverbal mannerisms and behaviors that are exhibited during the interview. Greater weight is given to the voice stylistics and observed psychomotor and other nonverbal behaviors than to the verbal reports, since many subjects have poor insight into their behaviors.

Adminstration of the SI should take the form of a challenge interview because Type A individuals respond to situational challenges more than do Type B individuals (Humphries, Carver, & Neumann, 1983). Thus interviewers are taught to ask questions in a mildly challenging manner and to interject spontaneous interruptions during the respondents' answers. Assessment of the intensity of the TABP is based on the various verbal responses and overt behaviors that are aroused in predisposed individuals in part by questions that were purposely designed to stimulate recall of salient milieu stressors, and in part by the challenging style and occasional interruptions of an adept interviewer.

The SI requires about 15 minutes for a trained interviewer to administer. Although it has not been changed substantially since its development (Rosenman et al., 1964), several questions that were found to be redundant have been eliminated. The idea that the SI might be used by other investigators was not considered at the time it was developed. When psychologists became interested in the TABP and sought training in the administration of the SI, many had difficulty with the concept of an interview that had been developed to provide a challenge and give the least weight to answer content. Accordingly, in order to avoid making the SI into a routinized question-and-answer interview, the method of instruction was modified to teach interviewers to provide greater challenge and to interrupt subjects at suitable times.

Although the assessments of behavior from the SI can provide a dichotomous or a multiple-point Type A–Type B classification (depending primarily on a subject's exhibiting a relatively greater or lesser degree of the respective patterns), it should be emphasized that the TABP is not a trait variable; moreover, Type A and Type B behavior patterns have both quantitative and qualitative differences, and they are the product of an interaction among several factors in a given subject. Thus the behavior pattern is a typology and as such does not provide a true continuum for statistical or other purposes.

The SI was tape-recorded in the WCGS for later assessment of the behavior patterns. Although a score sheet was available for the interviewers to describe nonverbal behaviors, a videotaped interview provides those who later assess the behavior patterns with a far more suitable methodology. Details of the methodology used for the administration of the SI and for the assessment of the behavior patterns are provided elsewhere (Rosenman, 1978).

When appropriately administered and scored by trained persons, the SI provides assessments of the Type A and B behavior patterns with a remarkably high degree of interrater agreement (Belmaker, Pollin, Jenkins, & Brensike, 1976; Blumenthal, O'Toole, & Haney, 1984; Friedman, Hellerstein, Jones, & Eastwood, 1968; Jenkins, Rosenman, & Friedman, 1968; Multiple Risk Factor Intervention Trial Group, 1979; Schucker & Jacobs, 1977). In a recent study of 282 adults whose behavior patterns were scored from the SI on a scale varying from 2 to 16 categories of behaviors, the assessments again showed a very high interrater agreement (Van Harrison et al., 1986).

When assessed by the SI, the TABP has been found to exhibit considerable stability over time (Blumenthal et al., 1984; Jenkins et al., 1968; Keith, Lown, & Stare, 1965; Van Harrison et al., 1986). This stability was found recently to extend over a 10-year period in a large population of adult, male twins (Carmelli, Rosenman, & Chesney, in press) who comprised a subset of the NHLBI Twin Study of Cardiovascular Risk Factors (Feinleib et al., 1977).

In this study, 80 percent of subjects who were initially rated as Type A by the SI were rated similarly a decade later.

The SI has been translated for use in France and Belgium (Kittel et al., 1978), Germany and Czechoslovakia (Horvath, personal communication, 1979), and China (Bo-yuan, 1983). Additionally, versions of the SI have been developed for use with females (Waldron, 1978a, 1987b), undergraduate students (Dembroski, MacDougall, Shields, Pettito, & Lushene, 1978; MacDougall, Dembroski, & Musante, 1979; Scherwitz, Berton, & Leventhal, 1977), adolescents (Butensky, Forelli, Heebner, & Waldron, 1976; Gerace & Smith, 1985; Matthews & Siegel, 1982; Siegal & Leitch, 1981; Siegel, Matthews, & Leitch, 1981), and children (Gerace & Smith, 1985).

## ASSESSMENT OF THE TYPE A BEHAVIOR PATTERN BY OTHER MEASURES

There has been an ongoing attempt to assess TABP by self-report questionnaires or other methods that would obviate the complexities involved with the SI. The first and most studied methodology is the Jenkins Activity Survey (JAS) (Jenkins, Rosenman, & Friedman, 1967; Jenkins, Zyzanski, & Rosenman, 1979), which was developed from an item pool based on the questions asked in the SI (Rosenman, 1978). The items were selected on the basis of their ability to discriminate Type A and Type B subjects in the WCGS (Rosenman et al., 1964), and the JAS was refined to yield a composite Type A scale and three factor-analytically derived subscales (i.e., Speed and Impatience, Hard Driving, and Job Involvement). In comparison with the SI, the JAS was found to be a weaker predictor of CHD in the WCGS (Brand, Rosenman, Jenkins, Sholtz, & Zyzanski, 1986) and other studies (Verhagen, Nass, Appels, van Bastelaer, & Winnubst, 1980). On the more positive side, however, the JAS has evidenced cross-cultural validity (Jenkins et al., 1979; Kittel et al., 1978) and good reliability (Johnston & Shaper, 1983). A large part of the JAS's ability to predict CHD in the WCGS was found to be related to its ability to mimic the SI, but the JAS added nothing to the predictive strength of the SI (Brand et al., 1986). The subscales of the JAS were not found to predict CHD in the WCGS (Brand et al., 1986; Jenkins, Rosenman, & Zyzanski, 1974), and the JAS inadequately measures the TABP characteristics of competitive drive, impatience, and potential for hostility that are captured by the SI and that were found to be particularly predictive of CHD incidence in the WCGS (Matthews, Glass, Rosenman, & Bortner, 1977).

The JAS was found to correlate with the Bortner Type A scale (Bortner, 1969) by Johnston and Shaper (1983). In addition, the JAS was found to correlate modestly with the Novaco Anger Scale by Katz and Toben (1986) although the JAS is generally considered not to assess adequately the potential for hostility and anger that is characteristic of Type A behavior (Matthews,

1982). The JAS has not been found to be related to anxiety (Smith, Houston, & Zurawski, 1983) and other measures of emotional distress (Chesney, Black, Chadwick, & Rosenman, 1981; Glass, 1977; Smith & O'Keefe, 1985; Wadden, Anderson, Foster, & Love, 1983), but it has been found to be positively correlated with depression (Dimsdale, Hackett, Block, & Hutter, 1978) and neuroticism (Irvine, Lyle, & Allon, 1982).

The JAS has been found to be less predictive of physiologic arousal than the SI (Dembroski et al., 1978; Houston, 1983; Katz & Toben, 1986; Smith & O'Keefe, 1985). Although the JAS is related to the core components of the TABP as measured by the SI (Smith & O'Keefe, 1985), it only provides an index of personality and behavioral predispositions and thus does not adequately assess the TABP (Ditto, 1982).

Some amplification may be warranted in regard to the differences in what the SI and the JAS measure. For example, the JAS does not measure the speech stylistics and other nonverbal psychomotor behaviors that are central to the Type A construct (Matthews, Krantz, Dembroski, & Mac-Dougall, 1982). Among other things, the Speed and Impatience subscale of the JAS taps time pressure (Matthews et al., 1982) but confounds speed with a sense of time urgency and impatience (Carmelli et al., in press). This JAS subscale is correlated positively with emotional distress (Chesney, Black, Chadwick, & Rosenman, 1981) and shows a much lower test–retest correlation than does the Activity scale of the Thurstone Temperament Schedule (Carmelli et al., in press). The JAS also appears to measure different attributes than the Framingham Type A Scale (Matthews et al., 1982; Scherwitz et al., 1977; Smith & O'Keefe, 1985).

Thus the JAS captures some of the relevant content of the SI answers, but not the behaviors observed during the SI that are essential to the Type A construct and its relevance for CHD (Anderson & Waldron, 1983; Brand et al., 1986). Not surprisingly, the JAS correlates poorly with the TABP as measured by the SI (Anderson & Waldron, 1983; Chesney, Eagleston, & Rosenman, 1981; Irvine et al., 1982; MacDougall et al., 1979; Matthews et al., 1982). It must be concluded, therefore, that the JAS cannot properly be used to assess the TABP (Matthews et al., 1982; O'Looney & Harding, 1985).

A second self-report method for measuring the TABP is the Bortner Rating Scale (Bortner, 1969; Bortner & Rosenman, 1967). This questionnaire, answered on a bar-type scale, provides an assessment of various Type A behaviors but fails to measure the hostility component of TABP. It has been found to correlate positively with the JAS in samples from both the United States (Bortner, 1969) and Europe (Defourny & Frankignoul, 1973), to have good test–retest reliability (Johnston & Shaper, 1983; Price, 1979), and to correlate with many Type A behaviors assessed in adolescents by a version of the SI (Siegel & Leitch, 1981). Although Bass (1984) found that scores on the Bortner Rating Scale correlated positively with anxiety and neuroticism, these findings may be questioned because of the use of an inadequate method of assessing TABP and because such correlations were observed in males but not in females. Moreover, even though Bass, Cawley, and Wade (1983) observed that neuroticism is correlated with functional chest pains that occur in the absence of significant coronary artery disease, the Bortner Rating Scale has been found to correlate with the prevalence and incidence of myocardial infarction in several studies (French-Belgian Collaborative Group, 1982; Heller, 1979) where neuroticism was not related to myocardial infarction.

In an attempt to develop a different self-report method of assessment of the TABP, the senior author included the Thurstone Temperament Schedule (TTS) (Thurstone, 1953) and the Adjective Checklist (ACL) (Gough & Heilbrun, 1975) in a study of two groups of subjects. One sample was a subset of adult male twins who participated in the NHLBI study of cardiovascular risk factors (Feinleib et al., 1977) and the second sample was white-collar, employed males. The senior author viewed the ACL as a self-report measure that might be completed by subjects with relative accuracy, and the TTS as a relatively unbiased measure of Type A pace of activities. Moreover, the Activity scale of the TTS had been found to be predictive of the incidence of CHD in an early prospective study (Brozek, Keys, & Blackburn, 1966).

The findings in the group of twin subjects (Rosenman, Rahe, Borhani, & Feinleib, 1976) were confirmed in the second group of subjects (Chesney, Black, Chadwick, & Rosenman, 1981; Herman, Blumenthal, Black, & Chesney, 1981). The adjectives and derived scales of the ACL that correlated with Type A as measured by the SI were all congruent with the TABP construct, including Self-Confidence, Aggression, Dominance, Autonomy, Achievement, Self-Control, and Exhibition. The same was found for the TTS. High scorers on the Activity scale of the TTS are said to enjoy rapid psychomotor pace even when this is inappropriate, which is an apt description of a prominent Type A behavior. Other TTS scales that correlated with the TABP were Impulsiveness, Dominance, and Sociability (Rosenman 1976; Rosenman, Swan, & Carmelli, in press). The findings for the ACL have been confirmed by others (Blumenthal et al., 1985).

The TTS Activity scale has been found to correlate positively with the JAS Type A scale and its Speed and Impatience subscale. It shows a high test–retest correlation over a span of many years, and has evidenced the highest test–retest correlation among a variety of purported TABP self-report questionnaires (Carmelli et al., in press). It has not been found to correlate with anxiety (Smith et al., 1983) and appears to be the most valid self-report questionnaire in correlating with the TABP as assessed by the SI (Carmelli et al., in press; MacDougall et al., 1979; Mayes, Sime, & Ganster, 1984; Rosenman, Rahe, Borhani, & Feinleib, 1976).

The Framingham Type A Scale (FTAS) (Haynes, Levine, Scotch, Feinleib & Kannel, 1978) that was administered to participants in the Framingham Heart Study is a short self-report inventory derived from an extensive questionnaire dealing with a wide variety of psychosocial factors. The items selected for the FTAS assessing the subject's pace of activity, impatience, and time urgency appeared to be relevant for the TABP. Some of the items dealt with drive, fatigue, and work satisfactions, and these may account for the correlation of the FTAS with perceived daily stress, emotional lability, tension, anxiety, neuroticism, and general emotional distress (Chesney, Black, Chadwick, & Rosenman, 1981; Haynes, Levine, Scotch, Feinleib, & Kannel, 1978; Smith et al., 1983; Smith & O'Keefe, 1985). However, the FTAS is not strongly correlated with the TABP as assessed by the SI (Chesney, Eagleston, & Rosenman, 1981; Meininger, 1985) and probably measures only a small part of the TABP (Chesney, Eagleston, & Rosenman, 1981). The FTAS also has different psychological correlates than does the JAS. For example, the FTAS, but not the JAS, was found to be correlated with trait anxiety (Smith & O'Keefe, 1985).

There have been considerable research and speculation concerning the correlates of the TABP. In this vein, Eysenck and Fulker (1982) suggested that the TABP is not a unitary phenomenon and that some of its behaviors correlate with extroversion and some with neuroticism, but that the two aspects of TABP are not related. In another study by Chesney, Black, Chadwick, and Rosenman (1981), extroversion and impulsivity as measured by the Eysenck Personality Inventory (EPI) (Eysenck & Eysenck, 1968) were found to correlate positively with the TABP as measured by the SI.

Glass (1977) found that there were small possible correlations of the TABP with (1) self-esteem, self-confidence, and dominance as measured by the Texas Social Behavior Inventory; (2) need for achievement as measured by the Edwards Personal Preference Schedule; (3) Active, Sociable, and Impulsive scales on the EASI Temperament Survey; and (4) internal orientation on Rotter's I-E Scale. The TABP has been found to correlate positively with the Self-Acceptance, Dominance, and Extroversion scales of the California Psychological Inventory (Gough, 1956; Rosenman 1976, Rosenman, Swan, & Carmelli, in press). Caffrey (1968, 1969) reports positive correlations between the TABP and the Warm, Outgoing, Self-Assured, Assertive, Alert, Adventurous, and Strong Emotional Control scales of the Cattell 16-Personality Inventory. No significant correlations have been found between the TABP and the SCL-90-R (Derogatis, 1977), the State-Trait Anxiety Inventory (Spielberger, Gursuch, & Lushene, 1970), or with the Type A scales developed by Vickers (1973) (Caplan, Cobb, French, Harrison, & Pinneau, 1975; Caplan & Jones, 1975). As might be expected, the TABP has been found to correlate with the use of self-referencing (Scherwitz, Graham, Grandits, Buehler, & Billings, 1986; Scherwitz, McKelvain, & Laman, 1983).

Attempts also have been made to assess TABP by a specially developed voice test (Friedman, Brown, & Rosenman, 1975) and by a polygraph recording of physiologic responses while subjects read a speech out loud that was designed to elicit impatience and other psychomotor Type A behaviors (Friedman & Rosenman, 1960). Finally, there has been an attempt to score the behaviors observed during a modified SI in order to provide a quantitative assessment of TABP. The numerical score on this Videotaped Structured Interview (VSI) (Friedman & Powell, 1984) is the sum of observed discrete signs and symptoms and provides a continuous scale. However, the VSI has not been validated by other investigators, and its interrater agreement, test–retest reliability, and usefulness as a measure of the TABP and as a predictor of CHD remain to be demonstrated. The VSI purports to observe and score behaviors that are exhibited independent of interviewer challenges. However, the approach of the VSI seems inadequate because, as discussed previously in this chapter, it is the challenging and provocative circumstances of life in general and the SI in particular that elicit the TABP (Byrne, Rosenman, Schiller, & Chesney, 1985; Rosenman, 1978).

The various self-report measures that have been described in this section all show acceptable reliability, but they exhibit only modest correlations among themselves and with the SI (Matthews, 1982). Thus although such scales purport to measure the TABP, they have only marginal overlap because they assess different behavioral characteristics. Self-reports are concerned largely with individual perceptions of attitudes, attributes, and activities, and as such they do not capture the stylistics and psychomotor behaviors that are essential to the construct and assessment of the TABP. The fact that the patterns of intercorrelations among the self-report measures are complex and variable may reflect that the TABP is not a unitary phenomenon but rather a complex composite of behaviors (Byrne et al., 1985).

Although the various self-report measures do not tap the TABP as well as the SI, it may be useful briefly to consider their relative merits. In this regard, the TTS is concerned with pace of activity and the Bortner Type A scale covers a larger range of behaviors than the TTS. Both emphasize self-observed behaviors and thus more closely parallel the Type A construct than do the JAS and FTAS, which tend more to measure attitudes and inclinations (Byrne et al., 1985).

In summary, the SI, by including judgments of actual Type A behaviors observed during administration of a challenging interview, extends the breadth and scope of assessment more closely to fit the construct that portrays TABP as a set of overt behaviors that occur in association with and in response to relevant situational stressors (Byrne et al., 1985; Matthews, 1982). Thus the SI is much less likely to be influenced by occupational and other characteristics than are measures of attitudes and values. Moreover, the self-reports not only have important psychological differences among measures (Smith, Houston, & Zurawski, 1985), but also suffer in cross-cultural studies because of limited generalizability across diverse cultures and populations of items that are content dependent (Powell, 1984). This limitation is emphasized by the lack of correlation between the content of answers and observed behaviors during the SI (Hecker, Chesney, Black,

& Rosenman, 1981; Scherwitz et al., 1977). Moreover, poor insight and self-appraisal, as well as response bias, actually suggest that self-reports may be much less objective than the SI when the interview is administered and assessed by properly trained persons. Indeed, the original formulation of the Type A construct emphasized that TABP is an overt syndrome that is best assessed by observing the presence or absence of its characteristics during a specially structured interview (Rosenman, 1978; Rosenman, et al., 1964).

Before closing this section on assessment of the TABP, measurement of the TABP in children needs to be addressed. The first attempt to measure TABP in children used the ratings of teachers on various adult Type A characteristics in the Matthews Youth Test for Health (MYTH) (Matthews, 1978; Matthews & Angulo, 1980; Matthews & Siegel, 1982; Murray & Bruhn, 1983). Another approach known as the Hunter-Wolf method of ratings is based on self-assessments that are believed to avoid the measurement errors that might be made by teachers (Hunter et al., 1982; Hunter et al., 1985; Wolf, Sklov, Wenzl, Hunter, & Berenson, 1982). This group of investigators found that the Hunter-Wolf self-assessments and the MYTH teacher ratings were not measuring the same variables and that, in subjects 8 to 17 years old, the MYTH tends to measure hyperactivity rather than TABP (Hunter et al., 1985). However, Murray, Matthews, Blake, Prineas, and Gillum (1986) recently provided further evidence for the construct validity of the MYTH method of assessment based on the ratings of teachers, and showed that there are considerable similarities between Type A behaviors in adults and in children. Yet another method of assessing the TABP in children is the Miami SI (Gerace & Smith, 1985), which was found to have cross-cultural validation and a 91 percent test–retest rate of agreement. Using this method, Smith, Gerace, Christakis, and Kafatos (1985) found that children identified as Type A via the Miami SI scored higher on ratings by the MYTH method.

Although Hunter and colleagues (1985) believe that research on TABP in children has suffered from problems of concept identification, clarification, refinement, and the use of multiple methods of measurement, it would appear that the TABP can be identified at early ages (Bortner, Rosenman, & Friedman, 1970; Matthews, 1978) and is stable over time. Related to this latter point, Bergman and Magnusson (1986) found that the Type A and Type B behavior patterns (including ratings of aggressiveness, overambitiousness, overachievement, and motor hyperactivity) assessed at age 13 in Swedish subjects predicted a large percentage of similar behaviors when measured in the same subjects at age 27. In a comment related to the issue of stability, Murray and colleagues (1986) concluded that the pattern in children is consistent with Glass's (1982) conceptualization of the Type A individual as one who actively seeks to control the environment through verbal aggression and who overreacts to threats to that control.

## PSYCHOPHYSIOLOGICAL RESPONSES OF TYPE A AND TYPE B SUBJECTS

In the WCGS the standard risk factors for CHD showed only small correlations with the TABP, indicating that the higher CHD risk exhibited by Type A as compared with Type B subjects was largely independent of such variables (Rosenman, Brand, Scholtz, & Friedman, 1976). This finding stimulated an ongoing search for the possible mechanisms by which the TABP confers an increased risk for CHD. It was initially found that, relative to Type B males, male subjects with well-defined, coronary-prone TABP exhibited a greater rise of plasma norepinephrine (NE) in response to a challenging, competitive, cognitive task (Friedman, St. George, Byers, & Rosenman, 1960) and a greater urinary NE excretion in their daily occupational milieu (Friedman, Byers, Diamant, & Rosenman, 1975) than did paired Type B men. These early findings led to a large number of studies of psychophysiological responses in which situational variables have been experimentally manipulated in order to investigate possible differences in catecholamine and cardiovascular responses of Type A and Type B children and adults of both sexes. It is not possible here to cite the substantial relevent literature (for reviews, see Glass & Contrada, 1983; Houston, Chapter 10, this volume; Krantz & Durel, 1983; Matthews, 1982; Rosenman, in press; Rosenman & Chesney, 1982). In addition, these studies also have provided a second approach to construct validation of the Type A concept by examining the degree to which Type A and B subjects differ in hard-driving and competitive behavior, time urgency and impatience, aggression and hostility, suppression of fatigue, and response to threats to personal control during a wide variety of mental and physical tasks.

A substantial number of these studies have provided supporting evidence for the Type A construct by finding that under appropriate stimulus conditions Type A individuals are more likely than Type B individuals to exhibit competitiveness, impatience, aggression, denial of fatigue, irritability, hostility, and heightened coping ability. Additionally, many of these studies have found that, although not differing in their baseline levels from Type B subjects, Type A persons respond to a variety of laboratory challenge stressors with high plasma catecholamines and associated elevations of heart rate and blood pressure. Moreover, the stylistic and behavioral components of TABP (i.e., competitiveness, hostility, and time urgency for cognitive processing that is involved in decision making or problem solving) that are found to be most strongly related to the prediction of CHD also appear to be particularly related to the enhanced psychophysiological responses of Type A subjects (Diamond et al., 1984; Houston, Smith & Zurawski, in press; Ward et al., 1986).

Contrary to the aforementioned studies, a number of studies have not found reliable Type A–Type B differences in physiological responses during performance of various tasks. This is not surprising given the complexities of these responses that not only differ according to the nature of the stressor but also are strongly influenced by a wide variety of individual characteristics that are related to heart rate and blood pressure levels. Catecholamine and cardiovascular reactivity are related to a multitude of factors, including age, sex, body build, lean body weight, distribution of excess adipose tissue, level of physical conditioning, amount of sleep, fatigue, blood volume, habitual and recent intakes of glucose, alcohol, caffeine, nicotine, electrolytes, pharmacological agents that affect receptor density and responsiveness, position during testing, and many psychological and emotional dimensions. Unfortunately, many of the studies of psychophysiological responses have been done without regard to the aforementioned factors that are related to cardiovascular reactivity.

An increased reactivity is commonly ascribed to an increased outflow of neural activity from the brain to the heart and vascular smooth muscle that is based only on cognitive perception. However, in any given individual, this reactivity variously may be due to one or more of the following: (1) an increased release of NE with each neural impulse (an increase resulting from its greater production because of a defect in catecholamine synthesis); (2) a decreased uptake of NE at nerve endings (which therefore makes it more available to stimulate receptors); (3) an increased number of receptors (which enhances the response to released NE); (4) an increased contribution by nerve terminal stimulation of receptors on nerve endings; and (5) an increased responsiveness of receptors on the myocardium and vascular smooth muscle (Rosenman, in press).

In consideration of these and probably other important factors, it is not surprising to observe diverse findings by investigators who have reported data on the cardiovascular reactivity of Type A and Type B subjects. In part, a diversity of findings also may result when the TABP is assessed by self-report questionnaires rather than the SI (Rosenman, 1978). Moreover, the pattern of physiological responses is different for various laboratory-type stressors, as well as for the different behaviors that comprise the global pattern. The TABP is not a fixed personality type and thus will often be elicited only by appropriate stimuli, that is, those that can bring out the specific behaviors that are accompanied by a hyperadrenergic response (Humphries et al., 1983), and particularly those stimuli that present the subject with a perceived personal challenge (Krantz & Durel, 1983).

In general, the greatest Type A–Type B differences in physiological reactivity are observed during tasks that are difficult, involve time pressure, and/or require competition. There are important psychological differences among various laboratory stressor procedures (Smith, Houston, & Zurawski, 1985); therefore, it is not surprising that the greatest Type A–Type B differences occur in responses to situational stressors that are perceived as relevant challenges (Glass & Contrada, 1983). Moreover, such eliciting situations must produce a certain degree of *psychological* challenge; thus it follows that differences in Type A–Type B reactivity may be greater for mental than for physical stressors (Dembroski, MacDougall, Herd, & Shields, 1979; Ward et al., 1986).

Taken together, the studies do not suggest that Type A as compared to Type B subjects have any intrinsic differences in cardiovascular reactivity; rather, it appears that Type A individuals' greater perception of challenge in relevant stressors is associated with an exaggerated psychophysiological response. This latter conclusion is supported by the finding that, during performance of a challenging task, Type A subjects exhibit greater electrocardiographic changes that are adrenergically mediated (Scher, Hartmen, Furedy, & Heslegrave, 1986; Van Egeren, Fabrega, & Thornton, 1983).

Schneider and colleagues (1986) employed an experimental methodology involving the fact that pupil size provides a measure of alpha-1 adrenergic tone outside the cardiovascular system and that platelets concentrate and store catecholamines both in vitro and in vivo and thus reflect average circulating plasma catecholamine levels. In a study of 33 healthy male adults whose behavior patterns were rated by the SI, Schneider and colleagues found that Type A as compared to Type B subjects consistently exhibited larger pupillary diameters and significantly greater platelet epinephrine content. These findings lend support to the belief that well-defined Type A individuals respond to their environmental milieus with enhanced sympathetic neural traffic.

Krantz and Durel (1983) hypothesized that the overt expression of TABP may be due to an underlying psychobiological factor that induces an excessive sympathetic neural response to milieu stressors. However, to date there is little empirical support for their hypothesis.

## CONSTRUCT VALIDATION OF THE TYPE A CONCEPT

Construct validation for the concept of the TABP has proceeded along two lines. One approach has been to correlate the components of TABP (Rosenman at el., 1964) with responses on self-report indices of behaviors, personality, and sociodemographic status. A second approach has been to study behavioral and psychophysiological differences between Type A and Type B persons who are subjected to situational manipulations in the experimental laboratory. In this latter vein, the results of selected studies were summarized earlier.

The assessments of the TABP from the SI are found to be in substantial agreement with the direct observations of others in several studies (Caffrey, 1968, 1969; Friedman & Rosenman, 1959; Rosenman & Friedman, 1961). Regardless of the problems of self-report measures described earlier, there is a remarkable consistency of the cluster of traits measured by the various self-report questionnaires in relation to the Type A construct (Byrne et al., 1985; Chesney, Black, Chadwick, & Rosenman, 1981; MacDougall et al., 1979; Matthews, 1982; Rosenman, Rahe, Borhani, & Feinleib, 1976). There are consistent findings that speech characteristics (Rosenman, 1978) differentiate Type A and Type B behavior patterns in both sexes (Guggisberg, Laederach, & Adler, 1981; Matthews, 1982; Scherwitz et al., 1977; Schucker & Jacobs, 1977; Sparacino, 1979; Sparacino, Hansell, & Smyth, 1979). Type A persons are found from self-reports to exhibit aggressiveness, dominance, self-confidence, impulsiveness, competitiveness, impatience, assertiveness, time consciousness and time urgency, a rapid pace of activity, self-control, achievement orientation, orderliness, alertness, a tendency to hurry through task performance, a high level of activity, strong vocational motivation, tension and poor ability to relax away from work, denial of fatigue, symptoms, and illness, irritability when frustrated, a preference for working alone when challenged, a propensity to be not easily distracted from task performance, an inclination to attempt to control the milieu, aggressive hostility during competitive task performance and when frustrated; and a tendency to experience more life conflicts, stresses, and dissatisfactions. Moreover, the remarkable consistency in the pattern of interrrelationships among Type A behaviors and self-reports prevails in different samples that vary by age, sex, geographic distribution, sites of administration of the SI, and the SI interviewers and scorers (Matthews, 1982).

Thus the empirical findings generally confirm that SI-categorized Type A subjects exhibit the component behaviors and responses that are consistent with the Type A construct. Even more striking, Type A individuals respond to frustrating, difficult, and competitive circumstances, including the SI, with characteristic speech stylistics, psychomotor behaviors, and physiological responses, but do not otherwise differ from Type B subjects in task performance (Matthews, 1982).

In the original formulation of the Type A construct it was believed that the TABP was not synonymous with anxiety, neuroticism, stress, or psychopathology. This belief has been confirmed by a number of studies (Chesney, Black, Chadwick, & Rosenman, 1981; Glass, 1977; Rosenman et al., 1964; Rosenman et al., in press; Wadden et al., 1983). Several other investigators purportedly have found that the TABP correlates positively with stress and tension (Dimsdale et al., 1978), with stress and emotional lability (Haynes et al., 1978), and with anxiety and psychopathology (Bass, 1984; Irvine et al., 1982). However, these studies used self-report measures that are now recognized to correlate poorly with the TABP as assessed by the SI. It may have been more appropriate and useful for these investigators to state that they found correlations of psychological and psychiatric symptomatology with their particular self-report measures, rather than with TABP.

## EVOLUTION OF TABP

One major shift in studies of theTABP has been to emphasize the use of psychophysiological test responses, some of which were reviewed previously in this chapter. There has been widespread acceptance of the belief that enhanced psychophysiological reactivity provides the major pathway by which TABP is related to the pathogenesis of CHD. However, it should be emphasized that this view is entirely hypothethical and that such augmented responsivity does not necessarily confer coronary proneness. For example, greater responsivity is not associated with a higher incidence of hypertension in Type A as compared with Type B subjects (Rosenman, in press). Moreover, although enhanced psychophysiological responsivity may be a marker for the TABP, there is remarkably little evidence to support the belief that it is responsible for accelerated coronary atherogenesis or higher incidence of CHD (Rosenman, 1985). One school of investigators (Dembroski, MacDougall, Eliot, & Buell, 1984) has consistently emphasized an old belief in the so-called "hot reactor," in which the magnitude of physiological arousal in response to the environment is considered to be the major factor leading to CHD. They imply that their new laboratory test of such responsiveness provides an objective means for the prediction of CHD and that this should replace the assessment of the TABP for prediction of CHD. Unfortunately, this rather simplistic approach to the complexities of the autonomic nervous system and its responses has long been applied in clinical as well as research investigations, but evidence in support of the hypothesis is lacking.

A second shift in methods of study has been to emphasize the components of the TABP (Rosenman et al., 1964) in order to identify the core Type A behaviors that are predictively related to the severity of coronary atherosclerosis and the incidence of CHD. This approach was initially suggested by two investigations based on the WCGS. Jenkins (1966) studied the relationship between component Type A behaviors assessed from the intake SIs of younger men who entered the WCGS with silent or clinically unrecognized myocardial infarction, and compared these men with controls matched for age, occupation, and behavior type. The results revealed that the subjects who entered the WCGS with a prior silent myocardial infarction scored higher than matched controls on most of the major Type A components in general, and the Type A Hostility dimension in particular.

It was therefore decided to examine the components of the TABP in a larger sample of WCGS subjects. For this purpose, Bortner was asked to do a blind rating of the SI responses of 62 initially healthy subjects who subsequently suffered CHD during follow-up, and to compare their responses with the responses of two control subjects matched for age and occupation with each CHD case. The untimely death of Bortner interrupted evaluation of the results, which were much later independently analyzed. The results revealed that, among the TABP components, those that related to competitive drive, impatience, and the potential for hostility particularly identified the coronary-prone subjects (Matthews et al., 1977).

Bortner did not provide details concerning how he rated the TABP components. However, two other methods of assessing hostility from the SIs have been developed. The methodology used by Dembroski and colleagues

(1978; MacDougall, Dembroski, & Van Horn, 1983) is based on the original formulation of the Type A concept and its component behaviors (Rosenman, 1978; Rosenman et al., 1964). The methodology developed by Hecker (Hecker et al., 1981) has not yet received construct validation. The results of an analysis of CHD cases and control subjects in the WCGS by the latter method are reported in Chapter 8 of this volume by Chesney, Hecker, and Black. However, it appears that the Hostility dimension assessed by this latter method differs from the TABP or the dimension that characterizes the TABP.

Considerable attention has been given to the so-called Hostility scale (Ho) derived from the MMPI by Cook and Medley (1954). Scores on this scale have been positively correlated with the incidence of CHD in several studies (Barefoot, Dahlstrom, & Williams, 1983; Shekelle, Gayle, Ostfeld, & Paul, 1983), as well as with the severity of coronary atherosclerosis observed in angiographic studies (Williams, Barefoot, & Skekelle, 1985). However, a more recent long-term study failed to confirm these findings (McCranie, Watkins, Brandsma, & Sisson, 1986). Megargee (1985) has pointed out that no studies of the Cook-Medley (1954) scale have provided construct validity for the belief that it measures hostility dimensions. Shekelle and colleagues (1983) and Barefoot and colleagues (1983) found that this scale assessed the quality and quantity of social supports rather than hostility. Nevertheless, Williams, Barefoot, and Shekelle (1985) have continued to emphasize their belief that the Cook-Medley scale is a measure of hostility, with two subscales that respectively measure Cynicism and Paranoid Alienation. However, a recent study by Costa, Zonderman, McCrae, and Williams (1986) found that neither of the two subscales measures anger, irritability, or aggression, and that both are strongly related to measures of psychopathology. They also found that the two subscales are highly intercorrelated and concluded that they are only different aspects of a single trait measured by the full Cook-Medley scale, which is substantially related to neuroticism and psychopathology. The findings are further confused by the fact that neuroticism and psychopathology are not known to be predictors of CHD (Bass et al., 1983; Costa, 1986). It is also difficult to reconcile the interpretation of this MMPI scale with the fact that, in the studies by Barefoot and colleagues (1983) and Shekelle and colleagues (1983), the Ho scale was found to be related not only to the incidence of CHD but also to mortality from all causes including cancer.

Data from a California subgroup of twins who participated in the NHLBI Twin Study (Feinleib et al., 1977) were recently analyzed and the results have been presented in part by Rosenman and colleagues (in press) and are described more fully elsewhere (Swan, Carmelli, & Rosenman, 1986). The subjects were treated as individuals because the Cook-Medley scale was not found to be heritable and a dependency assumption therefore was not violated. The various self-report questionnaires used in this study have been described previously (Rosenman, Rahe, Borhani, & Feinleib, 1976).

It was found that high scorers on the Cook-Medley Ho scale also score high on Anxiety, Need for Succorance, and Reflectiveness and low on Dominance, Ego Strength, Well-Being, Tolerance, Achievement Orientation, Stability, and Extroversion. Item overlap did not appear to account for these correlations with scales from the CPI, TTS, ACL, and MMPI inasmuch as only two or three items were found to overlap. With few exceptions, the two Ho subscales were found to mirror the intercorrelation pattern found for the full Ho scale. It also was found that the correlates of the TABP were all congruent with the Type A construct, but they generally were different from the correlates of the Ho scale. This pattern of results indicates that the TABP is independent of what is being measured by the Ho scale. Moreover, it was found that the Ho scale and its two subscales correlated strongly with measures of anxiety and negatively with MMPI scales and other scales that assess constructs that presumably involve hostility, for example, scales of paranoia.

These findings as well as those obtained by Costa and colleagues (1986) do not appear to substantiate the belief of Williams and colleagues (1985) that the Cook-Medley Ho scale measures hostility dimensions. Moreover, these findings raise serious questions about the interpretation of the Ho scale, as Megargee (1985) and others have noted. It also is evident from these results that the Ho scale is measuring different dimensions from the TABP or Type A Hostility component of the TABP. The relationship between the Ho scale and CHD found by some but not all investigators thus has not been clarified. For the present, it would appear wise not to view studies that relate the Ho scale to CHD as support for a particular relationship of hostility to either coronary atherosclerosis or the incidence of CHD. This caution is further supported by the finding that hostility may be confused with competitiveness in the SI (Chesney, Eagleston, & Rosenman, 1981) and that the cynicism purportedly measured by the Ho scale is not equivalent to aggressive or even hostile behaviors (Smith & Frohm, 1985).

Williams (1984) has refered to the TABP as an old concept that should be replaced by hostility as measured by the Cook and Medley scale and by measurements of cortisol and hyperresponsivity. The lack of support for the first premise has already been discussed. Evidence for the second premise also has not been obtained.

One is reminded, in the present context, of the words of Mark Twain when he read a mistaken account of his death. Twain's comment was: "The rumors of my demise are greatly exaggerated." The same could be said of the TABP.

## REFERENCES

Anderson, J. R., & Waldron, I. (1983). Behavioral and content components of the Structured Interview assessment of the Type A behavior pattern in women. *Journal of Behavioral Medicine, 6*, 123–134.

Barefoot, J. C., Dahlstrom, G., & Williams, R. B. (1983). Hostility, CHD incidence, and total mortality: A 25-year follow-up study of 255 physicians. *Psychosomatic Medicine, 45,* 59–63.

Bass, C. (1984). Type A behavior in patients with chest pain: Test–retest reliability and psychometric correlates of Bortner scale. *Journal of Psychosomatic Research, 28,* 289–300.

Bass, C., Cawley, R., & Wade C. (1983). Unexplained breathlessness and psychiatric morbidity in patients with normal and abnormal coronary arteries. *Lancet, 1,* 605–609.

Belmaker, R. H., Pollin, W., Jenkins, C. D., & Brensike, J. (1976). Coronary-prone behavior patterns in a sample of Type II hypercholesteremic patients. *Journal of Psychosomatic Research, 20,* 591–594.

Bergman, L. R., & Magnusson, D. (1986). Type A behavior: A longitudinal study from childhood to adulthood. *Psychosomatic Medicine, 48,* 134–142.

Blumenthal, J. A., Herman, S., O'Toole, L. C., Haney, T. L., Williams, R. B., & Barefoot, J. C. (1985). Development of a brief self-report measure of the Type A (coronary-prone) behavior pattern. *Journal of Psychosomatic Research, 29,* 265–274.

Blumenthal, J. A., O'Toole, L. C., & Haney, T. (1984). Behavioral assessment of the Type A behavior pattern. *Psychosomatic Medicine, 46,* 415–423.

Bortner, R. W. (1969). A short rating scale as a potential measure of Pattern A behavior. *Journal of Chronic Diseases, 22,* 87–91.

Bortner, R. W., & Rosenman, R. H. (1967). The measurement of Pattern A behavior. *Journal of Chronic Diseases, 20,* 525–533.

Bortner, R. W., Rosenman, R. H., & Friedman, M. (1970). Familial similarity in Pattern A behavior: Fathers and sons. *Journal of Chronic Diseases, 23,* 39–43.

Bo-yuan, Z. (1983). The feature of psychophysiological reaction in cardiovascular disease: I. A preliminary research on the arousal level and habituation of coronary heart disease. *Acta Psychologica Sinica, 2,* 206–210.

Brand, R. J., Rosenman, R. H., Jenkins, C. D., Sholtz, R. I., & Zyzanski, S. J. (1986). *Comparison of coronary heart disease prediction in the Western Collaborative Group Study using the Structured Interview and the Jenkins Activity Survey assessments of the coronary-prone Type A behavior pattern.* Manuscript to be submitted for publication.

Brozek, J., Keys, A., & Blackburn, H. (1966). Personality differences between potential coronary and non-coronary subjects. *Annals of the New York Academy of Sciences, 134,* 1057–1064.

Butensky, A., Forelli, V., Heebner, D., & Waldron, I. (1976). Elements of the coronary-prone behavior pattern in children and teenagers. *Journal of Psychosomatic Research, 20,* 439–444.

Byrne, D. G., Rosenman, R. H., Schiller, E., & Chesney, M. A. (1985). Consistency and variation among instruments purporting to measure the Type A behavior pattern. *Psychosomatic Medicine, 47,* 242–261.

Caffrey, B. (1968). Reliability and validity of personality and behavioral measures in a study of coronary heart disease. *Journal of Chronic Diseases, 21,* 191–204.

Caffrey, B. (1969). Behavior patterns and personality characteristics related to prevalence rates of coronary heart disease. *Journal of Chronic Diseases, 22,* 93–103.

Caplan, R. D., Cobb, S., French, J. R. P., Harrison, R. V., & Pinneau, S. R. (1975). *Job demands and worker health.* U.S. Department of Health, Education, and Welfare, Publication No. (NIOSH), 75–160. Washington, DC: U.S. Government Printing Office.

Caplan, R. D., & Jones, K. W. (1975). Effects of work load, role ambiguity, and Type A personality on anxiety, depression, and heart rate. *Journal of Applied Psychology, 60,* 713–719.

Carmelli, D., Rosenman, R. H., & Chesney, M. A. (in press). Stability of the Type A Structured Interview and related questionnaires in a 10 year follow-up of an adult cohort of twins. *Journal of Behavioral Medicine.*

Chesney, M. A., Black, G. W., Chadwick, J. H., & Rosenman, R. H. (1981). Psychological correlates of the coronary-prone behavior pattern. *Journal of Behavioral Medicine, 4,* 217–230.

Chesney, M. A., Eagleston, J. R., & Rosenman, R. H. (1981). Type A behavior: Assessment and intervention. In C. Prokop & L. Bradley (Eds.), *Medical psychology: Contributions to behavioral medicine.* New York: Academic.

Cook, W., & Medley, D. (1954). Proposed Hostility and Pharisaic-Virtue scales for the MMPI. *Journal of Applied Psychology, 38,* 414–418.

Costa, P. T. (1986). Is neuroticism a risk factor for CAD? Is Type A a measure of neuroticism? In T. Schmidt, T. Dembroski, & G. Blumchen (Eds.), *Biological and psychological factors in cardiovascular disease.* New York: Springer-Verlag.

Costa, P. T., Zonderman, A. B., McCrae, R. R., & Williams, R. B. (1986). Cynicism and paranoid alienation in the Cook and Medley Ho scale. *Psychosomatic Medicine, 48,* 283–285.

Defourny, M., & Frankignoul, M. (1973). A propos du comportement predisposant aux co-ronaropathies (overt pattern A) [Concerning the behavior predisposing to coronary disease (overt pattern A)]. *Journal of Psychosomatic Research, 17,* 219–230.

Dembroski, T. M., MacDougall, J. M., Eliot, R. S., & Buell, J. C. (1984). Moving beyond Type A. *Advances, 1,* 16–25.

Dembroski, T. M., MacDougall, J. M., Herd, J. A., & Shields, J. L. (1979). Effects of level of challenge on pressor and heart rate response in Type A and B subjects. *Journal of Applied Social Psychology, 9,* 208–228.

Dembroski, T. M., MacDougall, J. M., Shields, J. L., Pettito, J., & Lushene, R. (1978). Components of the Type A coronary-prone behavior pattern and cardiovascular responses to psychomotor performance challenge. *Journal of Behavioral Medicine, 1,* 159–176.

Derogatis, L. R. (1977). *SCL-90.* Baltimore: Johns Hopkins University.

Diamond, E. L., Schneiderman, N., Schwartz, D., Smith, J. C., Vorp, R., & DeCarlo Pasin, R., (1984). Harassment, hostility, and Type A as determinants of cardiovascular reactivity during competition. *Journal of Behavioral Medicine, 7,* 171–188.

Dimsdale, J., Hackett, T., Block, P., & Hutter, A. (1978). Emotional correlates of the Type A behavior pattern. *Psychosomatic Medicine, 40,* 580–585.

Ditto, W. B. (1982). Daily activities of college students and the construct validity of the Jenkins Activity Survey. *Psychosomatic Medicine, 44,* 537–543.

Eysenck, H. J., & Eysenck, S. B. G. (1968). *Eysenck Personality Inventory.* San Diego: Educational and Testing Service.

Eysenck, H. J., & Fulker, D. (1982). The components of Type A behavior and its genetic determinants. In M. Horvath & E. Frantik (Eds.), *Psychophysiological risk factors of cardiovascular diseases. Activitas Nervosa Superior* (Suppl. 3), 111–125. Prague: Basle Karger.

Feinleib, M., Garrison, R. J., Fabsitz, R., Christian, J. C., Hrubec, Z., Borhani, N. O., Kannel, W. B., Rosenman, R. H., Schwartz, J. T., & Wagner, J. O. (1977). The NHLBI Twin Study of Cardiovascular Disease Risk Factors: Methodology and summary of results. *American Journal of Epidemiology, 106,* 284–295.

French-Belgian Collaborative Group. (1982). Ischaemic heart disease and psychological patterns. Prevalence and incidence studies in Belgium and France. In H. Dendin (Ed.), *Psychological problems before and after myocardial infarction. Advances in Cardiology, 21,* 25–31. Basel: Eskarger.

Friedman, E. H., Hellerstein, H. K., Jones, S. E., & Eastwood, G. L. (1968). Behavior patterns and serum cholesterol in two groups of normal males. *American Journal of Medical Science, 255,* 237–244.

Friedman, M., Brown A. E., & Rosenman, R. H. (1975). Voice analysis test for detection of behavior pattern. *Journal of the American Medical Association, 208,* 828–836.

Friedman, M., Byers, S. O., Diamant, J., & Rosenman, R. H. (1975). Plasma catecholamine response of coronary-prone subjects (Type A) to a specific challenge. *Metabolism, 24,* 205–210.

Friedman, M., & Powell, L. H. (1984). The diagnosis and quantitative assessment of Type A behavior: Introduction and description of the Videotaped Structured Interview. *Integrative Psychiatry, 2,* 123–136.

Friedman, M., & Rosenman, R. H. (1959). Association of specific overt behavior pattern with blood and cardiovascular findings. *Journal of the American Medical Association, 169,* 1286–1296.

Friedman, M., & Rosenman, R. H. (1960). Overt behavior pattern in coronary diseases. *Journal of the American Medical Association, 173,* 1320–1325.

Friedman, M., St. George, S., Byers, S. O., & Rosenman, R. H. (1960). Excretion of catecholamines, 17-ketosteroids, 17-hydroxycorticoids, and 5-hydroxyindole in men exhibiting a particular behavior pattern (A) associated with high incidence of clinical coronary artery disease. *Journal of Clinical Investigation, 39,* 758–764.

Gerace, T. A., & Smith, J. C. (1985). Children's Type A interview: Interrater, test–retest reliability, and interviewer effect. *Journal of Chronic Diseases, 38,* 781–791.

Glass, D.C. (1977). *Behavior patterns, stress, and coronary disease.* Hillsdale, NJ: Erlbaum.

Glass, D. C. (1982). Psychological and physiological responses of individuals displaying Type A behavior. *Acta Medica Scandinavica* (Suppl. 660), 193–202.

Glass, D. C., & Contrada, R. (1983). Type A behavior and catecholamines: A critical review. In C.R. Lake & M. Ziegler (Eds.), *Norepinephrine: Clinical aspects.* Baltimore: Williams & Wilkins.

Goldband, S. (1980). Stimulus specificity of physiological response to stress and the Type A coronary-prone behavior pattern. *Journal of Personality & Social Psychology, 39,* 670–679.

Gough, H. G. (1956). *California Psychological Inventory.* Palo Alto: Consulting Psychologists Press.

Gough, H. H., & Heilbrun, A. B. (1975). *The Adjective Checklist.* Palo Alto: Consulting Psychologists Press.

Guggisberg, R., Laederach, K., & Adler, R. (1981). Formal speech stylistics and Type A behavior in 38 subjects during non stress interviews. *Psychotherapy & Psychosomatics, 36,* 86–91.

Haynes, S. G., Levine, S., Scotch, N., Feinleib, M., & Kannel, W. B. (1978). The relationship of psychosocial factors to coronary heart disease in the Framingham Study: I. Methods and risk factors. *American Journal of Epidemiology, 107,* 362–383.

Hecker, M.H.L., Chesney, M. A., Black, G. W., & Rosenman, R. H. (1981). Speech analysis of Type A behavior. In J. Darby (Ed.), *Speech evaluation in medicine.* New York: Grune & Stratton.

Heller, R. F. (1979). Type A behavior and coronary heart disease. *British Medical Journal, 2,* 368.

Herman, S., Blumenthal, J. A., Black, G. M., & Chesney, M. A. (1981). Self-ratings of Type A (coronary prone) adults: Do Type A's know they are type A's? *Psychosomatic Medicine, 43,* 405–413.

Houston, B. K. (1983). Psychophysiological responsivity and the Type A behavior pattern. *Journal of Research in Personality, 17,* 22–39.

Houston, B. K., Smith, T. W., & Zurawski, R. M. (in press). Principal dimensions of the Framingham Type A Scale: Differential relationships to cardiovascular reactivity and anxiety. *Journal of Human Stress.*

Humphries, C., Carver, C. S., & Neumann, P. G. (1983). Cognitive characteristics of the Type A coronary-prone behavior pattern. *Journal of Personality & Social Psychology, 41,* 177–187.

Hunter, S. M., Parker, F. C., Williamson, G. D., Downey, A. M., Weber, L. S., & Berenson, G. S. (1985). Measurement assessment of the Type A coronary prone behavior pattern and hyperactivity/problem behaviors in children: Are they related? The Bogalusa Heart Study. *Journal of Human Stress, 11*, 177–183.

Hunter, S. M., Wolf, T. M., Sklov, M. C., Webber, I. S., Watson, R. M., & Berenson, G. S. (1982). Type A coronary-prone behavior pattern and cardiovascular risk factor variables in children and adolescents: The Bogalusa Heart Study. *Journal of Chronic Diseases, 35*, 613–621.

Irvine, J., Lyle, R., & Allon, R. (1982). Type A personality as psychopathology: Personality correlates and an abbreviated scoring system. *Journal of Psychosomatic Research, 26*, 183–189.

Jenkins, C. D. (1966). Components of the coronary-prone behavior pattern: Their relation to silent myocardial infarction and blood lipids. *Journal of Chronic Diseases, 19*, 599–609.

Jenkins, C. D., Rosenman, R. H., & Friedman, M. (1967). Development of an objective psychological test for the determination of the coronary-prone behavior pattern in employed men. *Journal of Chronic Diseases, 20*, 371–379.

Jenkins, C. D., Rosenman, R. H., & Friedman, M. (1968). Replicability of rating the coronary-prone behavior pattern. *British Journal of Preventive Social Medicine, 22*, 16–22.

Jenkins, C. D., Rosenman, R. H., & Zyzanski, J. S. (1974). Prediction of clinical coronary heart disease by a test for the coronary-prone behavior pattern. *New England Journal of Medicine, 290*, 1271–1275.

Jenkins, C. D., Zyzanski, S. J., & Rosenman, R. H. (1979). *The Jenkins Activity Survey.* New York: Psychological Corporation.

Johnston, D. W., & Shaper, A. G. (1983). Type A behavior in British men: Reliability and intercorrelation of two measures. *Journal of Chronic Diseases, 36*, 203–207.

Katz, R. C., & Toben, T. (1986). The Novaco Anger Scale and Jenkins Activity Survey as predictors of cardiovascular reactivity. *Journal of Psychopathology & Behavioral Assessment, 8*, 149–155.

Keith, R. A., Lown, B., & Stare, F. J. (1965). Coronary heart disease and behavior patterns: An examination of method. *Psychosomatic Medicine, 27*, 424–434.

Kittel, F., Kornitzer, M., Zyzanski, S. J., Jenkins, C. D., Rustin, R. M., & Degre, C. (1978). Two methods of assessing the Type A coronary-prone behavior pattern in Belgium. *Journal of Chronic Diseases, 31*, 147–155.

Krantz, D. S., & Durel, L. A. (1983). Psychobiological substrates of the Type A behavior pattern. *Health Psychology, 2*, 393–411.

MacDougall, J. M., Dembroski, T. M., & Musante, L. (1979). The structured interview and questionnaire methods of assessing coronary-prone behavior in male and female college students. *Journal of Behavioral Medicine, 2*, 71–83.

MacDougall, J. M., Dembroski, T. M., & Van Horn, A. E. (1983). Component analysis of the Type A coronary-prone behavior pattern in male and female college students. *Journal of Personality & Social Psychology, 45*(5), 1104–1117.

Matthews, K. A. (1978). Assessment and developmental antecedents of the coronary-prone behavior pattern in children. In T. M. Dembroski, S. M. Weiss, J. L. Shields, S. G. Haynes, & M. Feinleib (Eds.), *Coronary-prone behavior.* New York: Springer-Verlag.

Matthews, K. A. (1982). Psychological perspectives on the Type A behavior pattern. *Psychological Bulletin, 91*, 293–323.

Matthews, K. A., & Angulo, J. (1980). Measurement of the Type A behavior pattern in children: Assessment of children's competitivesness, impatience–anger, and aggression. *Child Development, 51*, 466–475.

Matthews, K. A., Glass, D. C., Rosenman, R. H., & Bortner, R. W. (1977). Competitive drive, Pattern A, and coronary heart disease: A further analysis of some data from the Western Collaborative Group Study. *Journal of Chronic Diseases, 30,* 489–498.

Matthews, K. A., Krantz, D. S., Dembroski, T. M., & MacDougall, J. M. (1982). Unique and common variance in Structured Interview and Jenkins Activity Survey assessments of the Type A behavior pattern. *Journal of Personality & Social Psychology 42,* 303–313.

Matthews, K. A., & Siegel, J. M. (1982). The Type A behavior pattern in children and adolescents: Assessment, development, and associated coronary-risk. In A. Baum & J. Singer (Eds.), *Handbook of psychology and health* (Vol. 2). Hillsdale, NJ: Erlbaum.

Mayes, B. T., Sime, W. E., & Ganster, D. C. (1984). Convergent validity of Type A behavior pattern scales and their ability to predict physiological responsiveness in a sample of female public employees. *Journal of Behavioral Medicine, 7,* 83–108.

McCranie, E. W., Watkins, L. O., Brandsma, J. M., & Sisson, B. D. (1986). Hostility, coronary heart disease (CHD) incidence, and total mortality: Lack of association in a 25-year follow-up study of 478 physicians. *Journal of Behavioral Medicine, 9,* 119–125.

Megargee, E. I. (1985). The dynamics of aggression and their application to cardiovascular disorders. In M. A. Chesney & R. H. Rosenman (Eds.), *Anger and hostility in cardiovascular and behavioral disorders.* New York: Hemisphere.

Meininger, J. C. (1985). The validity of Type A behavior scales for employed women. *Journal of Chronic Diseases, 38,* 375–383.

The Multiple Risk Factor Intervention Trial Group (1979). The MRFIT behavior pattern study: I. Study design, procedures, reproducibility of behavior pattern judgments. *Journal of Chronic Diseases, 32,* 293–305.

Murray, D. M., Matthews, K. A., Blake, S. M., Prineas, R. J., & Gillum, R. F. (1986). Type A behavior in children: Demographic, behavioral, and physiological correlates. *Health Psychology, 5,* 159–169.

Murray, J. L., & Bruhn, J. G. (1983). Reliability of the MYTH scale in assessing Type A behavior in preschool children. *Journal of Human Stress, 9,* 73–78.

O'Looney, B. A., & Harding, C. M. (1985). A psychometric investigation of two measures of Type A behaviour in a British sample. *Journal of Chronic Diseases, 38,* 841–848.

Powell, L. H. (1984). Area review: Stress, Type A behavior, and cardiovascular disease. The Type A behavior pattern: An update on conceptual, assessment, and intervention research. *Behavioral Medicine Update, 6,* 7–10.

Price, K. P. (1979). Reliability of assessment of coronary-prone behavior with special reference to the Bortner Rating Scale. *Journal of Psychosomatic Research, 23,* 45–47.

Rosenman, R. H. (1978). The interview method of assessment of the coronary-prone behavior pattern. In T. M. Dembroski, S. M. Weiss, J. L. Shields, S. G. Haynes, & M. Feinleib (Eds.), *Coronary-prone behavior.* New York: Springer-Verlag.

Rosenman, R. H. (1985). Health consequences of anger and implications for treatment. In M. A. Chesney & R. H. Rosenman (Eds.), *Anger and behavior in cardiovascular and behavioral disorders.* New York: Hemisphere.

Rosenman, R. H. (in press). Type A behavior and hypertension. In S. Julius & D. R. Bassett (Eds.), *Handbook of hypertension (Behavioral factors in hypertension,* Vol. 10). Amsterdam: Jaap deVries.

Rosenman, R. H., Brand, R. J., Sholtz, R. I., & Friedman, M. (1976). Multivariate prediction of coronary heart disease during 8.5 year follow-up in the Western Collaborative Group Study. *American Journal of Cardiology, 37,* 903–910.

Rosenman, R. H., & Chesney, M. A. (1982). Stress, Type A behavior, and coronary disease. In L. Goldberger & S. Breznitz (Eds.), *Handbook of stress: Theoretical and clinical aspects.* New York: Free Press.

Rosenman, R. H., & Friedman, M. (1961). Association of specific behavior pattern in women with blood and cardiovascular findings. *Circulation, 24,* 1173–1184.

Rosenman, R. H., Friedman, M., Straus, R., Wurm, M., Kositchek, R., Hahn, W., & Werthessen, N. T. (1964). A predictive study of coronary heart disease: The Western Collaborative Group Study. *Journal of the American Medical Association, 189,* 15–22.

Rosenman, R. H., Rahe, R. H., Borhani, N. O., & Feinleib, M. (1976). Heritability of personality and behavior. *Acta Geneticae Medicae et Gemellologiae, 25,* 221–224.

Rosenman, R. H., Swan, G. E., & Carmelli, D. (in press). Some recent findings relative to the relationship of Type A behavior pattern to coronary heart disease. In S. Maes, P. Defores, I. Sarason, & C. Spielberger (Eds.), *Proceedings of First International Expert Conference on Health Psychology,* Tilburg University, Tilburg, The Netherlands, July 3-5, 1986.

Scher, H., Hartmen, L. M., Furedy, J. J., & Heslegrave, R. J. (1986). Electrocardiographic T-wave changes are more pronounced in Type A than in Type B men during mental work. *Psychosomatic Medicine, 48,* 159–166.

Scherwitz, L., Berton, K., & Leventhal, H. (1977). Type A assessment and interaction in the behavior pattern interview. *Psychosomatic Medicine, 39,* 229–240.

Scherwitz, L., Graham, L. E., Grandits, G., Buehler, J., & Billings, J. (1986). Self-involvement and coronary heart disease incidence in the Multiple Risk Factor Intervention Trial. *Psychosomatic Medicine, 48,* 187–199.

Scherwitz, L., McKelvain R., & Laman, C. (1983). Type A behavior, self-involvement and coronary atherosclerosis. *Psychosomatic Medicine, 45,* 47–57.

Schneider, R. H., Julius, S., Moss, G. E., Dielman, T. E., Zweifler, A. J., & Karunas, R. *New markers for Type A behavior: Pupil size and platelet epinephrine.* Manuscript submitted for publication.

Schucker, B., & Jacobs, D. R. (1977). Assessment of behavioral risk of coronary disease by voice characteristics. *Psychosomatic Medicine, 39,* 219–228.

Shekelle, R. B., Gayle, M., Ostfeld, A. M., & Paul, O. (1983). Hostility, risk of coronary heart disease and mortaility. *Psychosomatic Medicine, 45,* 109–114.

Siegel, J. M., & Leitch, C. J. (1981). Assessment of the Type A behavior pattern in adolescents. *Psychosomatic Medicine, 43,* 45–56.

Siegel, J. M., Matthews, K. A., & Leitch, C. J. (1981). Validation of the Type A interview assessment of adolescents: A multidimensional approach. *Psychosomatic Medicine, 43,* 311–321.

Smith, T. W., & Frohm, K. D. (1985). What's so unhealthy about hostility? Construct validity and psychosocial correlates of the Cook and Medley Ho scale. *Health Psychology, 4,* 503–520.

Smith, J. C., Gerace, T. A., Christakis, G., & Kafatos, A. (1985). A cross-cultural validation of the Miami Structured Interview-1 for Type A in children: The American-Hellenic Heart Study. *Journal of Chronic Diseases, 38,* 793–799.

Smith, T. W., Houston, B. K., & Zurawski, R. M. (1983). The Framingham Type A Scale and anxiety, irrational beliefs, and self-control. *Journal of Human Stress, 3,* 32–37.

Smith, T. W., Houston, B. K., & Zurawski, R. M. (1985). The Framingham Type A Scale: Cardiovascular and cognitive–behavioral responses to interpersonal challenge. *Motivation & Emotion, 9,* 123–134.

Smith, T. W., & O'Keefe, J. L. (1985). The inequivalence of self-reports of Type A behavior: Differential relationships of the Jenkins Activity Survey and the Framingham scale with affect, stress, and control. *Motivation & Emotion, 9,* 299–311.

Sparacino, J. (1979). The Type A behavior pattern: A critical assessment. *Journal of Human Stress, 5*(4), 37–51.

Sparacino, J., Hansell, S., & Smyth, K. (1979). Type A (coronary-prone) behavior and transient blood pressure change. *Nursing Research, 28,* 198–204.

Spielberger, C. D., Gorsuch, R. L., & Lushene, R. (1970). *State-Trait Anxiety Inventory.* Palo Alto: Consulting Psychologists Press.

Swan, G. D., Carmelli, D., & Rosenman, R. H. (1986). *The Cook and Medley Ho scale: I. Construct validity and relationship to Type A behavior pattern.* Manuscript to be submitted for publication.

Thurstone, L. L. (1953). *Temperament Schedule.* Chicago: Science Research Associates.

Van Egeren, L. F., Fabrega, H., & Thornton, D. (1983). Electrocardiographic effects of social stress on coronary-prone (Type A) individuals. *Psychosomatic Medicine, 45,* 195–203.

Van Harrison, R., Moss, G. E., Dileman, T. E., Harlan, W. K, Horvath, M., & Butchart, A. T. (1986). *Interrater reliability of the Structured Interview assessment of the Type A behavior pattern in a population-based sample.* Manuscript submitted for publication.

Verhagen, F., Nass, C., Appels, A., Van Bastelaer, A., & Winnubst, J. (1980). Cross-validation of the A/B typology in the Netherlands. *Psychotherapy & Psychosomatics, 34*(2–3), 178–186.

Vickers, R. A. (1973). *A short measure of the Type A personality.* Unpublished manuscript. Ann Arbor: University of Michigan, Institute for Social Research.

Wadden, T. A., Anderson, C. H., Foster, G. D., & Love, W. (1983). The Jenkins Activity Survey: Does it measure psychopathology? *Journal of Psychometric Research, 27,* 321–325.

Waldron, I. (1978a). The coronary-prone behavior pattern, blood pressure, employment and socioeconomic status in women. *Journal of Psychosomatic Research, 22,* 79–87.

Waldron, I. (1978b). Sex differences in the coronary prone behavior pattern. In T. M. Dembroski, S. M. Weiss, J. L. Shields, S. G. Haynes, & M. Feinleib (Eds.), *Coronary-prone behavior.* New York: Springer-Verlag.

Ward, M. M., Chesney, M. A., Swan, G. E., Black, G. W., Parker, S. F., & Rosenman, R. H. (1986). Cardiovascular responses in Type A and B men to a series of stressors. *Journal of Behavioral Medicine, 9,* 43–49.

Williams, R. B. (1984). Type A behavior and coronary heart disease: Something old, something new. *Behavioral Medicine Update, 6,* 29–33.

Williams, R. B., Barefoot, J. C., & Shekelle, R. B. (1985). The health consequences of hostility. In M. A. Chesney & R. H. Rosenman (Eds.), *Anger and behavior in cardiovascular and behavioral disorders.* New York: Hemisphere.

Wolf, T. M., Sklov, M. C., Wenzl, P. A., Hunter, S. M., & Berenson, G. S. (1982). Validation of a measure of Type A behavior pattern in children: Bogalusa Heart Study. *Child Development, 53,* 126–135.

# 3

## Interviewer Behaviors in the Western Collaborative Group Study and the Multiple Risk Factor Intervention Trial Structured Interviews

LARRY SCHERWITZ

## INTRODUCTION

### Literature Review

Type A behavior has captured more attention as a coronary heart disease (CHD) risk factor than any other psychosocial variable. The many exemplary efforts to characterize (Friedman, 1969; Friedman & Rosenman, 1974; Glass, 1977; Price, 1982; Rosenman, 1978), measure (Friedman, Brown, & Rosenman, 1969; Matthews, 1978; Powell & Thoresen, 1985; Scherwitz, Berton, & Leventhal, 1977; Schucker & Jacobs, 1977), study prospectively (Haynes, Feinleib, Levine, Scotch, & Kannel, 1978; Rosenman et al., 1975), theorize about (Glass, 1977; Price, 1982; Williams, 1978), and treat (Friedman et al., 1984; Roskies et al., 1979) Type A behavior show how widely considered it is as a CHD risk factor. It is safe to say that the Type A concept contributed much to the rapid rise of behavioral medicine research.

Recently, however, there have been several studies showing Type A behavior as measured by the Structured Interview (SI; see Rosenman, Swan, & Carmelli, Chapter 2, this volume) not to be associated with coronary artery disease (CAD) severity (Arrowood, Uhrich, Gomillion, Popio, & Raft, 1982; Blumenthal et al., 1985; Dembroski, MacDougall, Williams, Haney, & Blumenthal, 1985; Dimsdale et al., 1979; Krantz, Sanmarco, Selvester, & Matthews, 1979; Krantz et al., 1981; Scherwitz et al., 1983; Siegman, Feldstein, Ringel, & Tomasso, in press), as well as a major epidemiologic study showing SI-defined Type A behavior to be unrelated to CHD incidence (Shekelle et al., 1985). To assess whether there had been a slippage in the predictiveness of SI-defined Type A behavior, Booth-Kewley and Friedman (in press) conducted a metaanalysis of Type A behavior in studies that had measures of CHD outcomes. Using a simple Pearson correlation to assess effect size, they found that SI-defined Type A correlated .27 with all CHD disease outcomes before 1977 but dropped to a correlation of .17 during or after 1977. The relationship was significant for both time periods, but it may be getting weaker.

The studies relating Type A behavior and coronary artery disease severity before 1980 were overwhelmingly positive, and the studies after 1980 have been mostly negative. Others have offered explanations for the recent negative findings, and they will be discussed shortly. Unfortunately, there are too many explanations for a final conclusion, particularly with retrospective designs using clinical populations. Angiographic populations may all differ in how subjects are sampled, the patients' severity of disease, the physicians' aggressiveness in diagnosis and treatment, cardiovascular drug effects, and Type A assessment, among other factors. So there are many possible explanations for inconsistent findings.

To escape some of the shortcomings of retrospective designs, researchers have turned to prospective, epidemiological studies of Type A behavior and CHD incidence. There have been only two completed prospective studies of SI-defined Type A behavior and CHD incidence. The first project, the Western Collaborative Group Study (WCGS), found Type A behavior to be strongly predictive of CHD incidence, but the Multiple Risk Factor

This study was made possible due to the efforts of the original WCGS and MRFIT researchers who designed the studies and collected the Structured Interview data and the investigators who cooperated in providing the tape-recorded interviews. The ideas discussed in this chapter were fostered in collaboration with Dr. Lewis Graham. Credit also goes to the team of speech auditors for their many thousands of playbacks required to score the Structured Interviews accurately and to Greg Grandits, M. S., who conducted the statistical analyses on the MRFIT data. The project was funded by NHLBI Behavioral Medicine grant HL29573 and American Heart Association California Affiliate grant-in-aid #84-N149.

Intervention Trial (MRFIT), initiated 13 years later, found no association between Type A behavior and CHD (Shekelle et al., 1985). The purpose of the current study was to determine whether there were differences in the way the SIs were conducted that might help explain the discrepant findings between the WCGS and MRFIT studies.

With the cooperation of the MRFIT and WCGS principal investigators, the author and coworkers have systematically assessed SIs from both studies. The aims of the ancillary study reported here were to describe and compare how WCGS and MRFIT interviewers conducted the SIs, using objectively defined criteria. The SIs were compared on the pace and length of the interview, the type and number of questions asked, the different types of interruptions, and the quantity of nonstandard speech. These parameters are described in greater detail later in this chapter.

The substantial differences in speed, interruptions, and number of questions between the WCGS and MRFIT SIs that are described in this chapter provided grounds for theorizing about how interviewer behaviors could affect the predictive validity of Type A or hostility assessments. In the last section of this chapter, the author employs the conceptual framework of engagement–involvement from Singer (1974) to theorize about how the interviewer behaviors that were measured could increase or decrease the predictive validity of global SI Type A assessments. This theorizing goes far beyond the study results, and it calls for further research before we can come to conclusions about interviewer behaviors affecting the predictiveness of Type A assessments.

## Review and Explanations of Empirical Results

**Coronary Artery Studies.**   Two early angiography studies using SI-defined Type A (Blumenthal, Williams, & Kong, 1978; Frank, Heller, Kornfeld, Sporn & Weiss, 1978), a study using the thallium exercise stress test (Kahn et al., 1982), and an early autopsy study of coronary arteries (Friedman, Rosenman, Straus, Wurm, & Kositchek, 1968) found SI-defined Type A assessments to be linked with CAD severity. While the effect size of this association was modest, it was very consistent among published studies. However, beginning with Dimsdale and colleagues (1979), seven published studies, and one in press, have not found SI-defined Type A to be associated with CAD severity (Arrowood et al., 1982; Blumenthal et al., 1985; Dembroski et al., 1985; Dimsdale et al., 1979; Krantz et al., 1979; Krantz et al., 1981; Scherwitz et al., 1983; Siegman et al., in press).

In the first attempt at providing an explanation for the lack of association between Type A and CAD, Dimsdale and colleagues (1979) suggested that population differences could be responsible. Population differences remain a viable although not very interesting explanation for the recent negative findings, but, at least in one population, it is inconsistent with the results. Specifically, the study by Blumenthal and colleagues (1978) originally found Type A behavior to correlate positively with CAD severity using patients drawn from the Duke University sample, but two recent studies from this population, conducted by Dembroski and colleagues (1985), and by Blumenthal and colleagues (1985), showed no correlation between SI assessments and CAD severity.

Another possible reason that Type A has not been associated with CAD severity is the high prevalence of Type A behavior in coronary angiography patients, thus reducing the statistical power to detect true differences (Matthews & Haynes, 1986). While we cannot rule out this explanation, the prevalence of Type A in the studies with positive findings does not differ substantially from the prevalence of Type A in studies with negative findings. The studies by Frank and colleagues (1978) and Blumenthal and colleagues (1978) that found a positivie association between Type A and CAD severity contained 70 and 60 percent Type A's respectively, compared with the studies with negative findings: Krantz and colleagues (1981), 66 percent; Scherwitz and colleagues (1983), 70 percent; Siegman and colleagues (in press), 68 percent; and Dembroski and colleagues (1985), 63 percent.

Another possible reason is that the criteria for referral or the selection process for patients to undergo coronary catheterization may bias the findings (Matthews & Haynes, 1986). If Type A's selectively entered the studies in an earlier stage of disease, it could have biased the samples in the direction of the negative findings. Unfortunately, this is not testable with the existing studies because the process of patient referral and selection for angiography has not been systematically documented.

Another explanation is that SI-defined Type A behavior cannot be properly assessed during hospitalization, which is a time of high stress for all patients and is possibly a poor setting for conducting the SI. But the earlier studies by Frank and colleagues (1978) and Blumenthal and colleagues (1978) were also conducted upon hospitalized patients.

Yet another explanation concerns the differential use of beta-blocker drugs. Beta-blockers have been shown to reduce global Type A behavior (Krantz et al., 1982; Rosenman, 1978; Schmieder, Friedrich, Neus, Rüddel, & Von Eiff, 1983). It is possible that individuals who had more severe CAD were taking higher doses of beta-blockers, thus reducing their Type A behaviors. If the sicker subjects' behaviors were more subdued and interviewers focused upon those behaviors in making their assessments, then the Type A assessments could have been systematically biased by the drugs.

And yet another factor may be unreliable CAD severity estimates. Studies have indicated that nonquantitative estimates of lumen stenosis vary as much as Type A judgments, up to 31 percent (Bjork, Spindola-Franco, Van Houten, Cohn, & Adams, 1975; Brown, Bolson, & Dodge, 1982; DeRouen, Murray, & Owen, 1977; Detre, Wright, Murphy, & Takaro, 1975; Myers, Shulman, Saibil, & Naqvi, 1978; Zir, Miller, Dinsmore, Gilbert, & Harthorne, 1976). This could easily have added error variance to the estimates of disease severity, thus making it harder to detect true differences. There is no reason to suspect, however, that cardiologists' assessments of lumen stenosis were more accurate in the earlier studies than they were in the later studies.

A final explanation may be that Type A is no longer or never was a risk factor for atherosclerosis in certain populations. Alternatively, Type A behavior may have been a risk factor in the past, but may have disappeared due to cultural or life-style changes in the populations studied. Given the many alternative explanations just listed, and the many studies indicating an association between Type A behavior and some aspect of CHD, it is simply too early to rule out Type A as a risk factor for CAD.

**CHD Incidence Studies.**   In the WCGS, 3454 middle-aged males were interviewed at intake and the CHD status was monitored for 8.5 years (Rosenman et al., 1975). Before the intake screening began, the behavior type interviewers were trained over a period of months with actual subjects, many of whom had CHD. Both Dr. Friedman and Dr. Rosenman developed the interviewers' skills face to face as they sat in on the SIs. They also audited tape-recorded SIs, pointing out to interviewers Type A characteristics as well as giving feedback on the interviewing technique. The WCGS SIs were administered from June 1960 until December 1961 to employees of 11 participating business organizations, nine from the San Francisco Bay area and two from the Los Angeles area (Rosenman et al., 1964). The SIs were conducted and tape-recorded by a field team of four interviewers on the organizations' premises. Dr. Rosenman continued to audit the tape-recorded SIs and provide feedback to each of the interviewers throughout the screening period.

Dr. Rosenman made the final assessment of behavior pattern after "(1) audition of the tape-recorded personal interview, [and] (2) study of the interviewer's description and personal estimate of the subject's general behavior and motor actions during the interview" (Rosenman et al., 1964, p. 115). The results showed that Type A's were twice as likely to incur unrecognized myocardial infarction (MI), symptomatic MI, and angina pectoris as were Type B's; and the relationship between Type A behavior and CHD remained strong when statistically adjusted for parental history of CHD, current cigarette smoking, systolic blood pressure, and serum cholesterol (Rosenman, Brand, Sholtz, & Friedman, 1976).

The MRFIT was a randomized primary prevention trial to test the effect of a combined intervention program on mortality from CHD (MRFIT Group, 1982). Participants in the program were 12,866 men who volunteered for a series of three screening examinations in 22 clinics located in 18 U.S. cities. MRFIT participants were selected into the study if they were in the upper fifteenth percentile of risk (Framingham criteria) based upon their combined measures of diastolic blood pressure, serum cholesterol, and cigarette smoking. All participants had to agree to continue to be monitored for long-term follow-up and be willing to change their life-style if they were assigned to the special care group.

Eight of the 22 MRFIT clinics, located in Chicago, Minneapolis, Newark, San Francisco, and Davis, California, administered the SI to 3110 individuals eligible for this study. The MRFIT researchers appreciated the difficulty in assessing Type A behavior and they expended considerable effort in planning and implementing the procedures for selecting, training, monitoring, and assessing Type A behavior (MRFIT Group, 1973, 1979). The extensive procedures for maintaining quality control of the behavior type interviews have been described in a previous report (MRFIT Group, 1979). Because the MRFIT researchers recognized the methodological difficulties of assessing Type A behavior, they took steps to minimize the problems, including: (1) requiring the interviewers to meet certain standards of performance when recruited as candidates; (2) having the interviewers centrally trained and approved by Dr. Rosenman; (3) requiring 75 percent agreement on 100 audits before they were certified; (4) tape-recording all interviews and having them audited for global ratings centrally; (5) maintaining continuous surveillance over the frequency of disagreements between interviewers and auditors; (6) having Dr. Rosenman adjudicate SIs where there was a major disagreement (A vs. B) between the interviewer and auditor; and (7) having Dr. Rosenman make global assessments of a probability sample.

Interviewers were initially selected by the local MRFIT centers and sent to San Francisco to be trained in 5 days by Dr. Rosenman and coworkers (MRFIT Group, 1973, 1979). Relative to the WCGS, the interviewers had less training and experience with CHD patients before conducting the SI, and due to the distance from the training site and the logistics in copying and mailing the tape-recorded SIs, they could not be monitored closely nor taught in person as the intake interviews continued (Rosenman, Swan, & Carmelli, in press; Shekelle et al., 1985). Type A assessments were made by the interviewer and one of two auditors. Dr. Rosenman made a third assessment for a probability sample and when the auditor and interviewer disagreed in major category (A vs. B). The official Type A assessment was Dr. Rosenman's ratings when present; otherwise it was the auditors' ratings. Auditors based their A–B judgments upon the audio tape-recorded verbal characteristics and the interviewers' ratings of subjects' general demeanor, facial expression, and motor characteristics.

During the follow-up of 6 to 8 years, 129 individuals incurred their first major coronary event in the 8 clinical centers that conducted the SI. SI-defined Type A was not associated with risk of coronary death or with total mortality in usual care or special intervention groups, analyzed separately or together. When Type A (A1, A2) was compared with non-Type A (X, B), the crude relative risk ($RR$) was .92 (4.06 percent–4.40 percent), and the adjusted $RR$ was .87 (with 95 percent confidence interval .59–1.28) (Shekelle et al., 1985). Furthermore, when similar analyses were conducted separately with the interviewers', auditors', and Dr. Rosenman's behavior type ratings, the results were similar in showing no significant relationship between SI-defined Type A and CHD incidence.

The MRFIT findings are harder to dismiss than other recent negative findings that have been based on retrospective designs or only questionnaire measures of Type A (Case, Heller, Case, Moss, & Multicenter Post-Infarction Research Group, 1985; Ruberman, Weinblatt, Goldberg, & Chaudbury, 1984). Shekelle and colleagues (1985) have provided evidence to rule out several explanations for the failure of Type A behavior to predict CHD in the MRFIT study. They have maintained that there was adequate statistical power with the total sample (with 3110 there was a probability of .93 to detect a true $RR$ of 2.0). They also have suggested that differences in procedures between the WCGS and the MRFIT for identifying and classifying CHD endpoints could not explain the lack of predictiveness. And in their analyses, they statistically adjusted for possible effects of beta-blockers and alcohol intake.

Shekelle and colleagues addressed the explanation of whether Type A behavior is less predictive in individuals at high risk on other standard risk factors. Based upon findings from the WCGS (Brand, 1978) and the Framingham Study (Haynes, Feinleib, & Eaker, 1983), Type A alone is equally predictive of CHD at higher and lower levels of other risk factors. Thus if we can generalize from these findings, being at high risk on other risk factors probably did not reduce the risk of Type A behavior in MRFIT.

In addition, Shekelle and colleagues (1985) provided evidence that Type A's and Type B's were not simply misclassified. Most errors in misclassification are based upon individuals who are in the midrange of behavioral intensity. Thus if there is a dose–response relationship between degree of Type A behavior intensity and CHD, then one would expect the extreme Type A1's to have more CHD than the Type B's. But this was not the case; the analysis using the extremes (A1's vs. B's) shows the same lack of association as the total A versus B analysis.

A related though unlikely possibility is that being in MRFIT may have selectively alerted Type A's to alter their risk more than Type B's. This is not a very plausible explanation, for three reasons. First, there was no attempt to alter Type A behavior. Second, Type A's in the special intervention did not reduce their blood pressure, serum cholesterol, or smoking more than Type B's. And third, the lack of a relationship between Type A behavior and CHD was similar for the special intervention and the usual care groups.

There is yet another plausible explanation worth considering. The MRFIT study with its life-style change component was much more demanding than typical cardiovascular epidemiology studies that just involve follow-up measures. Thus it is possible that true coronary-prone* individuals who

*Coronary prone and Type A are not synonymous terms. Coronary prone is not yet clearly defined; it is more a hypothetical construct than a set of defined behaviors, but it is used to refer to a biobehavioral process that increases CHD risk. Type A behavior has been richly described and endlessly characterized; its assessment in the Structured Interview appears to rely upon clearly identified behavioral and speech expressions, although the scope and emphasis for particular characteristics may differ across interviewers.

may have been hostile to such intrusion in their lives did not volunteer for the study. If the true coronary-prone individuals (who were also Type A) did not volunteer, then one cannot expect Type A behavior to be associated with CHD.

## IN-DEPTH FOCUS UPON TYPE A ASSESSMENT

The many explanations for why Type A behavior has not been associated with CHD in recent studies prevent us from reaching any firm conclusions about whether Type A behavior remains a risk factor for CHD. Unfortunately, many of the explanations require new and in some cases prohibitively expensive projects. To add to this complexity, the author proposes yet another explanation—one, however, that is open to empirical research with existing data. This explanation is based upon Type A behavior assessment in the WCGS and MRFIT SIs. The following paragraphs will discuss our reasoning and the findings, beginning with how interviewers or auditors appraise Type A behavior in the MRFIT and then turning to how interviewers elicited Type A behavior in the WCGS and MRFIT SIs.

### Appraising Type A Behaviors

Although SI judgments of behavior type were not correlated with CHD incidence, either by the criterion measure or by individual rater, there is the possibility that the two auditors overlooked a behavioral component that correlated with CHD incidence in the MRFIT. To pursue this we began by auditing a large case-control sample from the MRFIT for four speech characteristics (SCs) including voice emphasis, speed of speaking, latency of answering, and answer content. Previous studies have shown these components to be correlated with global SI assessments (Anderson & Waldron, 1983; Blumenthal, O'Toole, & Haney, 1984; Hecker, Chesney, Black, & Rosenman, 1981; Howland & Siegman, 1982; Scherwitz et al., 1977; Scherwitz, Graham, Grandits, & Billings, 1987; Schucker & Jacobs, 1977). In another study in progress, Dembroski is assessing potential for hostility, and we must wait for his results before making any conclusions about the predictiveness of specific Type A components in the SI. But our analysis with the four SCs shows a statistically significant though very weak association between two of the SCs (voice emphasis and latency of answering) and all-cause CHD incidence.

While this does not rule out the possibility that other characteristics may have been associated with CHD, for example, hostility, it does suggest, somewhat equivocally, that the three raters did not commit gross errors in overlooking salient coronary-prone behaviors. It may be that the true coronary-prone behaviors were not elicited by these SIs. Perhaps the behaviors that reflect underlying risk for CHD are identifiable only under certain conditions or certain interpersonal situations.

### Eliciting Type A Behaviors

If coronary-prone behaviors existed in the MRFIT SIs, they were not identified and incorporated in making A–B judgments, and they were only weakly apparent in two components. So far as we know, appraising which behavioral components one uses in making a global A–B judgment was not a problem with the MRFIT SI assessments. There remained another possibility, the other half of the equation for how global assessments are derived—the way interviewers elicited and inhibited Type A expressions in their subjects. A major question to consider is: What is the interviewers' basic strategy for stimulating subjects' Type A behaviors?

From listening to the SIs, it was obvious that the WCGS differed from the MRFIT in length, pace, and degree of standardization. The WCGS interviews were slower paced, much longer, and somewhat more unstructured. The WCGS strategy seemed to be one of getting subjects to reflect upon their daily experiences, for example, experiences of irritating or frustrating situations. In contrast, though question content was the same, the MRFIT strategy seemed to be getting the subjects to react to the speed and delivery of the questions. Because these clinical observations were vaguely defined and open to bias, we developed an objective procedure to score the SI and make comparisons between the MRFIT and the WCGS on pace, length, type of question, and type of interruption. Following the design and procedures to be described, these interviewer behaviors will be compared.

### WCGS and MRFIT Ancillary Study Methods

Due to the large number of SIs in both the WCGS and the MRFIT, and the great detail in auditing interviewer SCs, only a' subset of interviews was audited from each study. The subset was chosen based upon other studies designed to identify Type A components that were most predictive of future CHD (Hecker, Frautschi, Chesney, Black, & Rosenman, 1985; Scherwitz, Graham, Grandits, Buehler, & Billings, 1986). Accordingly, in each ancillary study those who incurred CHD were compared with a matched sample of those who did not.

In the WCGS, during the 8.5 year follow-up period, 257 individuals incurred their first clinical manifestation of CHD. Of these 257, the SI audiorecordings were usable for 250 cases. Two CHD-free individuals were matched for each case (500) on age and company of employment. Of these 750 SIs, auditing has been completed for 702 SIs. The remaining 48 SIs were not available at the time of this analysis, but there is no reason to suspect that they differ from those already audited.

The design and subject selection criteria for the MRFIT are discussed in a previous study (Scherwitz, Graham, Grandits, Buehler & Billings, 1986). Briefly, the sample consisted of 577 males, 35 to 57 years old, who were drawn from 3087 individuals interviewed at the baseline MRFIT screening and for whom JAS and educational data were available. The sample included all 193 individuals who incurred a first cardiovascular event during the 7-year follow-up; specifically 60 CHD deaths, 31 nonfatal MIs, and 102 with a diagnosis of angina pectoris. Two control subjects who had remained free of CHD at the 7-year follow-up were matched with each case on age, education, clinical center, interviewer, and time of interview. Thus 577 SIs were available for the analysis, 498 of which we have completed for the preliminary analysis reported here. The remaining 79 SIs were being audited elsewhere and were not available for the preliminary analysis; there is no reason to suspect that they differ from those already audited.

## Interviewer Speech Characteristics

The author and coworkers have done considerable work to develop the current system to score interviewers' speech behaviors. First, choosing interviewer behaviors to score was a major concern. From the beginning, we looked for behaviors that reflected the interviewers' strategy of eliciting or inhibiting subjects' speech; this is a testable idea in that we have speech data on subjects. Furthermore, speech-eliciting and speech-inhibiting techniques have relevance to Singer's concept of engagement–involvement. While there are exceptions, for example, interviewers who interrupt out of enthusiasm or empathy with something the subject just said, generally interviewers who interrupt the subjects' speech are less engaging than interviewers who ask more questions and otherwise stimulate subjects to speak more. And if engagement–involvement can affect physiological reactivity and other biological processes as profoundly as the findings of Singer and associates suggest (Singer, 1974; Thaler-Singer, Reiser, & Weiner, 1957; Weiner, Singer, & Reiser, 1962), it could also affect the accuracy of Type A assessments. Consequently, work is in progress on developing an index of engagingness; it combines speed of speaking and asking questions, the number of questions, and amount of nonstandard speech.

The speech-auditing procedures were developed by listening to numerous SIs from the WCGS, MRFIT, the Recurrent Coronary Prevention Project, and samples from Seeman and Syme's (1987) and Williams and colleagues' (1980) angiography studies. We listened for interviewer behaviors that seemed to facilitate or inhibit the subjects' speech. From this first step we made a large list of behaviors and developed definitions and protocols for scoring them. Then we practiced independently scoring these behaviors, analyzed discrepancies, and refined the protocol, dropping behaviors that could not be scored reliably or interpreted clearly. This process was repeated and the protocol revised with three different SI populations.

Three features of interviewer behavior were scored, including speed factors (speed of speaking and asking latency), question probes that elicit speech, and interruptions that inhibit subject speech. The two interviewer Type A behaviors include speed of speaking and asking latency; these speed factors do much to control the pace of the interview. Both speed of speaking and asking latency were scored from 11 questions selected to be comparable in the MRFIT and WCGS. All other measures were scored for the entire SI. To measure speed of speaking we counted the syllables in the interviewer questions and, with a stopwatch, timed how long it took to ask the questions. To measure asking latency, speech auditors timed the latency period between the subject's completed answer and the beginning of the interviewer's next question.

Distinctions of how interviewers interrupt subjects may be important and should be discriminated in the scoring procedure. One distinction made is the type of question asked, and one can divide all the SI questions into three types: (1) primary question; (2) standard probe; and (3) nonstandard speech. Primary questions are the 25 or so numbered questions in the SI scripts. The interviewers ordinarily ask all or nearly all of these questions. The standard probe is also on the script, but it is a follow-up to the primary question. And because it is often related to something the subject just said, the standard probe is usually more engaging than a primary question. The nonstandard speech contains questions and comments that are not standard and that may be the most engaging, because such speech is not written into the script at all and it is usually tailored to something the subject has just said.

By considering question type we can crudely order interruptions by their "rudeness." Interrupting to ask the next primary question is the rudest form of interruption because it not only stops the subject, but it also changes the topic. Interrupting with a standard probe is less rude because at least it remains on the topic. And interrupting with an acknowledgment (e.g., "I see") or an interjection of some nonstandard comment or question (e.g., "That's amazing!") is usually least rude and in some cases can stimulate the subjects to speak more.

The interauditor reliability for all the interviewer behaviors is acceptable. As part of a completed phase of the project, speech auditors independently scored 69 SIs for the interviewers' asking latency, speed of speaking, and voice emphasis, with corresponding intraclass correlations of .88, .95, and .59. Voice emphasis was lower because it involves a subjective judgment in scoring.

We tested the interauditor reliability for the remaining components in a pilot study of 10 randomly selected MRFIT SIs using three speech auditors. The reliability coefficients for total standard probes varied from $r = .95$ to .96, for total nonstandard speech from $r = .99$ to 1.00, and for total interruptions from $r = .75$ to .94. The interruptions were more difficult to score in that they are harder to hear with mono audio-recordings because both interviewer and subject are speaking together. Also, the line between standard and nonstandard is clearly demarcated on the basis of the script content, whereas interrupting versus noninterrupting is often a judgment call based on form and interaction style, with no definite dividing line.

## Results: WCGS and MRFIT SI Comparisons

A simple t-test for independent means was conducted upon each SI characteristic; the results are presented on Table 3.1.

**Interview Questions.** It is clear that the WCGS interviewers asked more questions than the MRFIT interviewers. Including the primary questions (which are not in the table, as they did not need to be counted), the WCGS interviewers had a total average of about 82 questions and nonstandard speech compared with 60 for the MRFIT. The WCGS had six more primary questions, 11 more standard probes, and five more nonstandard speech utterances; all comparisons were significant beyond $p = .0001$ for both the total and individual type of question.

**Speed Factors.** The WCGS interviewers had a much longer latency in asking questions than the MRFIT interviewers: 1.84 versus 0.99 seconds. In contrast, the WCGS interviewers spoke rather more quickly than the MRFIT interviewers when asking questions: 5.9 versus 5.1 syllables per second.

**TABLE 3.1. WCGS AND MRFIT INTERVIEWER BEHAVIORS AND SI CHARACTERISTICS**

|  |  | WCGS (N = 702) | MRFIT (N = 498) |  |
|---|---|---|---|---|
| Total standard probes | Mean | 29.879 | 19.568 | T = 42.36 |
|  | SD | 5.064 | 2.332 | $p < .0001$ |
| Total nonstandard speech | Mean | 23.603 | 19.285 | T = 5.89 |
|  | SD | 10.706 | 14.687 | $p < .0001$ |
| Asking latency (seconds) | Mean | 1.838 | 0.994 | T = 26.71 |
|  | SD | 0.634 | 0.367 | $p < .0001$ |
| Speed of speaking (syllables per second) | Mean | 5.886 | 5.130 | T = 17.17 |
|  | SD | 0.908 | 0.443 | $p < .0001$ |
| Interrupting primary questions | Mean | 0.254 | 1.024 | T = −13.23 |
|  | SD | 0.633 | 1.348 | $p < .0001$ |
| Interrupting standard probes | Mean | 1.030 | 1.436 | T = −4.95 |
|  | SD | 1.222 | 1.618 | $p < .0001$ |
| Interrupting nonstandard speech | Mean | 2.726 | 3.538 | T = −4.33 |
|  | SD | 2.825 | 3.666 | $p < .0001$ |
| Polite standard probes | Mean | 28.967 | 18.102 | T = 38.83 |
|  | SD | 5.725 | 2.955 | $p < .0001$ |
| Polite nonstandard speech | Mean | 20.876 | 15.697 | T = 7.82 |
|  | SD | 10.015 | 12.914 | $p < .0001$ |
| Interview length (minutes) | Mean | 13.608 | 8.717 | T = 24.86 |
|  | SD | 3.744 | 2.719 | $p < .0001$ |

**Interruptions.** The MRFIT interviewers interrupted more than the WCGS interviewers with an average of seven per SI versus four for the WCGS. This difference is all the more significant when considering that WCGS SIs were longer than the MRFIT SIs; thus the rate of interrupting was much higher in the MRFIT than in the WCGS. And MRFIT interviewers had a higher percentage of ruder interruptions: 49 percent (of total interruptions) compared with 32 percent for the WCGS.

**Interview Length.** Given the many more questions, it is not surprising that the WCGS SIs were substantially longer than the MRFIT SIs. The WCGS average interview length was 13.6 minutes, compared with 8.7 for the MRFIT, a difference of 4.9 minutes. The four WCGS interviewers varied from an average of 12.5 to 18.0 minutes, compared with averages of 7.0 to 12.2 minutes for the MRFIT interviewers. Thus in terms of total SI time, the fastest WCGS interviewer took longer than the slowest MRFIT interviewer.

## SUMMARY AND INTERPRETATION OF INTERVIEWER DIFFERENCES

The WCGS interviewers asked many more questions than the MRFIT interviewers, and consequently, the interviews took a lot longer to complete. So the WCGS interviewers had more time to ask about, observe, and assess the subjects' behaviors. This could potentially affect the predictive validity of Type A assessments depending upon how much time is necessary to observe hypothetical coronary-prone behaviors and the relative skill of the interviewer in eliciting and observing them. For example, with more time a skilled interviewer could continue to develop rapport with subjects and consequently get them to express their feelings more openly.

The biggest difference in terms of the question type was the 11 more standard probes in the WCGS than in the MRFIT. In contrast to primary questions, follow-up probes can often have the direct effect of leading the subjects to evaluate their feelings, thoughts, and actions more deeply or more explicitly.

If it is considered rude to interrupt someone when he or she is answering a question (sometimes it is), then the MRFIT interviewers were relatively ruder than the WCGS; though the interviewers were professional in both studies, the MRFIT interviewers intentionally interrupted to provoke Type A behaviors. Not only were MRFIT subjects interrupted more overall, but a greater percentage of those interruptions were of the rudest type (interruptions with a primary question). The difference in interruptions in the MRFIT may be enough to have turned off those men most easily offended. In listening to SIs, we have observed that some subjects responded to an interrupting interviewer by clamming up, not expressing their feelings; others appear to let subsequent questions slide by with minimal answers.

Other researchers have observed that provocation with voice emphasis, speaking quickly, or interrupting tends to inhibit subjects from expressing their feelings (T. Haney, personal communication, 1985; J. Patterson, personal communication, 1985; J. A. Blumenthal, personal communication, 1985).

We are not trying to discredit provocation in general in the SI; it is needed, and so is an orderly proceeding throughout the interview. The WCGS interviewers were provoking in that, by their questions, they allowed the expression of more Type A behaviors than the MRFIT interviewers. Their more standard probes and nonstandard questions probably had the effect of getting subjects more involved in their previous experiences of Type A situations and feelings.

The WCGS interviewers spoke somewhat faster than the MRFIT interviewers. It is not clear what effect speaking 0.76 syllables faster per second has. The difference was fairly small and slightly increased the pace of the interview. But a short asking latency features very prominently in picking up the pace of an interview, and the MRFIT had an average latency of 0.99 seconds, which is very short. The WCGS interviewers took almost twice as long to ask the next question (1.8 seconds), partly because they paused to take notes. This could give the subjects an opportunity to amend and elaborate upon what they had just previously said; it also gave the interviewer a little more time to observe, weigh, and record the subjects' behaviors.

Beyond simple empirical results, there is another useful way to point out the differences in the WCGS and MRFIT: to take the speech auditors' perspective and focus upon the internal structure of the questions. Speech auditors preferred scoring MRFIT rather than WCGS interviews; the questions were asked in order, in the same way, with the emphasis in the expected places. The MRFIT SIs were fast, clean, and could be scored reliably with ease. For example, auditors who counted the syllables in the interviewers' questions could often use the values computed from the MRFIT script.

In contrast, the WCGS did not have a closely agreed-upon script; what is standard behavior and what is not is hard to determine at the level of detail that a speech auditor has to consider. WCGS interviewers had their own ways of asking certain questions, and they even varied from interview to interview in the way the questions were phrased. Thus WCGS interviewers took more liberties in the way they asked questions. If this reflects the interviewer's freedom to approach an interview script in the way he or she felt most comfortable, then it could have been more engaging for both interviewer and subjects.

The preliminary analysis indicated that there were many interviewer behavior differences between the MRFIT and WCGS SIs. The next step will be to combine the 11 interviewers from both studies and see whether interviewers differed in the *RR* ratios of their assessments for CHD incidence. If so, then we can ask whether the differences in predictiveness are related to differences in interviewer speech behaviors and engagement.

## Revisions in the SI

Do the differences between the WCGS and the MRFIT reflect more general changes in the way the interviewers were trained from the 1960s to the 1970s? One cannot say for sure without auditing and scoring a representative sample from other studies; however, the author has listened to SIs from four different research projects. The style of these interviewers, all trained by Dr. Rosenman and associates during the 1970s and the early 1980s, is more similar to the MRFIT than to the WCGS. It is crisp, with questions in order, delivered with emphasis on key words in a no-nonsense, professional manner. This may have been the primary interviewer style for the negative studies of SI-defined Type A and CAD severity (Dembroski et al., 1985; Krantz et al., 1981; Scherwitz et al., 1983). Each of these interviewers was trained by Rosenman and associates, who have been responsible for training the vast majority of SI interviewers conducting research in the mid- and late 1970s and early 1980s.

There are at least three reasons for changes in interview style. First, in an attempt to improve interinterviewer reliability and comparability across populations, the later interviewer training focused more on standardizing the question format and the stylistics designed to provoke or elicit Type A behaviors. In view of past concerns with assessment, this regimentation seemed necessary to meet the demands for using the SI in epidemiologic and clinical studies; while it did and does provide a more consistent stimulus across interviewers, it may have made the interview more mechanical.

Second, because expression of some important Type A components, for example, hostility, can be very subtle, interviewers were trained to become more aggressive to provoke these behaviors. Key words to be emphasized in the script questions were capitalized and interruptions were planned. These provoking sytlistics provide a defined stimulus, and they may elicit Type A behaviors better in socially extraverted subjects. On the other hand, stylistic provocation may inhibit Type A expressions in more passive–aggressive hostile subjects—a group that may be most coronary prone.

Third, because the time taken to conduct the early interviews was judged a disadvantage, the SI was "streamlined" and the pace was picked up. Questions regarding high school sports and leisure-time activities were dropped and interviewers were trained not to let the subjects "dawdle." While this new pace had an obvious speed advantage, it nevertheless reduced the time interviewers could use to develop rapport, and it definitely reduced the information interviewers could draw upon to make judgments.

One cannot conclude that interview style could affect the predictive validity simply from correlational studies because there are so many alternative explanations. Thus a key question is whether training interviewers to engage subjects will enhance the discriminative and predictive validity of behavior type judgments. We can ony suggest a clue here. As part of another project, the first author trained the Type A interviewers for a coronary angiography study conducted by Ragland, Syme, and coworkers at Pacific Presbyterian Medical Center in San Francisco (Ragland, personal communication, 1985). Interviewers were drilled on using nonstandard probes, coached on how to express interest, and generally taught the value of connecting with and engaging subjects. The results from this study show that Type A behavior, when controlled for income level, was significantly and positively correlated with number of diseased arteries. Because we did not experimentally vary interviewer engagement, we do not know whether the results would have been positive anyway.

A question raised by differences in the WCGS and MRFIT interviewers is whether coronary-prone behaviors are manifest only in context-dependent situations. If so, the interviewer may be just as important as the subject in determining whether a subject's behavior is risk predictive. Viewing risk behaviors as a transactional process (rather than a trait or intrapsychic process) would be more consistent with the original definition of Type A behavior as an interaction between the individual and the situation (Friedman, 1969).

Despite the support presented above, the author is still not convinced that the MRFIT interviewers' lack of engagement could completely account for the negative results on the association between Type A and CHD incidence. After all, the $RR$ of .87 was a long way from statistical significance, and there is a host of other plausible factors that could have reduced the association. More research is needed on the interpersonal process as a factor affecting predictive validity of behavioral assessments before we can know either the strength of the effects or the mechanisms mediating these effects.

## REFERENCES

Anderson, J. R., & Waldron, I. (1983). Behavioral and content components of the Structured Interview assessment of the Type A behavior pattern in women. *Journal of Behavioral Medicine, 6*, 123–134.

Arrowood, J., Uhrich, K., Gomillion, C., Popio, K. A., & Raft, D. (1982). New markers of coronary-prone behavior in a rural population [Abstract]. *Psychosomatic Medicine, 44*, 119.

Bjork, L., Spindola-Franco, H., Van Houten, F. X., Cohn, P. F., & Adams, D. F. (1975). Comparison of observer performance with 16 mm cinefluorography and 70 mm camera fluorography in coronary arteriography. *American Journal of Cardiology, 36*, 474–478.

Blumenthal, J. A., Herman, S., O'Toole, L. C., Haney, T. L., Williams, R. B., & Barefoot, J. C. (1985). Development of a brief self-report measure of the Type A (coronary-prone) behavior pattern. *Journal of Psychosomatic Research, 29*, 265–273.

Blumenthal, J. A., O'Toole, L. C., & Haney, T. H. (1984). Behavioral assessment of the Type A behavior pattern. *Psychosomatic Medicine, 46*, 415–423.

Blumenthal, J. A., Williams, R.B., & Kong, Y. (1978). Type A behavior pattern and coronary atherosclerosis. *Circulation, 58*, 634–639.

Booth-Kewley, S., & Friedman, H. (in press). Psychological predictors of heart disease: A quantitative review. *Psychological Bulletin*.

Brand, R. J. (1978). Coronary-prone behavior as an independent risk factor for coronary heart disease. In T. M Dembroski, S. M. Weiss, J. L. Shields, S. G. Haynes, & M. Feinleib (Eds.), *Coronary-prone behavior*. New York: Springer-Verlag.

Brown, B. G., Bolson, E. L., & Dodge, H. T. (1982). Arteriographic assessment of coronary atherosclerosis. Review of current methods, their limitations, and clinical applications. *Arteriosclerosis, 2*, 2–15.

Case, R. B., Heller, S. S., Case, N. B., Moss, A. J., & the Multicenter Post-Infarction Research Group (1985). Type A behavior and survival after acute myocardial infarction. *New England Journal of Medicine, 312*, 737–741.

Dembroski, T. M., MacDougall, J. M., Williams, R. B., Haney, T. L., & Blumenthal, J. A. (1985). Components of Type A, hostility, and anger-in: Relationship to angiographic findings. *Psychosomatic Medicine, 47*, 219–233.

DeRouen, T. A., Murray, J. A., & Owen, W. (1977). Variability in the analysis of coronary arteriograms. *Circulation, 55*, 324–328.

Detre, K. M., Wright, E., Murphy, M. L., & Takaro, T. (1975). Observer agreement in evaluating coronary angiograms. *Circulation, 52*, 979–986.

Dimsdale, J. E., Hackett, T. P., Hutter, A. M., Block, P. C., Catanzano, D. M., & White, P. J. (1979). Type A behavior and angiographic findings. *Journal of Psychosomatic Research, 23*, 273–276.

Frank, K. A., Heller, S. S., Kornfeld, D. S., Sporn, A. A., & Weiss, M. B. (1978). Type A behavior pattern and coronary angiographic findings. *Journal of the American Medical Association, 240*, 761–763.

Friedman, M. (1969). *Pathogenesis of coronary artery disease*. New York: McGraw-Hill.

Friedman, M., Brown, M. A., & Rosenman, R. H. (1969). Voice analysis test for detection of behavior pattern. *Journal of the American Medical Association, 208*, 828–836.

Friedman, M., & Rosenman, R. (1974). *Type A behavior and your heart*. New York: Knopf.

Friedman, M., Rosenman, R. H., Straus, R., Wurm, M., & Kositchek, R. (1968). The relationship of behavior pattern A to the state of the coronary vasculature: A study of 51 autopsied subjects. *American Journal of Medicine, 44*, 525–537.

Friedman, M., Thoresen, C. E., Gill, J. J., Powell, L. H., Ulmer, D., Thompson, L., Price, V., Rabin, D., Breall, W. S., Dixon, T., Levy, R., & Bourg, E. (1984). Alteration of Type A behavior and reduction in cardiac recurrences in postmyocardial infarction patients. *American Heart Journal, 108*, 237–248.

Glass, D. C. (1977). *Behavior patterns, stress, and coronary disease*. Hillsdale, NJ: Erlbaum.

Haynes, S. G., Feinleib, M., & Eaker, E. D. (1983). Type A behavior and the ten-year incidence of coronary heart disease in the Framingham Heart Study. In R. H. Rosenman (Ed.), *Psychosomatic risk factors and coronary heart disease*. Berne: Hans Huber.

Haynes, S. G., Feinleib, M., Levine, S., Scotch, N., & Kannel, W. B. (1978). The relationship of psychosocial factors to coronary heart disease in the Framingham Study: II. Prevalence of coronary heart disease. *American Journal of Epidemiology, 107(5)*, 384–402.

Hecker, M., Chesney, M., Black, G., & Rosenman, R. (1981). Speech analysis of Type A behavior. In J. K. Darby (Ed.), *Speech evaluation in medicine*. New York: Grune & Stratton.

Hecker, M., Frautschi, N., Chesney, M., Black, G., & Rosenman, R. (1985, March). *Components of the Type A behavior and coronary heart disease*. Paper presented at the meeting of the Society of Behavioral Medicine, New Orleans.

Howland, E. W., & Siegman, A. W. (1982). Toward the automated measurement of the Type-A behavior pattern. *Journal of Behavioral Medicine, 5*, 37–54.

Kahn, J. P., Kornfeld, D. S., Blood, D. K., Lynn, R. B., Heller, S. S., & Frank, K. A. (1982). Type A behavior and the thallium stress test. *Psychosomatic Medicine, 44*, 431–436.

Krantz, D. S., Durel, L., Davia, J. E., Shaffer, R. T., Arabian, J. M., Dembroski, T. M., &

MacDougall, J. M. (1982). Propranolol medication among coronary patients: Relationship to Type A behavior and cardiovascular response. *Journal of Human Stress, 8,* 4–12.

Krantz, D. S., Sanmarco, M. I., Selvester, R. H., & Matthews, K. A. (1979). Psychological correlates of progression of atherosclerosis in men. *Psychosomatic Medicine, 41,* 467–475.

Krantz, D. S., Schaeffer, M. A., Davia, J. E., Dembroski, T. M., MacDougall, J. M., & Shaffer, R. T. (1981). Extent of coronary atherosclerosis, Type A behavior, and cardiovascular response to social interaction. *Psychophysiology, 18,* 654–664.

Matthews, K. A. (1978). Assessment and developmental antecedents of the coronary-prone behavior pattern in children. In T. M. Dembroski, S. M. Weiss, J. L. Shields, S. G. Haynes, & M. Feinleib (Eds.), *Coronary-prone behavior.* New York: Springer-Verlag.

Matthews, K. A., & Haynes, S. G. (1986). Type A behavior pattern and coronary risk: Update and critical evaluation. *American Journal of Epidemiology, 123,* 923–960.

MRFIT Group (1979). The MRFIT behavior pattern study: I. Study design, procedures, and reproducibility of behavior pattern judgments. *Journal of Chronic Diseases, 32,* 293–305.

MRFIT Group (1982). The Multiple Risk Factor Intervention Trial: Risk factor changes and mortality results. *Journal of the American Medical Association, 248,* 1465–1477.

MRFIT Group (1973). *MRFIT behavior pattern study: Protocol.* Unpublished manuscript.

Myers, M. G., Shulman, H. S., Saibil, E. A., & Naqvi, S. Z. (1978). Variation in measurement of coronary lesions on 35 and 70 mm angiograms. *American Journal of Roentgenology, 130,* 913–915.

Powell, L., & Thoresen, C. (1985). Behavioral and physiologic determinants of long-term prognosis after myocardial infarction. *Journal of Chronic Diseases, 38,* 253–263.

Price, V. A. (1982). *Type A behavior pattern: A model for research and practice.* New York: Academic.

Rosenman, R. H. (1978). The interview method of assessment of the coronary-prone behavior pattern. In T. M. Dembroski, S. M. Weiss, J. L. Shields, S. G. Haynes, & M. Feinleib (Eds.), *Coronary-prone behavior.* New York: Springer-Verlag.

Rosenman, R. H. (1978). The role of the Type A behaviour pattern in ischaemic heart disease: Modification of its effects by beta-blocking agents. *British Journal of Clinical Practice, 32* (Suppl. 1), 58–90.

Rosenman, R. H., Brand, R. J., Jenkins, C. D., Friedman, M., Straus, R., & Wurm, M. (1975). Coronary heart disease in the Western Collaborative Group Study: Final follow-up experience of 8½ years. *Journal of the American Medical Association, 233,* 872–877.

Rosenman, R. H., Brand, R. J., Sholtz, R. I., & Friedman, M. (1976). Multivariate prediction of coronary heart disease during 8½ year follow-up in the Western Collaborative Group Study. *American Journal of Cardiology, 37,* 903–910.

Rosenman, R. H., Friedman, M., Straus, R., Wurm, M., Kositchek, R., Hahn, W., & Werthessen, N. T. (1964). A predictive study of coronary heart disease: The Western Collaborative Group Study. *Journal of the American Medical Association, 189,* 15.

Roskies, E., Kearney, H., Spevack, M., Surkis, A., Cohen, C., & Gilman, S. (1979). Generalizability and durability of treatment effects in an intervention program for coronary-prone (Type A) managers. *Journal of Behavioral Medicine, 2,* 195–207.

Ruberman, W., Weinblatt, E., Goldberg, J. D., & Chaudbury, B. (1984). Psychosocial influence on mortality after myocardial infarction. *New England Journal of Medicine, 311,* 552–559.

Scherwitz, L., Berton, K., & Leventhal, H. (1977). Type A assessment and interaction in the behavior pattern interview. *Psychosomatic Medicine, 39,* 229–240.

Scherwitz, L., Graham, L. E., Grandits, G., & Billings, J. (1986). *Speech characteristics and coronary heart disease incidence in the MRFIT.* Unpublished manuscript.

Scherwitz, L., Graham, L. E., Grandits, G., & Billings, J. (1987). Speech characteristics and behavior type assessment in the MRFIT Structured Interviews. *Journal of Behavioral Medicine, 10,* 173–195.

Scherwitz, L., Graham, L. E., Grandits, G., Buehler, J., & Billings, J. (1986). Self-involvement and coronary heart disease incidence in the Multiple Risk Factor Intervention Trial. *Psychosomatic Medicine, 48,* 187–199.

Scherwitz, L., McKelvain, R., Laman, C., Patterson, J., Dutton, L., Yusim, S., Lester, J., Kraft, I., Rochelle, D., & Leachman, R. (1983). Type A behavior, self-involvement, and coronary atherosclerosis. *Psychosomatic Medicine, 45,* 47–57.

Schmieder, R., Friedrich, G., Neus, H., Rüddel, H., & Von Eiff, W. (1983). The influence of beta-blockers on cardiovascular reactivity and Type A behavior pattern in hypertensives. *Psychosomatic Medicine, 45(4),* 417–423.

Schucker, B., & Jacobs, D. R. (1977). Assessment of behavioral risk for coronary disease by voice characteristics. *Psychosomatic Medicine, 39,* 219–228.

Seeman, T. E., & Syme, S. L. (1987). Social networks and coronary artery disease: A comparison of the structure and function of social relations as predictors of disease. *Psychosomatic Medicine, 49,* 341–354.

Shekelle, R., Hulley, S., Neaton, J., Billings, J. H., Borhani, N. O., Gerace, T. A., Jacobs, D. R., Lasser, N. L., Mittlemark, M. B., & Stamler, J., for the MRFIT Research Group (1985). The MRFIT behavior pattern study: II. Type A behavior and incidence of coronary heart disease. *American Journal of Epidemiology, 122,* 559–570.

Siegman, A. W., Feldstein, S., Ringel, N., & Tomasso, C. T. (in press). Expressive vocal behavior and the severity of coronary artery disease. *Psychosomatic Medicine.*

Singer, M. T. (1974). Presidential address—Engagement-involvement: A central phenomenon in psychophysiological research. *Psychosomatic Medicine, 36,* 1–17.

Thaler-Singer, M., Reiser, M. F., & Weiner, H. (1957). An exploration of the doctor–patient relationship through projective techniques. Their use in psychosomatic illness. *Psychosomatic Medicine, 19,* 228–239.

Weiner, H., Singer, M. T., & Reiser, M. F. (1962). Cardiovascular responses and their psychological correlates: I. A study in healthy young adults and patients with peptic ulcer and hypertension. *Psychosomatic Medicine, 24,* 477–498.

Williams, R. B. (1978). Psychophysiological processes, the coronary-prone behavior pattern, and coronary heart disease. In T. M. Dembroski, S. M. Weiss, J. L. Shields, S. G. Haynes, & M. Feinleib (Eds.), *Coronary-prone behavior.* New York: Springer-Verlag.

Williams, R. B., Haney, T., Lee, K. L., Kong, Y., Blumenthal, J., & Whalen, R. E. (1980). Type A behavior, hostility, and coronary atherosclerosis. *Psychosomatic Medicine, 42,* 539–549.

Zir, L. M., Miller, S. W., Dinsmore, R. E., Gilbert, J. P., & Harthorne, J. W. (1976). Interobserver variability in coronary angiography. *Circulation, 53,* 627–632.

# 4

# The Association of Type A Behavior with Cardiovascular Disease—Update and Critical Review

SUZANNE G. HAYNES AND KAREN A. MATTHEWS

## INTRODUCTION

During the past 20 years, a formidable body of information has accumulated on the association of Type A behavior and coronary artery disease. The importance of Type A as a risk factor for CHD was highlighted in 1978 by a distinguished panel of scientists, brought together by the

This research was completed during the tenure of Established Investigatorships to Drs. Haynes and Matthews from the American Heart Association. The opinions and interpretations of the data in this manuscript are those of the authors and not of the National Center for Health Statistics. The authors wish to thank Drs. Andrea LaCroix and Alice White for their assistance in the preparation of Tables 4.3 and Mrs. Charlotte Hinckley for the preparation of the manuscript.

National Heart, Lung, and Blood Institute (Dembroski, Feinleib, Haynes, Shields, & Weiss, 1978). The panel concluded:

> Type A behavior . . . is associated with an increased risk of clinically apparent coronary heart disease in employed, middle-aged U. S. citizens. This risk is greater than that imposed by age, elevated values of systolic blood pressure and serum cholesterol, or smoking, and appears to be of the same order of magnitude as the relative risk associated with the latter three of these factors. (Cooper, Detre, & Weiss, 1981, p. 1200)

Often in the course of scientific inquiry, positive findings of far-reaching importance, such as the Type A association, are followed by the publication of negative results. In recent years, data have been reported to suggest that the conclusion made by the 1978 panel should be reevaluated. A "turning point" in the Type A field has resulted from the publication of negative findings, particularly from angiography and secondary prevention trials.

As with all turning points in science, we are faced with a paradigm shift, that is, a profound change in the thoughts, perceptions, and values that form a particular vision of reality (Capra, 1982). Scientists are thinking more and more that Type A behavior is no longer a risk factor for coronary heart disease. It is thought that some element in the behavior pattern (measurement, study design, environment, coping style, etc.) has changed, so that the early findings from the Western Collaborative Group Study and Framingham Study no longer hold in other populations.

This chapter will focus on at least two of these factors, study design and work environment, to see whether changes in these elements have distorted recent findings and altered the original theory that helped us explain the Type A association. As with other major paradigm shifts in science, such as the shift in cholesterol research from total measures to measures of lipoprotein and apo lipoprotein, new inputs are likely to evolve from the refinement and challenge of the Type A theory.

Throughout the discussions presented in this book, it is important to think about the following questions regarding the cause of the recent paradigm shift:

1.  Has the strength of earlier scientific findings in white-collar men diminished because different subpopulations have been studied or because different study designs (case-control, clinical trial) have been used? If so, have methodological problems biased the findings from angiography studies and clinical trials?

2.  Have changes in the American work environment toward a Japanese style of management (i.e., greater cooperation, less individual competition, and more group participation) affected the behavior of Type A managers to the point of reducing their coronary risk?

3. Has the strength of Type A behavior as a coronary risk factor diminished because of widespread public awareness of the problem? In other words, has the scientific community succeeded in modifying Type A risk simply by its identification, resulting in changed behavior or in earlier medical intervention for Type A's?

The purpose of this chapter is to review and evaluate the available data related to Type A behavior and coronary heart disease. Particular focus is given to those data published since the 1978 conference and to a recently published review of the field by the present authors (Matthews & Haynes, 1986). Much of the material used in this chapter was derived from our recent review, although additional insights have been noted. The chapter is organized into three sections. The first section considers data from prospective studies of Type A behavior and coronary heart disease. Data from both population studies and studies of persons of high coronary heart disease risk are reviewed. The second section evaluates the evidence that Type A behavior is related to cardiovascular endpoints other than coronary heart disease: coronary atherosclerosis as measured by coronary arteriography and cerebrovascular accidents. In general, the data available for review in the second section are from cross-sectional and case-control studies. The third section will outline future directions in Type A research, with attention drawn to changes that may explain the recent paradigm shift.

## TYPE A AND CORONARY HEART DISEASE

Table 4.1 summarizes the major findings from prospective studies of coronary heart disease and global Type A behavior assessed by the four major assessment techniques or other techniques shown to relate to the Structured Interview assessment of Type A behavior. The findings from prevalence studies were reviewed by Jenkins (1983) and are not considered here because of the methodological and interpretative difficulties with prevalence data.

### Population-Based Studies

The first major prospective study designed to examine the coronary risk associated with the Type A behavior pattern was the Western Collaborative Group Study (Rosenman et al., 1975). Beginning in 1960, approximately 3200 employed men free of coronary heart disease were followed for a total of 8.5 years. The study was double blind, so that the Type A interviewer had no knowledge of the men's health status and the investigators assessing coronary heart disease risk had no knowledge of the men's Type A behavior. The final 8.5-year follow-up report showed that those men assessed as Type A by the Structured Interview at entry had a risk ratio of 2.2 for

## TABLE 4.1. TYPE A BEHAVIOR AND PROSPECTIVE FUNDINGS

| Reference | Study and Site | Selection and/or Exclusion Criteria | Sample Characteristics |
|---|---|---|---|
| Rosenman et al. (1975) | Western Collaborative Group Study, California | Employed in 1 of 10 firms; CHD-free at study entry; follow-up of 8½ years. | 3154 men; 39 to 59 years old at study entry. |
| Jenkins et al. (1974) | Western Collaborative Group Study, California | Employed in 1 of 10 firms; CHD-free at study entry; follow-up of 4 years. | 120 new cases of CHD compared to 524 healthy controls. |
| Haynes et al. (1980) | Framingham Heart Study, Framingham, MA | Members of Framingham cohort taking 8th or 9th medical exam; free of CHD; able to understand questions; 8-year follow-up. | 949 women, 725 men; 45 to 77 years old at study entry; white- and blue-collar men; housewives and working women. |
| Haynes et al. (1982) | Framingham Heart Study, Framingham, MA | Members of Framingham cohort taking 8th or 9th medical exam; free of CHD; able to understand questions; 10-year follow-up. | 750 women, 580 men; 45 to 64 years old at study entry. |
| Cohen et al. (1985) | Honolulu Heart Study | Out of 8006 men of Japanese descent, only those reporting for second exam in 1970 were in Type A study; followed for 8 years. | 2187 men; 51 to 70 years old. |
| French-Belgian Collaborative Study (1982) | French-Belgian Cooperative Heart Study, Brussels-Ghent, Belgium; Marseilles and Paris, France | Workers in factories in Belgium, follow-up, mean = 70.1 months for mortality, 65.5 months for morbidity; and in civil service in Marseilles, follow-up 96.7 and 74.1 months, respectively; and in Paris, follow-up of 53.5 months for both mortality and morbidity. | 836 men, mean age = 48.3 years from Brussels-Ghent; 791 men, mean age = 48.5 years from Marseilles; and 1,575 men, mean age = 45.9 years from Paris. |
| DeBaker et al. (1983) | Belgian Heart Disease Prevention Trial | Men free of AP or major electrocardiogram abnormalities at baseline; followed for 5 years. | 1958 men, 40 to 55 years old. |

*Source*: Adapted from Matthews & Haynes, 1986.

Abbreviations: SI, Structured Interview; JAS, Jenkins Activity Survey; VSI, Videotaped Structured Interview; CHD, coronary heart disease; AP, angina pectoris; MI, myocardial infarction.

| Type A Measure | Disease Categories | Findings |
| --- | --- | --- |
| SI; 50.4% Type A; 49.6% Type B. | Symptomatic MI; unrecognized MI; AP (without MI). | Incidence rates A/B; total CHD, 2.24; symptomatic MI, 2.16; unrecognized MI, 2.12; angina pectoris, 2.45. Associations significant in multivariate analyses. |
| JAS | Symptomatic MI; unrecognized MI; AP (without MI). | Type A scores higher among cases than controls. No multivariate results were presented. Not related to single manifestation. |
| Framingham Type A Scale. Median split within sex/age groups to form A–B groups. | MI; coronary insufficiency; AP; AP only; CHD death. | In men aged 45 to 64 years, Type A predicted total CHD and MI in multivariate analyses (due to white-collar men). In women aged 45 to 64 years, Type A predicted total CHD and AP in multivariate analyses for working women and univariate analyses for housewives. |
| Framingham Type A Scale. Median split within sex/age groups to form A–B groups. | MI only; complicated MI; AP only; CHD death; coronary insufficiency. | Type A women had greater risk for total CHD and AP only; $RR = 2.0$ and 2.6, respectively. Type A men had greater risk for total CHD ($RR = 2.4$) and MI complicated by angina (white-collar men only). |
| JAS-Form B | Definite MI; AP; coronary insufficiency; atherosclerosis scores from autopsy studies. | Type A not related to incidence of MI, angina, total CHD, and atherosclerosis, but related to prevalence of CHD in multivariate analyses. |
| Bortner Rating Scale | Hard events are fatal or nonfatal MI and sudden death; AP. | Type A predicted hard events and total CHD in multivariate analyses. |
| JAS | MI; sudden death. | Type A predicted total CHD. No significance tests were presented. Only 18 events occurred. |

development of coronary heart disease compared to Type B's. The risk associated with Type A persisted when simultaneous statistical adjustments were made for the other risk factors for coronary heart disease (adjusted risk ratios of 1.9 and 2.0 for the men 39 to 49 and 50 to 59 years old, respectively) (Rosenman et al., 1975). Review of these data by the present authors showed that Type A was less strongly associated with myocardial infarction (risk ratio = 2.1) than with angina pectoris occurring without myocardial infarction (risk ratio = 2.5) (Matthews & Haynes, 1986).

Analyses of all the participants who were free of coronary heart disease at the time of the Jenkins Activity Survey administration (N = 2750) showed a risk ratio of 1.8 for those with scores in approximately the upper third of the study distribution compared to those in the lower third (Jenkins, Rosenman, & Zyzanski, 1974). When simultaneous adjustments were made for other risk factors, Type A's with Jenkins Activity Survey scores above the Western Collaborative Group Study mean scores had a risk ratio of 1.3 ($p$ = .15) (Brand, Jenkins, & Rosenman, 1978).

The Framingham Heart Study has provided a rich source for testing the association of Type A behavior with coronary heart disease in a population quite different from the Western Collaborative Group Study. This population included women and men in both white-collar and blue-collar jobs. All had a thorough medical examination establishing that they were free from coronary heart disease at the beginning of the follow-up period. Multivariate analyses of the 8-year incidence data showed that Type A behavior measured by the Framingham Type A Scale was an independent predictor of coronary heart disease and myocardial infarction in men 45 to 64 years old and of coronary heart disease and angina in women of the same age (Haynes, Feinleib, & Kannel, 1980). Multivariate analyses showed that the significant effects were restricted to men in white-collar positions and were almost as strong in housewives and women employed over half of their adult years. Risk ratios for total coronary heart disease, myocardial infarction, and angina without myocardial infarction were 2.9, 7.3, and 1.8, respectively, in white-collar men and 2.1, 1.3, and 3.6, respectively, in women. Further analyses of the 10-year incidence data showed similar risk ratios (Haynes & Feinleib, 1982) of, respectively, 2.4, 7.9, and 1.8 in white-collar men and 2.0, 1.8, and 2.6 in women. Analyses of these data also suggested that the association between Type A behavior and coronary heart disease was most marked when the levels of other risk factors were elevated. Another distinctly different population in which the association of Type A behavior and coronary heart disease has been tested is the approximately 2200 men of Japanese descent enrolled in the Honolulu Heart Study (Cohen & Reed, 1985; Cohen, Syme, Jenkins, Kagan, & Zyzanski, 1979). These men were administered the Jenkins Activity Survey and followed for 8 years for the development of coronary heart disease. This sample was characterized by a low incidence of coronary heart disease, approximately 50 percent that of the incidence for U.S. Caucasians in the Framingham Heart Study. Subsequently, no relationship between Type A behavior and incidence of total coronary heart disease, myocardial infarction, and angina was observed (Cohen & Reed, 1985).

Two unusual features of these data deserve special attention:

1.  The very low prevalence of Type A behavior among Japanese men (18.7 percent as compared to approximately 50 percent in the U.S. population) (Jenkins, 1983)

2.  The very low prevalence and incidence of CHD in Japanese men as compared to Caucasian men (4.0 percent vs. 13 percent in the Framingham men 55 to 64) (Haynes, Feinleib, Levine, Scotch, & Kannel, 1978)

The first finding was explained by the fact that hard-driving and competitive behavior is discouraged in the Japanese culture, while social harmony, trust, and cooperation are encouraged at the expense of individual initiative (Cohen et al., 1979). The second finding could be explained by the first finding, or by the lower prevalence of other risk factor in the Japanese men. Given the recent and intense interest by American business in the Japanese style of management (Ouchi, 1981; Pascale & Athos, 1981) we might predict a reduction in Type A behavior over time in the United States. The Honolulu Heart Study findings suggest that such a reduction could lead to a decline in CHD rates and a lessening of Type A as a risk factor for CHD. At the present time, no studies are being conducted in the United States to test this intriguing hypothesis.

Relevant here are generally positive findings reported in several recent reports from ongoing prospective studies in European populations. The French-Belgian Collaborative Heart Study (1982) studied the predictors of incidence of coronary heart disease in 2811 male civil servants and factory workers in Brussels-Ghent, Belgium, and Marseilles and Paris, France. The men were free of coronary heart disease at entry and were enrolled in the study an average of 5 years and a minimum of 1 month. Type A scores by the Bortner Rating Scale (Bortner, 1969) were not significant predictors of coronary heart disease in each cohort taken separately, although they were always higher in the coronary heart disease group (French-Belgian Collaborative Heart Study, 1982). Multivariate analyses collapsing all cohort data together showed that Type A was a significant predictor of total coronary heart disease, as well as myocardial infarction and sudden death. The relative risk for total coronary heart disease among men in the top and bottom quartile of the distribution of Bortner scores was 1.8. Among men above and below the median score, the relative risk was 1.5. For myocardial infarction and sudden death combined, the comparable figures were 1.6 and 1.4, respectively.

The final prospective study to be reviewed here is a preliminary report by DeBacker, Dramaix, Kittel, and Kornitzer (1983) based on Jenkins Activity

Survey Type A data collected in the Belgian Heart Disease Prevention Trial. Among approximately 2000 men who passed a strenuous exercise test, trichotomized Jenkins Activity Survey scores were related in a linear fashion to total coronary heart disease (myocardial infarction or sudden death) during a 5-year follow-up period. The risk ratio was 1.9 for men whose Jenkins Activity Survey scores were in approximately the upper third compared to those whose scores were in the lower third of the distribution. No significance tests or multivariate analyses to control for other coronary heart disease risk factors were reported.

### Summary and Comment

On balance, the population-based studies show that Type A behavior is a risk factor for coronary heart disease. The one exception to this trend is the findings from the Honolulu Heart Study, which show no relationship between Jenkins Activity Survey Type A scores and coronary heart disease in a low-coronary-risk population.

Although it is dangerous to disqualify null results in reaching final conclusions, it is important to note that measurement and disease rate issues may account for the negative results from the Honolulu Heart Study. More specifically, the men in that study population had a low prevalence of Type A behavior and a low incidence of coronary heart disease relative to Caucasians, such as those in the Framingham Heart Study or the Western Collaborative Group Study. It may simply be the case that, in populations where Type A behavior is not part of the normative behavior patterns, it is not a risk factor. It may also be the case that Type A does not exert a pathogenic influence unless some other combination of risk factors is present (Haynes & Feinleib, 1982), a combination not currently present in the Japanese population.

### Studies of High-Risk Persons

There are six prospective studies of high-risk persons. The first study listed in Table 4.2 was by Jenkins, Rosenman, and Zyzanski (1976) on the predictors of the recurrence of myocardial infarction in the Western Collaborative Group Study population. In this study, the 267 men who had at least one coronary heart disease event (any coronary heart disease manifestation) either during or prior to the beginning of the Western Collaborative Group Study and who could be followed for at least 1 year prior to the end of the study were part of the study population. Of the 267, during the follow-up period 67 had a symptomatic myocardial infarction. Stepwise discriminant function analyses showed that the Jenkins Activity Survey Type A score was a significant predictor of recurrent myocardial infarction events, controlling for other coronary heart disease risk factors.

Three other prospective studies have investigated Type A behavior as assessed by the Jenkins Activity Survey as a predictor of new coronary disease events in coronary patients. Dimsdale, Block, Gilbert, Hackett, and Hutter (1981) studied predictors of new morbid events, that is, hospitalization, myocardial infarction, or death, in a group of 189 men who had undergone cardiac catheterization, usually for coronary symptoms, and were followed for 1 year. Contrary to expectations, the stepwise discriminant function analyses showed that Type B behavior was predictive of new morbidity. No risk ratios or recurrence rates were presented.

Case, Heller, Case, and Moss (1985) administered the Type A scale within 2 weeks of discharge from the coronary care unit to 63 percent of the 866 patients enrolled in the Multicenter Post-Infarction Program, a study aimed at identifying the risk factors that predict long-term survival after myocardial infarction. Those who did not participate in the Type A study had more severe cardiac disease as identified by four independent physiologic risk factors and higher mortality rates during follow-up than those who did participate. Survival analyses showed that Type A scores did not predict mortality that occurred during a subsequent follow-up period of 1 to 3 years. Shekelle, Gale, and Norusis (1985) investigated the predictors of recurrent myocardial infarction in a group of 244 female and 2070 male myocardial infarction patients enrolled in a 3-year clinical trial to assess the efficaciousness of aspirin for reducing risk of recurrent events. As with the absence of a positive effect of aspirin, Type A behavior had no value in predicting recurrence in women, men, or white-collar men alone. Risk ratios of high scorers as compared to low scorers were 0.40, 0.83, and 0.92 for women, men, and white-collar men, respectively.

The Multiple Risk Factor Intervention Trial population was used to test the hypothesis that Type A is a risk factor for coronary heart disease in men in the top decile of risk for coronary heart disease based on their levels of cigarette smoking, serum cholesterol, and blood pressure (Shekelle, Billings, et al., 1985). These men were initially coronary heart disease free at entry into the study and were followed for an average of 7 years. They were randomly assigned into a usual care group and a special care group. The latter group experienced interventions designed to reduce blood pressure by pharmacologic agents, serum cholesterol levels by diet, and cigarette smoking by behavioral interventions. All men were asked to complete the Jenkins Activity Survey and approximately one-fourth of the sample were also asked to complete the Structured Interview. In the latter group, 74 percent were Type A. Similar to the finding of an absence of a significant difference in either total mortality or coronary heart disease mortality between the usual care and special care groups (MRFIT Study Group, 1982), Shekelle, Billings, and colleagues (1985) reported that Type A's and Type B's assessed by either the Structured Interview or Jenkins Activity Survey did not have a differential first major coronary event experience. For the Structured

TABLE 4.2. TYPE A BEHAVIOR AND PROSPECTIVE FINDINGS OF

| Reference | Study and Site | Selection and/or Exclusion Criteria | Sample Characteristics |
|---|---|---|---|
| Jenkins et al. (1976) | Western Collaborative Group Study, California | All men who had at least one CHD event during or prior to Western Collaborative Group Study and could be followed for at least 1 year. | 67 men who had a second event of symptomatic MI and 220 men who did not. |
| Dimsdale et al. (1979) | Boston | Patients undergoing cardiac catheterization, usually for coronary symptoms; not for valvular disease, other interfering chronic disease; follow-up of 1 year. | 189 men; 18 to 70 years old; mean age = 50 years. 79 men had bypass surgery subsequent to catheterization. |
| Case et al. (1985) | Multicenter Post-Infarction Program | Survived acute MI. | 548 patients out of 866 in total sample. Demographic data presented in 516; 82% male, 69% $\leq$ 60 years; 73% employed; 13% $\leq$ 10th grade education. Participants were healthier than nonparticipants. |
| Shekelle, Gale, et al. (1985) | Aspirin Myocardial Infarction Study, 30 clinical centers | MI, no previous cardiac surgery; no other life limiting disease; 18 out of 30 centers participated; followed for 3 years. | 244 women, 2070 men, 29 to 69 years old; randomly assigned to aspirin or placebo group. |
| Shekelle, Billings, et al. (1985) | Multiple Risk Factor Intervention Trial, 22 clinical centers | Cigarette smoking, serum cholesterol and blood pressure at levels high enough to place in upper 10% of risk distribution based on Framingham data. No diabetes requiring treatment. No previous MIs, angina, lipid-lowering agents or too high blood pressure or cholesterol level. Followed for 7 years average. | 3110 men from 8 clinical centers; 35 to 57 years old; randomly assigned to special care or usual care. 12,772 men from all centers. |
| Friedman et al. (1986) | Recurrent Coronary Prevention Project, California | MI patients; aged $\leq$ 64 years; MI at least 6 months; not smoking for at least 6 months, no diabetes; followed for 4.5 years. | 1013 MI patients; mean age = 53 years; 90% male, 85% married; randomly assigned to Type A behavioral change or cardiologist-led treatment group. |

Source: Adapted from Matthews & Haynes, 1986.

Abbreviations: SI, Structured Interview; JAS, Jenkins Activity Survey; VSI, Videotaped Structured Interview; CHD, coronary heart disease; AP, angina pectoris; MI, myocardial infarction.

# CORONARY HEART DISEASE: STUDIES OF HIGH-RISK PERSONS

| Type A Measure | Disease Categories | Findings |
|---|---|---|
| JAS—34% of recurrent group took JAS after second event. | Symptomatic MI. | Type A score, higher in recurrence group. Association significant in stepwise discriminant function analysis. |
| JAS | New morbid event; i.e., hospitalization, MI, death. | Type B related to morbidity in total sample and in subsample of medically treated patients in stepwise discriminant function analysis. |
| JAS administered within 2 weeks after discharge from intensive care unit. | Mortality | No relation between Type A and mortality, left ventricular ejection fraction, time to death for nonsurvivors, duration of stay in coronary care unit. |
| JAS | Definite MI; fatal MI. | No relationship between recurrent event and Type A in total sample, men, women, and white-collar or blue-collar men. |
| SI; 35% A1; 39% A2; 9% X; 18% B. | Total mortality; mortality from CHD. | No relationship between Type A and mortality. |
| JAS-Form B | Total mortality; mortality from CHD. | No relationship between Type A and mortality. |
| VSI | Recurrent MI; sudden cardiac death. | Type A behavioral treatment group had lower recurrence rate (12.9%) after 4.5 years than did the control group (21.2%) or the comparison group not receiving any special treatment (24.2%). |

Interview, the A–B risk ratio of coronary heart disease death was 0.92, while for the Jenkins Activity Survey, the comparable risk ratio for men scoring in the top and bottom quintiles of the Jenkins scale was 0.82. It should be noted that the power to detect a statistical association between Type A and coronary heart disease in the usual group was low (.67), that is, less than the accepted level of .80 used in the design of studies.

## Type A Intervention Study

A sixth high-risk study of relevance, the Recurrent Coronary Prevention Project, was distinctly different from those summarized above (see Table 4.2). This study tested the hypothesis that interventions designed to alter Type A behaviors lower the risk of a recurrent event among myocardial infarction patients (Friedman et al., 1986). Of the 1013 male myocardial infarction study participants, 592 were randomly assigned to a behavioral intervention plus cardiology counseling group, 270 were assigned to the cardiology counseling only group, and 151 received no counseling of any kind. Results based on the first 4.5 years of the project have shown a significantly lower recurrence rate in the experimental group, 12.9 percent, relative to the cardiology counseling only group, 21.2 percent, or the control group, 28.2 percent. Subsidiary analyses showed that the latter effect was not restricted to nonfatal events, 7.6 percent versus 14.0 percent and 9.2 percent, respectively. By comparison, the percentages for fatal cardiac events were 5.2 versus 7.2 and 11.0 percent, respectively. Furthermore, although both groups experienced a significant decrease in self-reported Type A behaviors and in Videotaped Structured Interview scores, the decrease in the intervention group was greater. The report showed that the Type A behavioral counseling was statistically protective as early as the third year of the study. Thus the results from the Recurrent Coronary Prevention Project do provide support for viewing Type A behavior as a causal risk factor for coronary heart disease in a high-risk population.

## Summary and Comment

In contrast to the population-based studies, studies of high-risk persons, with the exception of the Recurrent Coronary Prevention Project, fail to support consistently the hypothesis that Type A behavior is a risk factor for recurrent events or for mortality in men at high risk for coronary heart disease because of risk factors other than Type A behavior. Two studies by Shekelle and colleagues (Shekelle, Billings, et al., 1985; Shekelle, Gale, & Norusis, 1985) and one by Case and colleagues (1985) found no effects of Type A behavior, whereas the study by Jenkins and colleagues (1976) showed a positive effect and that by Dimsdale and colleagues (1981) indicated a negative effect. Because these studies assessed Type A behavior by the

Jenkins Activity Survey, one might conclude that the inconsistent effects are due to measurement error in the behavior pattern. Since the Multiple Risk Factor Intervention Trial (Shekelle, Billings, et al., 1985) also assessed Type A behavior in a subsample by the Structured Interview and reported no association, it is unlikely that the negative effects are only due to the use of the Jenkins Activity Survey.

One explanation may lie in the enormous changes in health behaviors and treatment patterns that could have an impact on the risk associated with Type A behavior. Perhaps the most obvious behavior change is the tremendous decline in cigarette smoking among white-collar men, the group on which the Type A behavior concept was initially validated. In addition, awareness of the importance of exercise, reduction in stress levels, and early use of medical facilities is thought to have heightened. Perhaps these behaviors have interacted synergistically with Type A behavior so that in more recent studies changes in these behavioral styles have altered risk to Type A's. Furthermore, the widespread use of new clinical interventions in cardiovascular disease may have inadvertently benefited Type A patients more than Type B patients since Type A's tended to have the highest risk. For example, beta-blocking agents are clearly beneficial to many patients. We know from data reviewed elsewhere (Matthews & Haynes, 1986) that Type A men exhibited heightened cardiovascular responses to stressors that may be effectively blocked by such agents. These reactions to stressors are thought to be a mechanism through which Type A's incur their excess coronary risk.

A second explanation has to do with assessment of the behavior pattern itself. It has been assumed that Type A behavior is always stable over time. But this assumption may be naive in clinical trials in which there is a heightened awareness of the importance of health and changes in risk. We also have a concern about the appropriateness of the measures without further adaptation for populations other than white-collar men. Even within a sample of white-collar men, it appears that the associations between the Structured Interview and other Type A measures and changing (Matthews, Dembroski, Krantz, & MacDougall, 1982). This suggests that there might be some drift in the diagnostic criteria used in making the Structured Interview assessment of Type A behavior and that perhaps in earlier studies certain criteria, for example, hostility and anger, were emphasized that were more important for risk of coronary heart disease than the criteria currently emphasized. Chapter 8 of this volume, by Chesney, Hecker, and Black, should help to address this issue. A third explanation related to secular trends is also feasible (Type A behavior, anger, and hostility: Working Group Summary, 1985). The more negative studies were conducted and begun at a time when rates of coronary heart disease mortality were declining rapidly—1970 to 1983. This suggests the possibility that there were differences among the early population-based and late high-risk studies in the severity of the underlying coronary artery disease.

## TYPE A AND OTHER CARDIOVASCULAR ENDPOINTS

### Coronary Artherosclerosis

The increase in the number of medical centers performing coronary angiography and the tremendous numbers of patients undergoing this procedure for diagnosis of coronary artery disease have made it possible to examine the associations between risk factors such as Type A behavior and the extent of coronary atherosclerosis. Approximately 11.5 arteriograms per 10,000 population per year are being performed in the United States (Kennedy et al., 1980). Research on coronary risk factors, which once had to rely on crude outcome measures of coronary heart disease symptoms and major events, can now use refined outcome measures such as the degree of stenosis present in major coronary arteries.

Nonetheless, there are certain methodological and interpretative difficulties of angiography studies that limit their usefulness. The vast majority of the studies are cross-sectional, and thus it is not possible to determine the temporal relationships between risk factors and coronary artery disease. In addition, because of the cross-sectional nature of the studies, the characteristics of study participants are of crucial importance to the study interpretation. An essential characteristic of participants in angiography studies is that they have suspected coronary artery disease. Thus the findings cannot be generalized to populations without clinical symptoms. Referred patients may also have other cardiac diagnoses and medical history, for example, myocardial infarction, cardiomyopathy, or coronary artery bypass surgery, in addition to suspected coronary artery disease, which confound the results of risk factor research. Patients may also influence the referral process because of their personality and social characteristics. For example, individuals who complain frequently about symptoms, including chest pain, may be referred more often by their physicians, relative to more stoic individuals. To the extent that such characteristics are noncausally related to coronary artery disease, they also confound the results.

Despite these disadvantages, 16 investigations have been conducted on the association of Type A behavior and atherosclerosis. These studies are described in Table 4.3 in approximate order of publication.

### Global Type A

In the first of these investigations, Zyzanski, Everist, Flessas, Jenkins, and Ryan (1976) studied 94 men, who had been referred by private cardiologists to the Boston University Medical Center for angiography. The results showed that men with 50 percent or greater occlusion in two or more vessels had significantly higher Jenkins Activity Survey scores on the Type A scale as well as the three-factor scores than those with less disease. The angina intensity rating, from Class 1 (occurring never) to Class 4 (occurring at rest), showed no significant associations with Jenkins Activity Survey scores. However, men with more severe angina tended to score higher on the Type A scale: 1.2 for Class 1; 0.7 for Class 2 and 3; and 4.7 for Class 4 ($p < .09$). Further analyses of these data combined with additional data on 78 women and 11 men collected by Silver, Jenkins, Melidossian, and Ryan (1980) showed that after controlling for sex of the patient only Jenkins Activity Survey factor J, Job Involvement, was related to the diagnosis subsequently given to the patients, that is, coronary artery disease versus valve and other. Factor J was related to coronary artery disease positively in men but negatively in women.

Frank, Heller, Kornfeld, Sporn, and Weiss (1978) studied 124 male and 23 female patients referred because of clinical symptoms of coronary artery disease. A large proportion of men, 73 percent, were classified as Type A by the Structured Interview. Multivariate analyses showed that, after controlling for cholesterol, sex, age, smoking, and high blood pressure, Type A behavior was associated with the number of vessels occluded 50 percent or more.

A series of studies has emanated from the Duke University Medical Center in Durham, North Carolina. In the first of these studies (Blumenthal, Kong, Schanberg, Thompson, & Williams, 1978), a sample of 80 male and 62 female patients was administered both the Structured Interview and Jenkins Activity Survey. A total coronary index was developed as a measure of atherosclerosis. First, each vessel was assessed on a 4-point scale where 0 = no occlusion; 1 = < 75 percent occlusion; 2 = 75 to 99 percent occlusion; and 3 = 100 percent occlusion. Then scores for each of the four major arteries were summed and patients were divided into three groups on the basis of the total score. The results showed that the prevalence of Structured Interview Type A behavior rose with coronary artery disease scores: 44 percent (0 to 3), 69 percent (3 to 6); and 93 percent (7+) Type A's. However, no differences were observed in the prevalence of Type A behavior as measured by the Jenkins Activity Survey.

A second study, by Williams, Haney, and Lee (1980) studied the association among Type A behavior, the Cook-Medley Hostility Scale, and coronary artery disease in the same population, combined with additional patients totaling 307 men and 117 women. The above protocol for assessment of Type A behavior was followed, but only the Structured Interview results were reported. Significantly more of the Type A group (71 percent) had at least one vessel with 75 percent or more occlusion than the Type B group (56 percent). In addition, men had more occlusion than women, and hostile men and women had more occlusion than less hostile men and women.

The most recent work from the Duke series by Blumenthal and colleagues (1987) showed that Type A behavior, as measured by the Structured Interview, was associated with the number of vessels occluded 75 percent or more. The provocative findings of this study, however, were that Type A's who experienced a supportive environment from both peers and family were

## TABLE 4.3. TYPE A BEHAVIOR AND FINDINGS FROM CORONARY

| Reference | Referral Site | Selection and/or Exclusion Criteria | Sample Characteristics |
|---|---|---|---|
| Zyzanski et al. (1976) | Boston University Medical Center | Men referred with angina, ECG changes, congestive heart failure, aortic stenosis, mitral valve disease, cardiomyopathy. Prior bypass surgery excluded. | 94 men; 26 to 68 years old; 50% between 45 and 55 years; 49% had prior MI. |
| Silver et al. (1980) | Boston University Medical Center | Consecutive admissions referred with clinical symptoms of CHD and diagnosis of CAD, valvular heart disease, cardiomyopathy, chest pain of unknown origin. | 105 men, 78 women; 25 to 68 years old; males: 76.3% CAD, 30.2% valve disease; females: 23.7% CAD, 69.8% valve disease; 77% men—history of MI, 23% women—history of MI. |
| Frank et al. (1978) | Columbia Presbyterian Medical Center, New York | Presence of clinical symptoms consistent with CAD; consecutive admissions. | 124 men, 23 women; 29 to 65 years old; mean age = 51.7 years; 54% pervious MI; 83% typical angina; 12% atypical angina; 19% congestive heart failure; 32% hypertensive; 27% < 275 mg/dl cholesterol; 70% smokers. |
| Blumenthal et al. (1978) | Duke University Medical Center, Durham, NC | 142 consecutive patients; valve disease patients eliminated. | 80 men, 62 women; 15 to 69 years old; mean age = 47 years. |
| Williams et al. (1980) | Duke University Medical Center, Durham, NC | Patients referred to Duke between 5/76 and 4/77 with clinical history and/or laboratory evidence of CHD; valvular disease and cardiomyopathy excluded. | 307 men and 117 women. |

## ANGIOGRAPHY STUDIES

| Type A Measure and Time of Administration | Disease Categories | Findings |
|---|---|---|
| Before catheterization. 50% Type A by JAS. | Number of vessels obstructed ≥50%; 0 or 1 (N = 36) compared to >2 (N = 55). | JAS significantly related to CAD (p < .01). Also, objective measures of anxiety and depression related. |
| Before catheterization. Males more Type A (means 0.552 vs. −2.832) and more hard driving (7.433 vs. 3.340) than females, JAS. | Compared CAD patients to those with valve and other related disease. | Job involvement of the JAS and anxiety of the Minnesota Multiphasic Personality Inventory significantly related to CAD in men positively and in women negatively. |
| Before catheterization. SI; 51% A1; 22% A2; 20% B3; 5% B4. | Number of major arteries occluded ≥50%. | Type A significantly related to mean number of arteries stenosed, r = .24, p = .05. Association significant after controlling for cholesterol, sex, age, smoking, and hypertension. |
| After catheterization. 60% Type A by SI; JAS. | Coronary index where each vessel is scored on a 4- point scale. 3 = total occlusion; 2 = 75–99%; 1 = < 75%; 0 = no occlusion. 3 groups of patients based on index; <3 mild (N = 78); 3–6 moderate (N = 36); <6 severe (N = 28). | Type A significantly related to atherosclerosis, p < .001, independent of age, sex, blood pressure, cholesterol, and smoking. No association between any scales of the JAS with disease severity. |
| After catheterization. 75.2% Type A by SI; Cook–Medley Hostility Scale also administered. | At least one artery with stenosis ≥75% vs. no arteries with stenosis ≥75%. | Positive, significant association between Type A behavior and having at least one artery with ≥75% occlusion, p < .01. Sex and hostility interacted with Type A to predict atherosclerosis; males > females, high hostility > low hostility. |

*(Table continues on p. 68.)*

**TABLE 4.3.** (Continued)

| Reference | Referral Site | Selection and/or Exclusion Criteria | Sample Characteristics |
|---|---|---|---|
| Dimsdale et al. (1978) | Massachusetts General Hospital, Boston | Patients with clinical evidence of CAD or chest pain of uncertain origin. Excluded those with valvular heart disease, other critical conditions. | 99 men, 10 women; 18 to 70 years old; mean age = 49 years; 65% history of MI; 55% exertional angina, functional; classes II–IV. |
| Dimsdale et al. (1979) | Massachusetts General Hospital, Boston | Male patients with symptoms of CAD; valve disease patients eliminated. | 103 male patients; 18 to 70 years old; mean age = 50 years. |
| Krantz et al. (1981) | Walter Reed Army Medical Center, Washington, DC | Patients referred because of prior MI, chest pain, EKG abnormality; excluded CHF, aortic insufficiency, mitral stenosis, stroke, other valve disorders. | 76 men, 7 women; 30 to 67 years old; mean age = 49.3 years. |
| Sherwitz et al. (1983) | St. Luke's Episcopal Hospital, Houston | 156 male patients referred from 2 cardiology practices based on clinical symptoms or positive angiographic findings; exclusions: valvular heart disease, previous bypass surgery, serious non-cardiovascular illness, non-English speaking, non-US residents. | 150 men; 35 to 69 years old; mean age = 55 years; 59% previous MI, 72% history of angina, 52.4% ≤3 arteries occluded >50%, 69% eventually underwent coronary artery bypass graft. |
| Krantz et al. (1979) | Rancho Los Amigos Hospital, Downey, CA | Male cardiac outpatients who had repeat angiographs within 2 years; no bypass patients. | 67 men, mean age = 47.3 years. |

| Type A Measure and Time of Administration | Disease Categories | Findings |
|---|---|---|
| Before catheterization. JAS. | Number of vessels with ≥50% narrowing in diameter. | No association between mean JAS scores and number of diseased vessels. Comparing 0 and 1 vessels to 2 or more vessels diseased, those with mild disease had higher JAS scores (mean JAS 4.79 vs. 0.47, $p < .03$). |
| Before catheterization. 64% Type A by SI; JAS. | Number of vessels with ≥50% narrowing in diameter. Compared 0 vs. some and 0 + 1 vs. >2. | No association between mean JAS score or SI and number of vessels occluded. Comparing none vs. some, the nonoccluded group had significantly higher JAS scores (7.51 vs. 1.47, $p < .02$). Excluding those who were not extreme A's or B's, there was still no association. |

| Vessels | % Type A by SI |
|---|---|
| 0 | 62.5 |
| 1 | 68.2 |
| 2 | 61.5 |
| 3 & 4 | 64.1 |

| Type A Measure and Time of Administration | Disease Categories | Findings |
|---|---|---|
| Before catheterization. 74.7% Type A, by SI. | Severity index (4 point scale); 0 = no occlusion; 1 = ≤75%; 2 = 75–99%; 3 = total occlusion. Also examined number of coronary vessels occluded >50%. | No association between Type A and levels of disease severity. No association with number of vessels occluded >50%. |
| Before catheterization. SI, 70% Type A. | 1) Simple count of 4 main coronary arteries with 50% occlusion. 2) Severity index, range 0–27; 0 = no lesion; 1 = 50%; 2 = 50 to 74%; 3 = 75–100% and summed across 9 segments of arteries. Correlations of two methods = 0.85. | No correlation of behavior type with number of occluded arteries or disease severity. Stratified by previous MI, the results were the same. |
| SI, JAS; Type A measures given to 31% after and to 69% prior to repeat catheterization, 66% Type A by SI. | Number of vessels ≥70% narrowing; progression = increase of 25% occlusion or total occlusion in one vessel. | SI Type A, not JAS Type A, related to number of vessels occluded at first catheterization, $p < .07$; patients who progressed in CAD were more likely to be extreme JAS Type A's and unlikely to be Type B's, $p < .07$. |

(*Table continues on p. 70.*)

**TABLE 4.3.** (Continued)

| Reference | Referral Site | Selection and/or Exclusion Criteria | Sample Characteristics |
|---|---|---|---|
| Bass et al. (1982) | King's College Hospital, London, England | Consecutive patients under age 65 years; excluded perious MIs, valvular heart disease, cardiomyopathy and CHF. | 67 men, 32 women; aged 31 to 65 years; Caucasian; 21.2% taking antihypertensives; 56.5% smokers; 43.4% nonmanual workers; 56.6% manual workers; 35.3% previous emergency admissions for chest pain. |
| Kornitzer et al. (1982) | Two university hospitals, Brussels, Belgium | Male patients; excluded aortic or mitral valve lesion patients. | 117 male patients, 21 to 64 years old; median age = 49.0 years; 54% previous MI; 85% typical or atypical chest pain; 38% blue-collar, 5% clerks, 11% executives; 46% self-employed. |
| Pearson et al. (1983) | Johns Hopkins Hospital, Baltimore | 792 white men and women. | Caucasian, many more females with normal arteries. |
| Young et al. (1984) | Milwaukee, WI, Cardiovascular Registry | Referred because of clinical symptoms of CAD. | 2451 male patients. |
| Blumenthal et al. (1987) | Duke University Medical Center, Durham, NC | 113 consecutive patients. | 86 men, 27 women; 34 to 79 years old; mean age = 53 years. |

**TABLE 4.3.** (*Continued*)

| Type A Measure and Time of Administration | Disease Categories | Findings |
|---|---|---|
| After catheterization. Bortner Rating Scale. | Three groups of patients; I, no obstructive disease; II, obstruction in at least 1 vessel <50% stenosis; III, obstruction in at least 1 vessel with >50% stenosis. | Negative association between Type A and CAD group. Group I patients had highest Bortner scores, Group III the lowest (nonsignificant). Stratified by sex, the above was significant for males, no differences observed for females. |
| Before catheterization. Bortner Rating Scale. | Coronary score; each artery scored: 0 (normal), 1 (<50%), 2 (one stenosis of 50%), 3 (several stenoses of 50% or one between 50 to 90%), 4 (one stenosis of 90% or more), or 5 (complete occlusion). Dichotomized at median for analyses. Also number of coronary arteries with a lesion of ⩾50%. | No association of Bortner score with summary score of lesions or with number of coronary arteries with significant stenosis. |
| Bortner Rating Scale. | Number of vessels with >50% narrowing of arterial lumen. | Type A scores slightly higher in those with CAD, but did not increase with number of diseased vessels. When stratified by chest pain, a similar Type A score was found in those with and without CAD. |
| Before catheterization. Ten items from subjective and quantitative scales that predict both SI and JAS assessment. | Occlusion scale, 0–300. 0 = no occlusion; 300 = >90% in all 3 main coronary arteries; 0–49 = low; 50–149 = moderate; 150–300 = severe. | Type A items were not associated with occlusion, but were associated with diagnoses of angina. |
| After catheterization 63% Type A by SI. Also used perceived social support scale. | Number of vessels with 75% or greater nominal narrowing. | Type A significantly related to atherosclerosis, $p < .05$. Levels of CHD decreased for Type A's as the level of social support increased ($p = .031$), but there was no such relationship for Type B's. Results were similar for peer and family social support. |

(*Table continues on p. 72.*)

**TABLE 4.3.** (Continued)

| Reference | Referral Site | Selection and/or Exclusion Criteria | Sample Characteristics |
|---|---|---|---|
| Seeman & Syme (1987) | Six Bay Area hospitals | Patients referred with a diagnosis of angina pectoris, coronary artery disease, recent myocardial infarction (within 6 months) or asymptomatic coronary artery disease. | 119 men, 40 women; 30 to 70 years old. |

Source: Adapted from Matthews & Haynes, 1986.

less likely to have atherosclerosis than Type A's who did not have such support. One cannot help but refer again to the earlier discussion in this chapter on the Honolulu Heart Study and the lack of association of Type A behavior to CHD incidence in the more supportive Japanese environment.

The interaction of Type A and social support was not found in another study by Seeman and Syme (1987), although different measures of social support (structural and emotional) were used. In this study, feelings of being loved and network support were significantly associated with the extent of atherosclerosis. Both studies also reported that Type A behavior, assessed by the Structured Interview, had more coronary artery disease than Type B's after adjustment for the traditional coronary risk factors.

Dimsdale, Block, Catanzano, Hachett, and Hutter (1978) and Dimsdale and colleagues (1979) at Massachusetts General Hospital in Boston have also published a series of reports on the Type A behaviors of patients undergoing coronary arteriography. In the first of these studies (Dimsdale et al., 1978) 99 men and 10 women were administered the Jenkins Activity Survey on the day prior to angiography. The results showed no relationship between the Jenkins Activity Survey scores and the number of vessels occluded 50 percent or more. In fact, Jenkins Activity Survey scores were higher among those patients with one or no vessels occluded 50 percent than among patients with more than one vessel occluded. Furthermore, among those patients with no significant occlusion in any vessel, the Jenkins Activity Survey scores were higher in the group suffering from Class 3 and 4 angina than in the group suffering from Class 1 and 2 angina. Although the number of patients in the latter group was limited, this pattern of results does suggest that Type A behavior might be related to the severity of angina, independent of underlying coronary artery disease.

Another report by Dimsdale and colleagues (1979) on men in the sample just discussed plus 4 more patients, examined the association of both the Structured Interview and Jenkins Activity Survey measures of Type A

**TABLE 4.3.**  (*Continued*)

| Type A Measure and Time of Administration | Disease Categories | Findings |
| --- | --- | --- |
| Day before cardiac catheterizations. Type A by SI. Also administered structural, instrumental, and emotional support questions. | Mean atherosclerosis scores, continuous scores. | Type A significantly related to level of atherosclerosis ($p < .05$). Network instrumental support and feelings of being loved also significant, independent of Type A. |

behavior and number of vessels occluded 50 percent or more. As reported above, there were either no relationships or inverse relationships between the Jenkins Activity Survey scores and the various indices of atherosclerosis, and there were no significant relationships between the Structured Interview Type A assessments and atherosclerosis.

Three recent studies classified individuals according to the Structured Interview and examined the association of Type A behavior and degree of occlusion. Krantz and colleagues (1981) reported no association between Type A behavior and severity of disease (number of vessels occluded 50 percent or more) in a sample of 76 men and 7 women referred because of prior myocardial infarction, chest pain, or electrocardiogram abnormalities. Seventy-five percent were assessed as Type A. Scherwitz, McKelvain, and Laman (1983) found no significant correlations between Type A behavior and number of arteries occluded 50 percent or more or a severity index in 156 men younger than 70 years. Seventy percent were assessed as Type A. In addition, two self-report measures correlated with Structured Interview Type A assessment—the Thurstone Temperament Schedule Activity scale (Thurstone, 1949) and specific items (McDougall, Dembroski, & Musante, 1979) from the Gough Adjective Checklist (Gough & Heilbrun, 1975)—did not discriminate disease and disease-free groups, whereas self-involvement indexed by the number of *I's*, *me's*, and *my's* during the Structured Interview did. In regard to the latter observation, Scherwitz and colleagues suggest that self-involvement is a more valid measure of coronary proneness than is Type A behavior, but evaluation of this construct is beyond the scope of this chapter. Another study, by Krantz, Matthews, Sanmarco, and Selvester (1979), did show a positive, albeit marginal ($p < .07$), association of Structured Interview Type A, but not Jenkins Activity Survey Type A and the number of vessels occluded 70 percent or more in a sample of 67 men referred for angiograms. A unique feature of this study is that to be in the study population all patients had to have a second angiogram within an average of 17 months of the initial angiogram. Twenty patients (30 percent) progressed to total occlusion or increased in occlusion by 25 percent in any one artery during the course of study; these patients were assessed as more Type A by the Jenkins Activity Survey, but not by the Structured Interview, than those patients who did not progress.

The Bortner Rating Scale has been used in far fewer angiography studies than has either the Structured Interview or the Jenkins Activity Survey. Nonetheless, the findings from these studies are unequivocal in failing to support an association between Type A behavior and coronary artery disease. In a study of 67 male and 32 female patients at King's College Hospital, London, referred for chest pain, Bass and Wade (1983) found that persons with no obstructive disease had higher Bortner Rating Scale scores than patients with obstruction in at least one vessel greater than 50 percent stenosis. Subsidiary analyses showed that this effect was restricted to males. Significantly more patients in the no disease or slight disease groups were admitted to the hospital through emergency medicine than were patients in the severe disease groups. Kornitzer and colleagues (1982) reported that, among 117 patients referred for catheterization at two university hospitals in Brussels, no associations were found between Bortner Rating Scale scores and number of arteries occluded more than 50 percent. Pearson (1983) studied 792 white men and women. Persons with stenosis greater than 50 percent in any one vessel were slightly more Type A than those without disease, but there was no association between Type A and number of vessels involved. In the absence of underlying disease, Type A scores of men with chest pain were higher than those of the men without chest pain. Pearson suggests that the presence of Type A behavior may increase the likelihood of clinical recognition of coronary artery disease because of patient and physician awareness of Type A behavior as a risk factor for coronary heart disease, particularly in the presence of anginal chest pain.

Young, Anderson, Barboriak, and Hoffman (1980, 1984) reported the results of analyses from a large sample of 2451 male patients. The men were administered a lengthy questionnaire including ratings of the extent and frequency of a patient's competitive, hard-driving, ambitious, and angry behaviors. The total of these ratings was shown to be related significantly to Type A behavior assessments by both the Structured Interview and Jenkins Activity Survey in a separate sample of 45 healthy men. Results showed no relationship between this Type A score and the extent of occlusion in any age group. However, they did show that the Type A scores were highly associated with diagnoses of angina, but not with diagnoses of myocardial infarction, independent of the major risk factors for coronary heart disease. The authors concluded that Type A behavior is related to angina independent of underlying coronary artery disease. Furthermore, they suggest that, because patients referred for angiography are already selected partially on the basis of chest pain, the relationships of Type A behavior and coronary occlusion, angina, and myocardial infarction should be different in such patient groups than in the general population.

The final paper to be reviewed in this section, by Stevens, Turner, Rhodewalt, and Talbot (1984) (not included in Table 4.3), differs from the other papers in two ways. It reports the relationship of Type A behavior and atherosclerosis in carotid arteries measured by Doppler ultrasonography. The patient population was 44 men and women referred for noninvasive evaluation of carotid and peripheral arterial stenosis. Associations between Jenkins Activity Survey scores and no (< 25 percent), mild (25 to 75 percent), and severe (> 75 percent) carotid artery disease scores were significant ($p < .04$), so that those with mild disease had higher Type A scores than those with no disease. Patients with severe disease were indistinguishable from either the mild or no disease groups.

### Summary and Comment

The results for the 16 angiography studies are not consistent. Two-thirds of studies using the Structured Interview demonstrate positive associations between the Structured Interview Type A and extent of disease. The majority of studies using the Jenkins Activity Survey to classify individuals report no effects, with the interesting exception of the progression study by Krantz and colleagues (1979). The Bortner Rating Scale and other less traditional paper-and-pencil tests of Type A behavior are not related to coronary artery disease. In sum, it might be concluded that Type A behavior is associated with coronary artery disease only if measured by interview and not by self-reported paper-and-pencil techniques.

We noted above several methodological and interpretative difficulties due to the cross-sectional nature of angiography studies and unknown biases resulting from patient characteristics. There are additional difficulties specific to the Type A studies. The first difficulty is that, with few exceptions, the Type A angiography studies have small sample sizes. As a consequence, the power of the statistical tests is low, given an estimated relative risk of 2.0 for Type A behavior.

A second difficulty is the high prevalence of Type A's (60 to 75 percent) in studies using the Structured Interview. (This was also the case in the Multiple Risk Factor Intervention Trial [Shekelle, Billings, et al., 1985].) Pearson (1984) suggests that a signal detection bias may have caused an overrepresentation of Type A's without underlying coronary artery disease to be included in the angiography studies. He argues that Type A behavior is related to chest pain (independent of coronary atherosclerosis), which leads physicians to refer proportionately more Type A patients for tests including coronary angiography that aid in diagnosis of coronary artery disease. According to Criqui (1979), the overrepresentation of a risk factor such as Type A behavior influences the validity of relative risk estimates when the disease rates in the study groups are also unrepresentative of the target population. Because angiography studies do not have population-based control groups, the ability of such studies to detect an association between Type A behavior and coronary artery disease is weakened by the unrepresentative preponderance of Type A's and coronary cases. An analogy to this situation is found in the diet–heart disease literature, where numerous studies have found no association of dietary intake of fats with serum cholesterol levels or with coronary heart disease (McGill, 1979). An explanation of these results lies in the low variability of fat intake in the United States in combination with the high levels of fat consumption in the western diet (McGill, 1979).

A third difficulty stems from the use of self-report measures. In a majority of those studies the Type A assessment occurred immediately prior to angiography when patients would understandably be anxious and preoccupied. How such states affect the reliability and validity of the behavior pattern assessment is unknown.

Despite these methodological difficulties, the data do point to the interesting possibility that Type A may be related to the diagnosis of angina, independent of underlying atherosclerosis. This possibility suggests that physicians may consider complaints of chest pain by their Type A patients more seriously and more conservatively than complaints by their Type B patients because they recognize Type A behavior as a risk factor for coronary heart disease. In addition, Type A patients may perceive and act upon their symptoms in a manner different from that of Type B patients. For example, because of their aggressive natures, Type A patients may be more insistent when reporting symptoms to their physicians than are Type B patients.

## Cerebrovascular Accidents and Other Health Outcomes

Although the overwhelming majority of studies published on Type A behavior have concentrated on coronary heart disease outcomes, some studies have examined the relationship of Type A behavior with other atherosclerotic diseases, such as stroke. In recent reports from the Framingham Heart Study, no clear association was observed among men between Type A behavior and the 10-year incidence of stroke (Eaker, Feinleib, & Wolf, 1983). However, in women there was a significant association. Type A women aged 45 to 64 years and free of cardiovascular disease prior to the follow-up period were five times more likely to develop cerebrovascular disease during the subsequent 10 years than were Type B women. The Framingham analysis was unable, however, to differentiate among the various types of stroke occurring in women (i.e., thrombosis, or subarachnoid hemorrhage) because of diagnostic limitations and modest sample sizes.

In addition to the prospective studies mentioned above, two small case-control or case series (Adler, Engel, & MacRitchie, 1971; Gianturco et al., 1974) have suggested that a pressured pattern characterized by extremes of aggressiveness, ambition, and achievement striving was predominant among men with cerebral infarction. These studies can be faulted, however, by limited sample sizes and a failure to control for the presence of coronary artery disease in the analysis.

There is only one investigation to our knowledge on the relationship of Type A behavior and peripheral vascular disease. Cottier and colleagues (1983) studied three groups of 13 patients each with the following diagnoses: intermittent claudication; intermittent claudication and coronary artery disease; and disease other than vascular disease. The Bortner Rating Scale was administered to these patient groups. Results showed that the groups were different in their Type A behavior ($p < .05$). Patients with intermittent claudication and coronary artery disease were significantly more Type A than the patient control group. The patients with intermittent claudication and no coronary artery disease were similar to the patient group in their Type A behavior scores.

Type A behavior has also been related to accidents and acute symptoms. Elevated Jenkins Activity Survey Type A scores (mean = 3.4) were observed for accidental and violent deaths in the Western Collaborative Group Study (Zyzanski, 1978). Among college students, Type A's have reported experiencing upper respiratory infections, headaches, and allergies more often than Type B's (Barton, Brautigam, Fogle, Freitas, & Hicks, 1982; Hicks & Campbell, 1983; Stout & Bloom, 1982), although they do see themselves as being healthier (Hart, 1983). Other studies have found no association between Type A behavior and acute symptoms (Lundberg & Paludi, 1981). This discrepancy may be explained by findings that Type A's are significantly more likely to ignore fatigue and symptoms, more likely to work when suffering from symptoms, and less likely to take medications than Type B's, but only when in challenging circumstances (Carver, Coleman, & Glass, 1976; Matthews, Kuller, Siegel, Thompson, & Varat, 1983; Weidner & Matthews, 1978). When in nonchallenging circumstances, no A–B differences typically appear. Type A's are thought to ignore symptoms because they believe that illness might interfere with the completion of various tasks; they ignore anything that might interfere with task performance, and illness may be labeled by Type A's as a weakness, thus threatening their control over their environment (Matthews & Brunson, 1979).

## Future Directions in Type A Research

1.  At the present time, there are relatively few estimates of the prevalence of Type A behavior in men or women over time, making secular trend analyses impossible. Therefore, we recommend that ongoing

population-based surveys should include multiple measures of Type A behavior, along with Type A methods research, in their design.

2. The absence of data regarding the association of Type A behavior and coronary heart disease in women, Blacks, Hispanics, and young adults underscores the importance of investigations in these underresearched groups. Prior to initiating these investigations, however, innovative adaptations of the current ways to measure Type A behaviors must be developed.

3. We recommend that in future research investigators take special precautions to draw population-based samples or samples of Type A's and B's in proportion to the distribution of Type A–B in "normal" populations. In this way, the high prevalence of Type A's found in angiography and other studies of high-risk persons could be avoided. Given that Type A's and Type B's may volunteer to serve in clinical trials to a different extent, we also recommend that the health behaviors of Type A's be studied. For example, the extent to which Type A's perceive chest pain and choose to self-diagnose and treat their symptoms may be quite informative for understanding why Type A's report angina symptoms, perhaps independent of underlying coronary artery disease. These health behaviors may also explain why studies of high-risk populations have a high prevalence of Type A's and why Type A's might delay medical attention until pain becomes quite severe.

4. Finally, we should design studies to look at a multiplicity of factors rather than a unicausal "magic bullet" that explains the Type A risk of CHD. Such factors include:
   a. The structure and elements of the work environment, with specific focus on job demands, job control, the Japanese cooperative work environment versus the competitive American work environment, job satisfaction, competition with others, and so on.
   b. Individual characteristics other than Type A that can modify risk, such as perceived social support, trust of others, cooperation, anger expression (outward, inward), anger frequency, hostility, and feminine versus masculine characteristics.
   c. The structure and elements of the family environment, with specific focus on marital discord, work environment of both spouses, children, and overall social support and how it is used.

Research in this field will continue until the current shift has been achieved. The years 1987 to 1990 will be the turning point for Type A theory, research, and intervention. The ongoing controversy and discussion over Type A have been constructive, stimulating, challenging, and difficult. However, the answers provided in the next few years will play an important role in deciphering the behavioral etiology of coronary artery disease.

# REFERENCES

Adler, R., Engel, G., & MacRitchie, K. (1971). Psychologic processes and ischemic stroke. *Psychosomatic Medicine, 33,* 1–29.

Barton, S., Brautigam, M., Fogle, G., Freitas, R. C., & Hicks, R. A. (1982). Type A-B behavior and the incidence of allergies in college students. *Psychological Reports, 50,* 566.

Bass, C., & Wade, C. (1982). Type A behavior not specifically pathogenic. *Lancet, 2,* 1147–1149.

Blumenthal, J. A., Burg, M. M., Barefoot, J., Williams, R. B., Haney, T., & Zimet, G. (1987). Social support, Type A behavior, and coronary artery disease. *Psychosomatic Medicine, 49,* 331–340.

Blumenthal, J. A., Kong, Y., Schanberg, S. M., Thompson, L. W., & Williams, R. B. (1978). Type A behavior and coronary atherosclerosis. *Circulation, 58,* 634–639.

Bortner, R. W. (1969). A short rating scale as a potential measure of Pattern A behavior. *Journal of Chronic Diseases, 22,* 87–91.

Brand, R. J., Jenkins, C. D., Rosenman, R. H. (1978). Comparison of coronary heart disease prediction in the Western Collaborative Group Study using the Structured Interview and the Jenkins Activity Survey assessments of the coronary-prone Type A behavior pattern. [Abstract]. *American Heart Association Cardiovascular Disease Epidemiology Newsletter, 24.*

Capra, F. (1982). *The turning point.* New York: Bantam.

Carver, C. S., Coleman, A. E., & Glass, D. C. (1976). The coronary-prone behavior pattern and the suppression of fatigue on a treadmill test. *Journal of Personality and Social Psychology, 33,* 460–466.

Case, R. B., Heller, S. S., Case, N. B., & Moss, A. J. (1985). Type A behavior and survival after acute myocardial infarction. *New England Journal of Medicine, 312,* 737–741.

Cohen, J. B., & Reed, D. (1985). Type A behavior and coronary heart disease among Japanese men in Hawaii. *Journal of Behavioral Medicine, 8,* 343–352.

Cohen, J. B., Syme, S. L., Jenkins, C. D., Kagan, A., & Zyzanski, S. J. (1979). Cultural context of Type A behavior and risk for CHD: A study of Japanese American males. *Journal of Behavioral Medicine, 2,* 375–384.

Cooper, T., Detre, T., & Weiss, S. M. (1981). Coronary prone behavior and coronary heart disease: A critical review. *Circulation, 63,* 1199–1215.

Cottier, C., Adler, R., Gerber, R., Hefer, T., Hurny, C., & Vorkauf, H. (1983). Pressured pattern or Type A behavior in patients with peripheral arteriovascular disease: Controlled retrospective exploratory study. *Psychosomatic Medicine, 45,* 187–193.

Criqui, M. H. (1979). Response bias and risk ratios in epidemiologic studies. *American Journal of Epidemiology, 109,* 394–399.

DeBacker, G., Dramaix, M., Kittel, F., & Kornitzer, M. (1983). Behavior, stress, and psychosocial traits as risk factors. *Preventive Medicine, 12,* 32–36.

Dembroski, T. M., Feinleib, M. F., Haynes, S. G., Shields, J. L., & Weiss, S. M. (Eds.). (1978). *Coronary-prone behavior.* New York: Springer-Verlag.

Dimsdale, J. E., Block, P. C., Catanzano, D. M., Hackett, T. P., & Hutter, A. M. (1978). Type A personality and extent of coronary atherosclerosis. *American Journal of Cardiology, 42,* 583–586.

Dimsdale, J. E., Hackett, T. P., Hutter, A. M., Block, P. C., Catanzano, D. M., & White, P. J. (1979). Type A behavior and angiographic findings. *Journal of Psychosomatic Research, 23,* 273–276.

Dimsdale, J. E., Block, P. C., Gilbert, J., Hackett, T. P., & Hutter, A. M. (1981). Predicting cardiac morbidity based on risk factors and coronary angiographic findings. *American Journal of Cardiology, 47,* 73–76.

Eaker, E. D., Feinleib, M., & Wolf, R. (1983). Psychosocial factors and the ten-year incidence of cerebrovascular accident in the Framingham Heart Study [Abstract]. *American Heart Association Cardiovascular Disease Epidemiology Newsletter, 33*, 54.

Frank, K. A., Heller, S. S., Kornfeld, D. S., Sporn, A. A., & Weiss, M. B. (1978). Type A behavior and coronary angiographic findings. *Journal of American Medical Association, 240*, 761–763.

French-Belgian Collaborative Group (1982). Ischemic heart disease and psychological patterns: Prevalence and incidence studies in Belgium and France. *Advances in Cardiology, 29*, 25–31.

Friedman, M., Thoresen, C. E., Gill, J. J., Ulmer, D., Powell, L. H., Price, V. A., Brown, B. B., Thompson, L., Rabin, D. D., Breall, W. S., Bourg, E., Levy, R., & Dixon, T. (1986). Alteration of Type A behavior and its effect on cardiac recurrences in post myocardial infarction patients: Summary results of the recurrent coronary prevention project. *American Heart Journal, 112*, 653–665.

Gianturco, D. T., Breslin, M. S., Gentry, W. D., Heyman, A., Jenkins, C. D., & Kaplan, B. (1974). Personality patterns and life stress in ischemic cerebrovascular disease: 1. Psychiatric findings. *Stroke, 5*, 453–460.

Gough, H. H., & Heilbrun, A. B. (1975). The Adjective Checklist. Palo Alto: Consulting Psychologists Press.

Hart, K. E. (1983). Physical symptom reporting and health perception among Type A and B college males. *Journal of Human Stress, 17*, 22.

Haynes, S. G., & Feinleib, M. (1982). Type A behavior and the incidence of coronary heart disease in the Framingham Heart Study. *Advances in Cardiology, 29*, 85–95.

Haynes, S. G., Feinleib, M., & Kannel, W. B. (1980). The relationship of psychosocial factors to coronary heart disease in the Framingham Study: III. Eight-year incidence of coronary heart disease. *American Journal of Epidemiology, 111*, 37–58.

Haynes, S. G., Feinleib, M., Levine, S., Scotch, N., & Kannel, W. B. (1978). The relationship of psychosocial factors to coronary heart disease in the Framingham Study: II. Prevalence of coronary heart disease. *American Journal of Epidemiology, 107*, 384–402.

Hicks, R. A., & Campbell, J. (1983). Type A-B behavior and self-estimates of the frequency of headaches in college students. *Psychological Reports, 52*, 912.

Jenkins, C. D. (1983). Psychosocial and behavioral factors. In N. M. Kaplan & J. Stamler (Eds.), *Prevention of coronary heart disease: Practical management of the risk factors*. Philadelphia: Saunders.

Jenkins, C. D., Rosenman, R. H., & Zyzanski, S. J. (1974). Prediction of clinical coronary heart disease by a test for the coronary prone behavior pattern. *New England Journal of Medicine. 23*, 1271–1275.

Jenkins, C. D., Rosenman, R. H., & Zyzanski, S. J. (1976). Risk of new myocardial infarction in middle-aged men with manifest coronary heart disease. *Circulation, 53*, 342–347.

Kennedy, R. H., Frye, R. L., Giuliani, E. R., Kennedy, M. A., Nobrega, F. T., Pluth, J. R., Ritter, D. G., & Smith, H. C. (1980). Use of the cardiac catheterization laboratory in a defined population. *New England Journal of Medicine, 303*, 1213–1217.

Kornitzer, M., Magotteau, V., Degre, C., Kittel, F., Struyven, J., & van Thiele, E. (1982). Angiographic findings and the Type A pattern assessed by means of the Bortner scale. *Journal of Behavior Medicine, 5*, 313–320.

Krantz, D. S., Davia, J. E., Dembroski, T. M., MacDougall, J. M., Shaffer, R. T., & Schaeffer, M. A. (1981). Extent of coronary atherosclerosis, Type A behavior, and cardiovascular response to social interaction. *Psychophysiology, 18*, 654–664.

Krantz, D. S., Matthews, K. A., Sanmarco, M. E., & Selvester, R. H. (1979). Psychological correlate of progression of atherosclerosis in men. *Psychosomatic Medicine, 41*, 467–475.

Lundberg, P. K., & Paludi, M. A. (1981). Type A/B behavior patterns and the reporting of lifetime symptomatology A-B. *Perceptual Motor Skills, 52,* 473–474.

MacDougall, J. M., Dembroski, T. M., & Musante, L. (1979). The Structured Interview and questionnaire methods of assessing coronary-prone behavior in male and female college students. *Journal of Behavioral Medicine, 2,* 71–83.

Matthews, K. A., & Brunson, B. I. (1979). Allocation of attention and the Type A coronary prone behavior patterns. *Journal of Personality & Social Psychology, 39,* 2081–2090.

Matthews, K. A., Dembroski, T. M., Krantz, D. C., & MacDougall, J. M. (1982). Unique and common variance in Structured Interview and Jenkins Activity Survey measures of the Type A behavior pattern. *Journal of Personality & Social Psychology, 42,* 303–313.

Matthews, K. A., & Haynes, S. G. (1986). Type A behavior pattern and coronary disease risk. *American Journal of Epidemiology, 123,* 923–960.

Matthews, K. A., Kuller, L. H., Siegel, J. M., Thompson, M., & Varat, M. (1983). Determinants of decisions to seek medical treatment by patients with acute myocardial infarction symptoms. *Journal of Personality & Social Psychology, 44,* 1144–1156.

McGill, H. C. (1979). The relationship of dietary cholesterol to serum cholesterol concentrations and to atherosclerosis in man. *American Journal of Clinical Nutrition, 32,* 2644–2702.

MRFIT Study Group (1982). Multiple Risk Factor Intervention Trial: Risk factor changes and mortality results. *Journal of American Medical Association, 248,* 1465–1477.

Ouchi, W. G. (1981). *Theory Z.* Reading, MA: Addison-Wesley.

Pascale, R. T., & Athos, A. G. (1981). *The art of Japanese management.* New York: Simon & Schuster.

Pearson, T. A. (1983). *Risk factors for arteriographically defined coronary artery disease.* Doctoral dissertation from the Johns Hopkins University. #83-16989. Ann Arbor, MI: University Microfilms International.

Pearson, T. A. (1984). Coronary arteriography in the study of the epidemiology of coronary artery disease. *Epidemiologic Reviews, 6,* 140–166.

Rosenman, R. H., Brand, R. J., Jenkins, C. D., Friedman, M., Straus, R., & Wurm, M. (1975). Coronary heart disease in the Western Collaborative Group Study: Final follow-up experience of 8½ years. *Journal of the American Medical Association, 233,* 872–877.

Scherwitz, L., McKelvain, R., & Laman, C. (1983). Type A behavior, self-involvement, and coronary atherosclerosis. *Psychosomatic Medicine, 45,* 47–57.

Seeman, T. E., & Syme, S. L. (1987). Social networks and coronary artery disease: A comparison of the structure and function of social relations as predictors of disease. *Psychosomatic Medicine, 49,* 341–354.

Shekelle, R. B., Billings, J. H., Borhani, N. O., Gerace, T. A., Hulley, S. B., Jacobs, D. R., Lasser, N. L., Mittlemark, M. B., Neaton, J. D., & Stamler, J. (1985). The MRFIT behavior pattern study: II. Type A behavior and incidence of coronary heart disease. *American Journal of Epidemiology, 122,* 559–570.

Shekelle, R. B., Gale, M., & Norusis, M. (1985). Type A score (Jenkins Activity Survey) and risk of recurrent coronary heart disease in the Aspirin Myocardial Infarction Study. *American Journal of Cardiology. 56,* 221–225.

Silver, L., Jenkins, C. D., Melidossian, C., & Ryan, R. J. (1980). Sex differences in the psychological correlates of cardiovascular diagnosis and coronary angiographic findings. *Journal of Psychosomatic Research, 24,* 327–334.

Stevens, J. H., Turner, C. W., Rhodewalt, F., & Talbot, S. (1984). The Type A behavior pattern and carotid artery atherosclerosis. *Psychosomatic Medicine, 46,* 105–113.

Stout, C. W., & Bloom, L. J. (1982). Type A behavior and upper respiratory infections. *Journal of Human Stress,* June 4-7.

Thurstone, L. L. (1949). *Thurstone Temperament Schedule.* Chicago: Science Research Associates.

Working Group Summary: Type A behavior, anger, and hostility (1985). In A. M. Ostfeld, E. D. Eaker (Eds.), *Psychosocial variables in epidemiologic studies of cardiovascular disease.* Bethesda, MD: NIH, 199–206. (NIH publication no. 85-2270.)

Weidner, G., & Matthews, K. A. (1978). Reported physical symptoms elicited by unpredictable events and the Type A coronary-prone behavior pattern. *Journal of Personality & Social Psychology, 36,* 1213–1220.

Williams, R. B., Haney, T. L., & Lee, K. L. (1980). Type A behavior, hostility, and coronary atherosclerosis. *Psychosomatic Medicine, 42,* 539–549.

Young, L. D., Anderson, A. A., Barboriak, J. J., & Hoffman, R. G. (1980). Attitudinal and behavioral correlates of coronary heart disease. *Journal of Psychomatic Research, 24,* 311–318.

Young, L. D., Anderson, A. J., Barboriak, J. J., & Hoffman, R. G. (1984). Coronary-prone behavior attitudes in moderate to severe coronary artery occlusion. *Journal of Behavior Medicine, 7,* 205–215.

Zyzanski, S. J. (1978). Coronary-prone behavior pattern and coronary heart disease: Epidemiological evidence. In T. M. Dembroski, M. F. Feinleib, S. G. Haynes, J. L. Shields, & S. M. Weiss (Eds.), *Coronary-prone behavior.* New York: Springer-Verlag.

Zyzanski, S. J., Everist, M., Flessas, A., Jenkins, C. D., & Ryan, T. J. (1976). Psychological correlates of coronary angiographic findings. *Archives of Internal Medicine, 136,* 1234–1237.

# 5

## Type A Behavior and Coronary Heart Disease in Women: Fourteen-Year Incidence from the Framingham Study

ELAINE D. EAKER AND WILLIAM P. CASTELLI

Although the rate of coronary heart disease (CHD) morbidity and mortality for women is only one-half to one-fourth that of men, CHD is nonetheless the leading cause of death among women in the United States. For this reason it is important to determine the biological and psychological risk factors for CHD in women. Studies that have examined the Type A behavior pattern as a risk factor for CHD have consisted almost exclusively of men, and at least three studies have shown the positive relationship between various measures of Type A behavior and the development of CHD in men (French-Belgian Collaborative Group, 1981; Haynes & Feinleib, 1981; Rosenman et al., 1975).

The Type A behavior pattern was described by its originators as an action–emotion complex that is exhibited by those individuals who are engaged in a relatively chronic struggle to obtain a limited number of poorly defined things from their environment in the shortest period of time and, if necessary, against the opposing efforts of other things or other persons in the same environment (Friedman & Rosenman, 1974). The overt manifestations of the behavior pattern include extremes of competitiveness, an easily aroused hostility, a sense of time urgency, and aggression. Contemporary western society may foster this behavior pattern by offering special rewards and opportunities to those who can think, perform, and play more rapidly and aggressively than their peers (Matthews, 1985). The extent to which this behavior is encouraged in women by our society and whether it is a risk factor for coronary heart disease in women remain to be clarified.

Previous reports of the association of the Framingham Type A Scale with the 8-year incidence of total coronary heart disease (myocardial infarction, coronary insufficiency, angina pectoris, and CHD death) indicated a positive relationship among women 45 to 64 years of age at the baseline examination (Haynes, Feinleib, & Kannel, 1980). Employment status (working woman or housewife) did not affect the association of behavior type to coronary heart disease or angina pectoris with or without myocardial infarction. The linking of Framingham Type A behavior to the 10-year incidence of CHD was associated only with coronary diagnoses in which angina pectoris symptoms were present (Haynes & Feinleib, 1981). Data presented in this chapter are from the Framingham Study and include the 14-year incidence of coronary heart disease. Data from this extended follow-up make it possible to examine the associations of Type A behavior to the different CHD endpoints.

## METHODS

There are a variety of ways to assess Type A behavior: structured interviews, peer nominations and ratings, self-report inventories, and behavioral tests (see Rosenman, Swan, & Carmelli, Chapter 2, this volume). In the Framingham Study, a longitudinal study of cardiovascular disease and its risk factors in a community-based cohort of men and women, a self-report inventory, developed by Haynes and colleagues from data collected by Drs. Levine and Scotch between 1965 and 1967, has been described and presented as the Framingham Type A Scale (Haynes, Levine, Scotch, Feinleib, & Kannel, 1978). The scale is based on ten questions derived from a 300-item questionnaire that was administered by interviewers in the Framingham Study. The scale has six items related to general feelings (the trait-related subscale), such as feeling pressed for time, being competitive, and eating too quickly (see Table 5.1). The trait-related subscale was answered by all people. There are also four questions related to one's regular line of work (the job-related subscale) that include either (1) questions related to job activities for men and women employed outside the home during most of their adult years (see Table 5.2), or (2) questions related to housework for

**TABLE 5.1.   FRAMINGHAM TYPE A SCALE, TRAIT-RELATED ITEMS (ALL MEN AND WOMEN)**

Do the following traits describe you:
  very well
  fairly well
  somewhat
  not at all
Being bossy or dominating
Having a strong need to excel (be best) in most things
Usually feeling pressed for time
Being hard driving and competitive
Eating too quickly
Upset when have to wait for anything (yes/no)

women who had not worked outside the home during most of their adult years (see Table 5.3). The Framingham Type A Scale assesses both perceived general personal characteristics and perception of one's regular line of work. Scale scores are derived by averaging the responses to the questions; if any item in the scale is missing for an individual then the scale is defined as missing and not calculated.

The following analyses will include associations of the Framingham Type A Scale and, in contrast to previous reports, the associations of the trait- and job-related subscales to the 14-year incidence of CHD. Because of the recent interest in the relationship between various components of Type A scales and CHD, the separate items that make up the Framingham Type A scales will also be examined in relation to the development of CHD in women.

For these analyses, the population under study included 749 women in the Framingham cohort, aged 45 to 64 years of age and free of CHD at the baseline medical examination. A number of psychosocial questions were asked in the 300-item questionnaire along with questions concerning demographic characteristics. In addition, measures of various physiological

**TABLE 5.2.   FRAMINGHAM TYPE A SCALE, JOB-RELATED ITEMS (EMPLOYED MEN AND WOMEN)**

How have you generally felt at the end of an average day in your regular line of work? (yes/no):
  Often felt very pressed for time
  Work often stayed with you so that you were thinking about it after working hours
  Work often stretched you to the very limits of your energy and work capacity
  Often felt uncertain, uncomfortable, or dissatisfied with how well you were doing in regular line of work

## TABLE 5.3.　FRAMINGHAM TYPE A SCALE, JOB-RELATED ITEMS (HOUSEWIVES)

With regard to your housework (yes/no):
Often felt very pressed for time
Often had a feeling of dissatisfaction
Work often stayed with you so thinking about it all day long
In general do (did) you find housework a big strain?

variables were collected at the same time, such as blood pressure, cholesterol, cigarette-smoking behavior, Framingham relative weight (ratio of the subject's body weight at examination to the median weight of the appropriate sex–height group at examination 1), and alcohol intake. Frequency of alcohol consumption was defined by the question: How often do you take alcoholic beverages (beer, whiskey, wine)?

Women indicating they had been employed outside the home for more than half their adult years (age 18 years and over) were classified as working women; otherwise they were classified as housewives. Working women were further classified into white-collar, clerical, or blue-collar occupations. In Framingham, women employed in white-collar jobs were generally teachers, nurses, or librarians and blue-collar jobs usually included factory or service workers.

Participants free of any manifestation of CHD at the baseline examination were followed for 14 years to detect the development of coronary heart disease. The criteria for coronary heart disease include any of the following diagnoses: myocardial infarction, angina pectoris, coronary insufficiency, CHD death (sudden or nonsudden). The definitions of the clinical manifestations of CHD are as follows:

Myocardial infarction (MI) required the demonstration of unequivocal serial changes in the electrocardiogram (ECG) when compared to previous tracings, or diagnostic elevation of serum enzymes indicating myocardial muscle necrosis, or both.

Angina pectoris (AP) was diagnosed from symptoms of substernal discomfort of short duration (less than 15 minutes), distinctly related to exertion or excitement and relieved by rest or nitroglycerin. Angina pectoris only (APO) was defined when these symptoms were the initial manifestation of CHD and when no other manifestation of CHD (myocardial infarction, coronary insufficiency, or CHD death) occurred during the 14 years of follow-up. AP includes all cases of angina, regardless of the development of other clinical manifestations of CHD.

Coronary insufficiency syndrome (CI) was diagnosed when a history of prolonged ischemic chest pain was accompanied by transient ischemic S-T segment and T-wave abnormality in the electrocardiographic tracing, but not accompanied by development of Q-wave abnormality or by serum myocardial enzyme changes characteristic of muscle necrosis.

CHD death, nonsudden, was diagnosed if available information (prior and current clinical illness) implied that the cause of death was probably CHD, if the terminal episode lasted longer than 1 hour, and if no other cause could be ascribed; CHD death, sudden, was diagnosed if the subject, apparently well, was observed to have died within a few minutes (operationally documented as under 1 hour) from the onset of symptoms, and if the cause of death could not reasonably be attributed to some potentially lethal disease other than CHD.

For these analyses coronary heart disease excluding angina pectoris was considered definite CHD and included myocardial infarction, coronary insufficiency, or CHD death where the first occurrence of these manifestations did not appear in conjunction with angina pectoris during the 2-year interval between exams.

To test the associations of CHD to Type A behavior, several statistical tests were used. When the Type A scale is used as a continuous variable, mean scale scores of persons developing CHD were compared with mean scale scores of people not developing CHD by Student's $t$-test. Relative risks were computed for scales such as the Framingham Type A Scale by comparing the coronary incidence rates among persons scoring above and below the median. The significance of these associations was determined by a chi-square test as were the associations between individual scale items and the incidence of CHD. A multiple logistic regression function analysis was used to assess the probability of persons developing CHD in relation to the Type A scale, the two subscales, or individual items while taking into account other known risk factors for CHD.

## RESULTS

In Figure 5.1 the 14-year incidence rates for coronary heart disease are presented among women who were 45 to 64 years old at the examination in which the Framingham Type A questions were administered. For this sample of women, 12.3 percent developed some form of coronary heart disease over the 14 years of follow-up, and 7.1 percent experienced CHD in which the first manifestation of CHD was not accompanied by angina pectoris during the 2-year interval between examinations; moreover, 5.4 percent of these women experienced angina pectoris that was the only manifestation of CHD over the 14-year interval. It is important to examine these various manifestations of CHD separately in women because the occurrence of angina pectoris alone may not be a true reflection of underlying coronary disease in women in Framingham. In this sample, only 6 percent of those women diagnosed as having angina pectoris only as the first

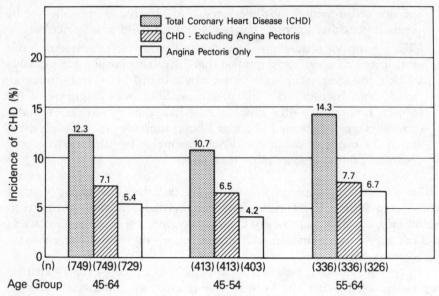

**FIGURE 5.1.**    Fourteen-year incidence of coronary heart disease among women 45 to 64 years old (Framingham study).

manifestation of CHD went on to develop definite CHD, that is, MI, CI, or CHD death, in the 14-year interval.

It has been shown previously that employment status is not related to total coronary heart disease incidence in women in Framingham. In Figure 5.2 are presented the incidence rates of CHD in women categorized by whether they worked inside or outside the home for most of their adult years. As can be seen from this figure, employed women have a slightly higher incidence rate compared to housewives (13.2 vs. 11.1 percent). The rate for CHD excluding angina was virtually identical for employed women and housewives. Employed women had a slightly higher rate of angina pectoris. None of these differences were statistically significant.

When employed women were stratified by occupational status, 2.6 percent of the white-collar workers, 7.8 percent of the clerical workers, and 8.4 percent of women employed in blue-collar occupations developed CHD (excluding AP) over the 14 years of follow-up. The association between CHD (excluding AP) and occupational status did not reach statistical significance.

The relationships of various characteristics measured at baseline with Type A and Type B behavior in women stratified by 10-year age groups are presented in Table 5.4. Framingham relative weight was the only characteristic that significantly differentiated Type A women from Type B women; Type A women were significantly heavier than Type B women, and this was true for both the younger and older age groups. Framingham relative

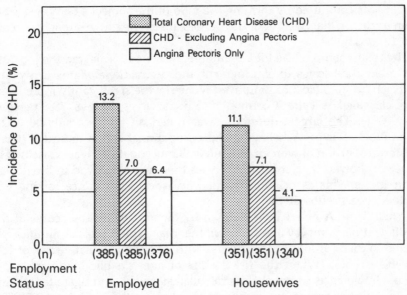

**FIGURE 5.2.** Fourteen-year incidence of coronary heart disease among women 45 to 64 years old stratified by employment status (Framingham study).

**TABLE 5.4. MEAN RISK FACTOR LEVELS FOR FRAMINGHAM TYPE A AND TYPE B BEHAVIOR PATTERN AMONG WOMEN 45 TO 64 YEARS OLD**

| | Age Group | | | | Total | |
| | 45 to 54 | | 55 to 64 | | | |
| Characteristic | Type B (206) | Type A (207) | Type B (166) | Type A (170) | Type B (372) | Type A (377) |
|---|---|---|---|---|---|---|
| Age (years) | 50.2 | 49.9 | 59.3 | 58.7 | 54.3 | 53.9 |
| Systolic blood pressure (mm Hg) | 131.5 | 131.7 | 140.4 | 140.8 | 135.5 | 135.8 |
| Diastolic blood pressure (mm Hg) | 81.3 | 81.7 | 81.5 | 84.1 | 81.4 | 82.8 |
| Serum cholesterol (mg/100 ml) | 231.6 | 234.8 | 249.0 | 252.0 | 239.4 | 242.6 |
| Framingham relative weight | 101.9 | 105.4* | 100.6 | 105.5** | 101.3 | 105.5*** |
| Cigarette smoking (%) | 8.3 | 9.0 | 7.2 | 5.3 | 7.8 | 7.4 |
| Glucose intolerance (%) | 3.8 | 6.7 | 4.8 | 5.9 | 4.3 | 6.4 |
| Alcohol intake | 2.6 | 2.6 | 2.5 | 2.5 | 2.5 | 2.5 |
| Blood pressure (%) medication | 10.2 | 14.1 | 20.7 | 17.2 | 14.9 | 15.5 |

* $.01 < p \leqslant .05$
** $.001 < p \leqslant .01$
*** $p \leqslant .001$

weight was computed by forming the ratio of the subject's body weight at exam to the median weight of the particular sex–height group at examination 1.

The relationship of the total Framingham Type A Scale and the job- and trait-related subscales to employment and occupational status in women is presented in Table 5.5. Employed women were significantly more likely to be classified as Type A compared to housewives (59.8 vs. 38.8 percent; $p = .0001$). The largest difference was noted on the trait subscale. The association of Type A behavior and occupational status indicates that a greater proportion of women in white-collar occupations were classified as Type A followed by clerical workers and women employed in blue-collar occupations. This association reached statistical significance for the job-related Type A subscale.

When Type A behavior is defined by dichotomizing the scores at the median cutoff point (by age and sex), the total Type A scale is significantly related to total coronary heart disease with a univariate relative risk of 1.73 (see Figure 5.3). When the risk factors of age, systolic blood pressure, glucose intolerance, serum cholesterol, relative weight, and cigarette smoking are taken into account, the multivariate relative risk is 1.76 ($p \leq 0.5$). The same relationship exists for both the job-related and the trait-related Type A subscales.

The same analyses as those described in the previous paragraph, but using coronary heart disease excluding the diagnosis of angina pectoris as the endpoint, are shown in Figure 5.4. Women defined as Type A on the total Framingham Type A Scale and the two subscales had slightly higher rates of CHD than did Type B women, but none of these reached statistical significance. There were 51 cases of definite coronary heart disease. Stratifying women by age group or employment status made no difference in these results. When the incidence of angina pectoris only is compared for Type A and Type B women (see Fig. 5.5), it can be seen that in both the univariate

**TABLE 5.5.   PREVALENCE OF TYPE A BEHAVIOR BY EMPLOYMENT STATUS AND OCCUPATION OF EMPLOYED WOMEN 45 TO 64 YEARS OLD**

|  | Framingham Type A | | Job Related | | Trait Related | |
|---|---|---|---|---|---|---|
|  | Percentage | p-value | Percentage | p-value | Percentage | p-value |
| **Employment** | | | | | | |
| Employed (385) | 59.8 | .0001 | 42.6 | .17 | 58.4 | .0001 |
| Housewife (351) | 38.8 | | 37.6 | | 41.6 | |
| **Occupation** | | | | | | |
| White collar (77) | 63.6 | .13 | 57.1 | .006 | 64.9 | .36 |
| Clerical (141) | 54.2 | | 40.8 | | 57.0 | |
| Blue collar (166) | 49.7 | | 35.8 | | 55.5 | |

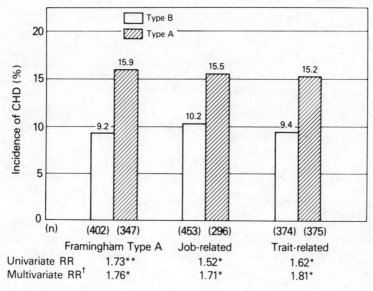

FIGURE 5.3. Fourteen-year incidence of total CHD among women 45 to 64 years old by Framingham Type A and job and trait subscales (Framingham study).

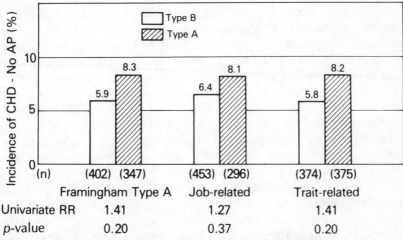

FIGURE 5.4. Fourteen-year incidence of CHD (no angina pectoris) among women 45 to 64 years old by Framingham Type A and job and trait subscales (Framingham study).

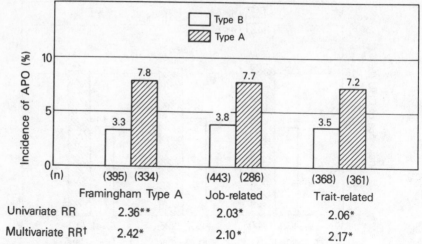

| | Framingham Type A | Job-related | Trait-related |
|---|---|---|---|
| Univariate RR | 2.36** | 2.03* | 2.06* |
| Multivariate RR† | 2.42* | 2.10* | 2.17* |

† Adjusted for age, systolic blood pressure, glucose intolerance, serum cholesterol, relative weight, cigarette smoking.
* 0.01 < p ≤ 0.05
** 0.001 < p ≤ 0.01

**FIGURE 5.5.** Fourteen-year incidence of angina pectoris only among women 45 to 64 years old stratified by Framingham Type A behavior and job and trait subscales (Framingham study).

and multivariate analyses Type A women have a risk of more than twice that of Type B women. There were 39 cases of angina pectoris only over the 14 years of follow-up.

When Type A is treated as a continuous variable, cases of total CHD consistently experienced a higher mean scale score on the total Framingham Type A and the two subscales than did the noncases, but none of these differences reached statistical significance. When angina pectoris only was examined as the endpoint for the association with the continuous Type A scores, the cases scored significantly higher than the noncases on the total scale score and on the two subscales.

These results confirm that the relationship of the total Framingham Type A Scale and the two subscales to CHD is stronger when angina pectoris is included in the diagnosis. The relative risks were not significant when angina was excluded from the diagnosis of CHD.

Recent research has led to the hypothesis that there may be certain elements or components of the Type A pattern that are more strongly related to the occurrence of coronary heart disease than other components of the total score; hostility is reported to be one such element (see Chesney, Hecker, & Black, Chapter 8; Williams & Barefoot, Chapter 9, this volume). The Framingham Type A Scale does not have a hostility component, but the two subscales and the individual items reflect different behavior complexes and perceptions. The following analyses examine the individual items to the various CHD endpoints and should be considered exploratory in nature.

TABLE 5.6.    TRAIT-RELATED TYPE A SCALE ITEMS AND 14-YEAR INCIDENCE OF CHD AMONG WOMEN 45 TO 64 YEARS OLD

| Item | Incidence of: Total Coronary Heart Disease[a] | | | | |
| | Not at All | Somewhat | Fairly Well | Very Well | p-value (chi-square test) |
|---|---|---|---|---|---|
| Bossy/dominating | 12.5 | 12.0 | 13.3 | 8.6 | .90 |
| Strong need to excel | 10.8 | 10.9 | 16.2 | 11.8 | .33 |
| Pressed for time | 5.7 | 13.4 | 17.4 | 12.9 | .01 |
| Hard driving/ competitive | 11.2 | 13.0 | 11.9 | 18.9 | .45 |
| Eating too quickly | 9.1 | 11.8 | 10.3 | 18.5 | .03 |
| Upset when wait (Y/N) | 11.1 | | | 15.0 | .18 |

[a]Cases = 92; noncases = 656.

The relationship of the trait-related Type A Scale items to the 14-year incidence of CHD among women 46 to 64 years old are shown in Table 5.6. The two items that were significantly related to the occurrence of total CHD were being pressed for time and eating too quickly. Women who reported that being pressed for time did not describe them at all had a particularly low rate of CHD (5.7 percent), but there was no clear gradient of risk as exposure to this variable increased. For the item eating too quickly there is a trend for greater risk among those who respond that this trait does not describe them well to describing them very well. When angina

TABLE 5.7.    TRAIT-RELATED TYPE A SCALE ITEMS AND 14-YEAR INCIDENCE OF CHD AMONG WOMEN 45 TO 64 YEARS OLD

| Item | Incidence of: CHD Excluding Angina Pectoris[a] | | | | |
| | Not at All | Somewhat | Fairly Well | Very Well | p-value (chi-square test) |
|---|---|---|---|---|---|
| Bossy/dominating | 8.6 | 5.5 | 9.2 | 0.0 | .13 |
| Strong need to excel | 7.7 | 6.8 | 6.7 | 7.1 | .98 |
| Pressed for time | 5.2 | 7.3 | 9.4 | 6.7 | .53 |
| Hard driving/ competitive | 6.4 | 7.8 | 8.3 | 7.5 | .87 |
| Eating too quickly | 6.3 | 3.6 | 5.2 | 13.0 | .002 |
| Upset when wait (Y/N) | 6.7 | | | 7.9 | .55 |

[a]Cases = 53; noncases = 694.

## TABLE 5.8. MULTIPLE LOGISTIC REGRESSION EQUATIONS OF 14-YEAR INCIDENCE OF TOTAL CHD AND CHD (NO ANGINA PECTORIS) AMONG WOMEN 45 TO 64 YEARS OLD AT BASELINE

| | | | Total CHD | | | |
|---|---|---|---|---|---|---|
| | CHD–No AP | | All Women | | Employed Women | |
| Variable | Unstnd Coefficient | Z | Unstnd Coefficient | Z | Unstnd Coefficient | Z |
| Age in Years | 0.04 | 1.19 | 0.05 | 2.06* | 0.06 | 1.87 |
| Systolic blood pressure (mm Hg) | 0.01 | 1.13 | 0.00 | 0.39 | 0.00 | 0.56 |
| Cigarette smoking (yes/no) | 0.02 | 1.33 | 0.02 | 2.06* | 0.02 | 1.62 |
| Serum cholesterol | 0.01 | 2.44* | 0.01 | 3.03** | 0.00 | 0.95 |
| Framingham relative weight | −0.00 | −0.02 | 0.02 | 2.86** | 0.02 | 1.91 |
| Glucose intolerance | 2.32 | 5.79*** | 1.64 | 4.37*** | 1.40 | 2.76** |
| Eating too quickly | 0.83 | 2.08* | | | | |
| Pressed for time | | | 0.88 | 2.59** | | |
| Stretched to limits | | | | | 0.56 | 1.71 |
| Cases = | 51 | | 90 | | 50 | |
| Noncases = | 708 | | 708 | | 362 | |

*.01 < $p$ ≤ .05
**.001 < $p$ ≤ .01
***$p$ ≤ .001

## TABLE 5.9. JOB-RELATED TYPE A SCALE ITEMS AND 14-YEAR INCIDENCE OF CHD AMONG WOMEN 45 TO 64 YEARS OLD

| | Incidence of: Total Coronary Heart Disease | | | | | |
|---|---|---|---|---|---|---|
| | Employed Women[a] | | | Housewives[b] | | |
| Item | No | Yes | p-Value | No | Yes | p-Value (chi-square test) |
| Pressed for time | 10.9 | 15.5 | .18 | 9.8 | 12.2 | .49 |
| Work stays with you | 11.7 | 15.9 | .24 | 10.0 | 17.0 | .13 |
| Dissatisfaction (uncertain, uncomfortable) | 13.9 | 11.0 | .49 | 9.1 | 14.0 | .16 |
| Stretched to limits (big strain) | 10.7 | 19.1 | .02 | 11.0 | 11.1 | .98 |

[a]Cases = 51; noncases = 334.
[b]Cases = 38; noncases = 307.

TABLE 5.10. JOB-RELATED TYPE A SCALE ITEMS AND 14-YEAR INCIDENCE OF CHD AMONG WOMEN 45 TO 64 YEARS OLD

| | Incidence of: CHD Excluding Angina Pectoris | | | | | |
|---|---|---|---|---|---|---|
| | Employed Women[a] | | | Housewives[b] | | |
| | | | | | | p-Value |
| Item | No | Yes | p-Value | No | Yes | (chi-square test) |
| Pressed for time | 7.3 | 6.7 | .83 | 6.7 | 7.2 | .87 |
| Work stays with you | 7.1 | 6.9 | .94 | 6.2 | 11.3 | .29 |
| Dissatisfied (uncertain, uncomfortable) | 7.3 | 6.1 | .71 | 7.2 | 6.6 | .83 |
| Stretched to limits (big strain) | 5.9 | 9.6 | .20 | 6.7 | 8.9 | .81 |

[a] Cases = 27; noncases = 358.
[b] Cases = 24; noncases = 321.

pectoris was excluded from the diagnosis of CHD (see Table 5.7), eating too quickly was still significantly related to the definite CHD endpoints, but pressed for time was not.

When the standard risk factors of age, systolic blood pressure, cigarette smoking, serum cholesterol, relative weight, and glucose intolerance were controlled for in a multiple logistic analysis (see Table 5.8), eating too quickly was found to be a significant independent risk factor for CHD excluding angina pectoris at the $p \leq .05$ level. Being pressed for time was related to total CHD among all women after controlling for the standard risk factors (but not to CHD excluding angina pectoris).

For the analysis of the job-related Type A Scale items, women were stratified by employment status. As can be seen in Table 5.9, the only item related to total CHD was being stretched to the limits among employed women; none of the job-related items were related to CHD among homemakers. After controlling for the standard risk factors (Table 5.8), being stretched to the limits was no longer significantly related to total CHD among employed women in the multivariate analysis. In addition, when angina pectoris was excluded from the criteria for CHD (Table 5.10), being stretched to the limits was no longer related to the 14-year incidence of definite CHD in the univariate analysis.

## SUMMARY

Data from women in the Framingham Study who completed the Framingham Type A Scale when they were 45 to 64 years of age and were followed for 14 years for the development of coronary heart disease indicate that at baseline Type A women were 4 percent higher on the Framingham relative weight scale than Type B women. Women who were employed outside the home most of their adult years were more likely to be classified as Type A than housewives. When the Framingham Type A Scale and the trait and job subscales were dichotomized at the median cut points, it was found that women classified as Type A were more likely to develop (1) coronary heart disease where angina pectoris was included in the criteria, or (2) angina pectoris without any other manifestation of CHD over the 14 years. When the Type A scales were treated as continuous variables, it was shown that cases of angina pectoris only had significantly higher mean scale scores than noncases of angina pectoris.

Of the ten individual questions that make up the total Framingham Type A Scale, only one—eating too quickly—was significantly related to definite coronary heart disease after taking into account the standard risk factors of age, systolic blood pressure, serum cholesterol, cigarette smoking, and glucose intolerance. The three individual questions that were related to the manifestation of angina pectoris only were (1) being pressed for time in general, (2) being pressed for time either at work or at housework, and (3) feeling stretched to the limits of one's capacity at work or for housework.

It can be concluded from these results that the Type A scales are related only to angina pectoris among women in the Framingham cohort and this manifestation of CHD in this population of women does not carry a serious prognostic outcome over the 14 years of follow-up. The individual questions were analyzed only in an exploratory attempt to see whether any of the items might be independently related to definite CHD. It was found that eating too quickly was associated with the 14-year incidence of definite CHD after controlling for the standard risk factors. Because, however, 20 comparisons were made in these item analyses, one would expect one significant result by chance alone. Therefore, the finding related to eating too quickly may be spurious. The search for an explanatory interpretation would be inappropriate. A study now underway in the Framingham offspring population is examining various measures of Type A behavior to the eventual occurrence of CHD with the intent better to understand the relationship of Type A and its components to various disease endpoints.

The evidence from the present study indicates that Type A behavior in women and the items that make up each of the Framingham Type A subscales are related to pain in a woman's chest and not to definite coronary heart disease. This is not to imply that a "coronary-prone" behavior does not exist in women. It may be a mistake, however, to assume that a behavior such as Type A, which is thought to be related to atherosclerotic heart disease in men, automatically applies to women. In order to determine what behaviors or stresses relate to disease in women, research and standardization of psychosocial scales must be performed among women.

# REFERENCES

French-Belgian Collaborative Group (1981). Ischemic heart disease and psychological patterns. Prevalence and incidence studies in Belgium and France. In H. Denolin (Ed.), *Advances in cardiology, Vol. 29: Psychological problems before and after myocardial infarction*. Basel: S. Karger.

Friedman, M., & Rosenman, R. H. (1974). *Type A behavior and your heart*. New York: Knopf.

Haynes, S. G., Levine, S., Scotch, N., Feinleib, M., & Kannel, W. B. (1978). The relationship of psychosocial factors to coronary heart disease in the Framingham Study: I. Methods and risk factors. *American Journal of Epidemiology, 107*, 362–383.

Haynes, S. G., Feinleib, M., & Kannel, W. B. (1980). The relationship of psychosocial factors to coronary heart disease in the Framingham Study: III. Eight-year incidence of coronary heart disease. *American Journal of Epidemiology, 111*, 37–58.

Haynes, S. G., & Feinleib, M. (1981). Type A behavior and the incidence of coronary heart disease in the Framingham Heart Study. In H. Denolin (Ed.), *Advances in cardiology, Vol. 29: Psychological problems before and after myocardial infarction*. Basel: S. Karger.

Matthews, K. A. (1985). Assessment of type A behavior, anger, and hostility in epidemiological studies of cardiovascular disease. In A. M. Ostfeld & E. D. Eaker (Eds.), *Measuring psychosocial variables in epidemiologic studies of cardiovascular disease*. DHHS, Bethesda, National Institutes of Health, NIH Publication No. 85-2270.

Rosenman, R. H., Brand, R. J., Jenkins, C. D., Friedman, M., Straus, R., & Wurm, M. (1975). Coronary heart disease in Western Collaborative Group Study: Final follow-up experience of 8½ years. *Journal of the American Medical Association, 233*, 872–877.

# 6

## Exploring the Type A Behavior Pattern in Children and Adolescents

CARL E. THORESEN AND JERRY R. PATTILLO

The growing scientific and public interest in the origins of the Type A behavior pattern has given rise to an expanding number of studies focused on younger people. Considerable controversy surrounds the Type A construct as it concerns adults (Booth-Kewley & Friedman, 1987; Friedman & Booth-Kewley, 1987a; Matthews, 1982; Matthews & Haynes, 1986; Thoresen & Ohman, 1986). These issues center on how best to conceptualize, assess, and modify this pattern. Similar and equally controversial issues can also be raised about Type A in younger people,* including such topics as: (1)

---

*In this chapter the term *Type A* is used to denote the Type A behavior pattern. In doing so we do not imply that Type A is a fixed personality trait or type, nor do we contend that the Type A pattern in children is identical with that identified in adults. Type A children and adolescents can be thought of as those who demonstrate "Type A-like" behaviors and characteristics. We also note that current measures of Type A in younger people do not always assess the same behaviors and characteristics that are labeled as Type A.

the nature versus nurture argument (i.e., Does the behavior pattern stem primarily from one's genetic heritage or from one's experiences, especially those during early childhood?); (2) the predictive disease relationship issue in terms of Type A in the young and clinical disease endpoints as adults (i.e., Are Type A children at higher risk as adults for myocardial infarctions, severe cerebral–vascular accidents, or coronary arrhythmias?); (3) the psychosocial–physiologic mechanisms issue (i.e., What evidence exists that Type A children manifest different physiologic reactivity patterns currently implicated in coronary artery disease?); and (4) the personality trait versus situation argument (i.e., Is Type A best thought of as an enduring and highly generalized personality trait or is it primarily a dispositional tendency only elicited by selected situational variables?).

These and other issues have been raised in the health field whenever a relationship, often an implied cause and effect relationship, has been advanced between psychosocial and physiologic variables (cf. Henry & Stephens, 1977; Weiner, 1977). However, unlike other psychosocial factors, Type A holds a unique position. This uniqueness is based, in part, on the cumulative results of several controlled prospective studies establishing Type A as an independent predictive risk factor for coronary heart disease, especially in more general population studies for White male adults (Booth-Kewley & Friedman, 1987; Matthews & Haynes, 1986). Further, the predictive validity of Type A as a single risk factor is comparable to that of other risk factors such as elevated serum cholesterol and hypertension (Cooper, Detre, & Weiss, 1981). As Feurstein, Labbe, and Kuczmierczyk (1986) recently noted, "this behavior pattern represents the first well-defined *psychological* or *behavioral* risk factor in the history of risk factor research in health and illness" (p. 317).

Perhaps of greater significance, Type A represents the first psychosocial risk factor that has been directly associated with reduction of clinical disease (namely, recurrence of myocardial infarction or cardiac death). That is, when Type A was modified within a controlled experiment, the rate of recurring infarctions (fatal and nonfatal) was significantly reduced (Friedman et al., 1986; see also Price, Chapter 12, this volume). Further, the magnitude of reduced cardiovascular morbidity and mortality for those receiving Type A modification treatment was substantial: Roughly 40 percent fewer cardiac recurrences took place in those receiving Type A modification compared to those receiving cardiologic treatment or no special treatment (Friedman et al., 1986). Finally, evidence of a dose–response relationship was observed; the greater the reduction in Type A, the fewer coronary events occurred (Friedman et al., 1986).

Results linking Type A to increased cardiovascular risk via prospective studies and the recent experimental data showing reduced cardiac morbidity and mortality in postinfarct patients and reduced severity of Type A in healthy adult males (Gill et al., 1985; Roskies et al., 1986) have raised questions about how this behavior pattern develops in people. Are Type

A characteristics primarily inherited or do children generally learn them? If learned, how and when are these characteristics acquired? Are these characteristics transmitted by social modeling and reinforcement manifested by parents, siblings, peers, as well as the mass media? As is often the case in probing "nature–nurture" questions, answers to the origins of Type A probably lie in a dynamic combination of genetic, constitutional, and social cognitive factors.

Studies of children and adolescents hold promise of further clarifying our understanding of the Type A syndrome. For example, global assessment of Type A has been recognized as being too imprecise to identify with needed sensitivity those people who are at risk for premature cardiovascular disease as adults (Matthews & Haynes, 1986; Thoresen & Ohman, 1986). Conceivably one or more subgroups of children with Type A-like characteristics may emerge via prospective studies as being at higher risk for disease as adults. Further, exploring Type A in children may highlight the need to restrict the designation of Type A to a more limited number of people, thereby allowing more focused and sensitive appraisal of the Type A construct.

Why might Type A in children eventually be related to increased health risk, such as CHD risk, as adults? One answer involves the relative consistency and stability of risk-related characteristics in young people. When young children have been assessed repeatedly over several years for physiologic risk factors such as blood pressure, serum lipids and lipoproteins, and body weight, the relative status of higher-risk children compared to their peers has often not significantly changed. Thus obese children usually remain obese as teenagers and adults. In one major study, the correlations for relative body fat level (skinfold measurements) over 5 years in over 1000 children (initially ranging from 2 to 14 years old) were in the range of .65 to .80. For systolic blood pressures the correlations ranged between .44 and .59, for total serum cholesterol they ranged between .59 and .69, and for low-density lipoproteins (LDL) they ranged between .63 and .76 (Webber, Cresanta, Voors, & Berenson, 1983). In general, children, especially those in the higher ranges for risk behaviors or characteristics, retain that risk status as they become adults.

In a recent *New England Journal of Medicine* editorial, Glueck (1986), prompted by the new autopsy findings of a strong positive relationship ($r = .67$) between serum cholesterol level and coronary artery disease [degree of fatty streaks and plaques] in children and adolescents [mean age = 18] (Newman et al., 1986), observed that "the behavioral patterns [cigarette smoking, and dietary habits leading to elevated LDL cholesterol levels and to obesity] underlying major risk factors for coronary heart disease are initiated in childhood and become incorporated into adult habits" (p. 176). He cautioned that research in children of *any* risk factor associated with heart disease in adults should not be confused with direct evidence of overt "disease" for children at that point in time. Still, he argued that careful long-term study of the behavior and physiologic patterns of children as they develop is extremely crucial in providing us with the basis for effective primary prevention programs.

Currently, no risk factor for cardiovascular disease present in children has been directly associated in prospective research with clinically significant disease endpoints during adulthood. Yet it seems plausible, even prudent, to hypothesize that children who evidence markedly high levels of risk factors (e.g., children in the top 20 percent of their gender and age cohort) may continue to demonstrate higher risk-factor levels compared to their peers as they move into adolescence and young adulthood. More specifically, if young children are assessed as being clearly in the highest segment of their cohort in terms of Type A, then they may indeed remain elevated in these behaviors and characteristics, *possibly* predisposing them for premature cardiovascular disease via accelerated pathophysiologic processes.

Some contend that the most prudent course of action is to take steps now to reduce risk-factor-related behaviors in younger people, despite the lack of clear-cut evidence (e.g., Parker et al., 1986). Thus children should be educated, for example, to avoid cigarettes, modify diets, reduce high blood pressure, and alter behavior patterns. An important and unacknowledged question emerges if one conjectures that markedly elevated Type A characteristics in children may be associated with ongoing pathophysiologic processes that subsequently lead to increased premature risk as adults. Would substantial reductions of Type A in younger people be associated with reduced *pathopsychogenic* processes, leading to improved social, behavioral, and emotional status as well as physical health status in later adolescence and adulthood?

Some of the studies to be reviewed here clearly seem to link Type A characteristics in children with various physiologic, social, and emotional symptoms and problems. The focus of most Type A studies with subjects of all ages has been restricted to cardiovascular-related variables. Generally ignored has been how Type A may relate to other physical disease markers as well as social–emotional problems and "mental" disorders (Margolis, McLeroy, Runyan, & Kaplan, 1983). Scientific inquiry concerning Type A needs to move in at least two major directions: (1) toward finer-grained studies that examine very specific relationships and mechanisms (e.g., differential changes in catecholamine levels in response to specific stimulus events or specific changes in perceptual–cognitive processing, such as certain perceived attributions in structured social interactions); and (2) toward broadly based "macro" studies focused on selected contextual issues (e.g., differences in school settings, parental modeling of Type A behavior, cultural values, and beliefs).

In this chapter we attempt to place the Type A construct as it relates to younger people into a broad context, one that goes beyond the important yet limited Type A–cardiovascular connection. We agree with Margolis and colleagues (1983) that theory and research in Type A have been seriously hampered by the failure to recognize contextual factors, such as interpersonal and institutional contexts (e.g., peer group and family). Initially we suspected from clinical and research experience with adults that the Type A pattern probably originates in childhood, perhaps early childhood, and that this pattern is intimately tied to the quality of the parent–child relationship. We also suspected that children and young adolescents with higher levels of Type A may also reveal other social and cognitive characteristics, including various social and emotional problems.

In this chapter we examine the available studies concerning Type A and younger people.* Studies have been organized into two major categories: Assessment studies and descriptive studies. (No treatment or intervention studies have been reported.) Several studies have understandably focused on how to assess Type A with some attention to validating measures. Among what we have termed *descriptive* studies, the following subcategories have been used: heritability, family, person–environment (including cognitive), and physiologic studies. After examining some of these studies, we discuss under the general heading of "Conceptual Connections and Concerns" the need for a broadly based conceptual framework, giving an example from another area of inquiry. Using a developmental perspective, we suggest that other areas of theory and research, namely, attachment theory, narcissistic personality disorders, and work in social–cognitive processes, merit attention. Concepts and findings from these areas are briefly presented, with discussion focused on the possible relevance to understanding Type A. The chapter closes with some concluding comments concerning Type A in children.

## LITERATURE REVIEW

### Assessment Studies

As a complex syndrome, Type A defies a simple and dichotomous categorization. Yet often a single measure of Type A in children, using a median split procedure to classify children as A or B, has been employed with the assumption that the Type A construct has been accurately assessed. This dichotomous and oversimplified assessment strategy has probably contributed to the problem of too many children being rated as Type A, thereby diluting its construct validity. Until a reliable and valid multiple measures strategy can be developed that more accurately and consistently assesses Type A, the literature will continue to suffer from confusion, contributing to problems of replication and meaningful comparisons between different research studies.

---

*Due to space limitations, a detailed table summarizing approximately 50 research studies concerned with children and young adolescents has been omitted. Readers may request copies from the first author, c/o School of Education, Stanford University, Stanford, CA 94305.

Notably lacking in studies of Type A in children have been well-documented clinical case studies. Such work characterized in part the initial work by Friedman and Rosenman in identifying the Type A syndrome in adults (see Friedman & Rosenman, 1974). The history of medical disorders and clinical psychopathology illustrates the essential contributions made by well-documented case histories in fostering theory development, including assessment strategies (Murphy, 1976; Weiner, 1977). Currently missing from the children's Type A literature are rich descriptive data, the kind of qualitative and quantitative information that allows creation of a comprehensive portrait of a Type A child. Such portraits, if they are developed, could help investigators understand better the experiences and expressions that have been termed *Type A.*

An example of the utility of such data concerns context. Several well-documented case histories, including a blend of retrospective self-reports, reports by significant others, and prospective self-monitoring, would be useful. In this way selected behaviors and feelings and thoughts could document the frequency, intensity, and duration of Type A–related characteristics in various social contexts (e.g., classroom, home, and neighborhood). If such data consistently revealed marked variability of the experience and expression of Type A behaviors, dependent on certain contexts, then subsequent studies using group designs could pursue this issue, seeking to clarify the contribution of context. As it stands we know very little about the role of social contexts, in part because we lack the kind of data provided by controlled case descriptions.

Presently, the most widely used instrument for assessing Type A is the teacher-rated Matthews Youth Test for Health (MYTH) (Matthews & Angulo, 1980). The MYTH has two principal components: Competitive Achievement–Striving (e.g., "This child is competitive" and "This child is a leader in various activities") and Impatience–Aggression (e.g., "This child does things in a hurry" and "This child interrupts others"). The importance of considering different loadings on these two components of the MYTH can be presented by example. Suppose that two children have the same total MYTH scores. One child has a moderate Competitiveness score and a very high Impatience–Aggression score while the other is very high in Competitiveness but only moderate in Impatience–Aggression. In a global sense both are classified as Type A, but clearly a different picture emerges for each child. The MYTH Competitiveness component represents a more prosocial value (Steinberg, 1987) and has been related, understandably, to higher school grades and achievement scores as well as ratings of being seen as a good athlete, leader, and popular (Whalen & Henker, 1986). By contrast, the MYTH Impatience–Aggression component has been related to more antisocial indicators (Steinberg, 1987), such as teacher-rated hyperactivity and ratings of having serious problems and being intense, noisy, and socially aggressive. It is interesting to note the very modest relationship ($r = .10$) in one study (Whalen & Henker, 1986) between the MYTH Competitiveness and Impatience–Aggression subscales. (Note that this particular correlation could be in error if the investigators computed the coefficient after varimax rotation, because such a procedure minimizes the covariance between factors.) An important question arises: Is it sufficient to be classified as Type A if a child is rated as highly competitive, but not time-urgent or aggressive?

The MYTH has demonstrated high internal consistency (.90) and test–retest reliability over 3 months (.82) and 1 year (.55) (Matthews & Avis, 1983). When the same teacher has rerated the child, the relationship has been robust (e.g., $r = .99$—Corrigan & Moskowitz, 1983). Even when the same teacher has rated the same child using two different measures of Type A (the MYTH and the modified Hunter-Wolf) the relationship remains strong ($r = .84$—Hunter et al., 1985). However, when different teachers rate the same child on the MYTH, lower reliability estimates ($r = .64$—Corrigan & Moskowitz, 1983; $r = .55$—Matthew & Avis, 1983) have been reported. Further, little agreement has been found when a teacher and a parent use the MYTH to rate the same child ($r = .20$). In this case mothers tended to rate their children as Type A more often while teachers tended to rate males higher on the MYTH Competitiveness and the Impatience–Aggression subscales (Murray, Bruhn, & Bunce, 1983). Significantly, MYTH scores appear unrelated or only slightly related to such measures as the self-report Student Type A Behavior Scale (STABS) ($r = .01$—Kirmil-Gray et al., 1987); the Hunter-Wolf Type A Scale ($r = .22$—Bishop, Hailey, & Anderson, 1987; $r = .27$—Hunter et al., 1985; $r = .21$—Jackson & Levine, 1987), the Bortner Type A behavioral interview ($r = .30$—Lawler, Allen, Critcher, & Standard, 1981), and the Behavior ($r = .24$ to .40) and Content ($r = -.02$ to .13) components of the Student Structured Interview (SSI) (Kirmil-Gray et al., 1987). Thus the MYTH has generally been shown to have high test–retest reliability but scant relationships to self-report measures and modest relationships to behavioral measures of Type A. Exclusive use of the MYTH to classify children raises a conceptual question: Can the Type A syndrome or Type A-like behaviors and characteristics be adequately assessed by a teacher without considering the child's own self-perception as well as the child's behavior as observed by others?

The descriptive and explanatory power of self-report measures lies in the assessment of children's perceptions of their own behavior and their own world. Clearly, we need to understand how children perceive themselves as well as how teachers and parents view them. Two self-report measures are currently being used. One is the Hunter-Wolf Type A Scale (HW) (Wolf, Sklov, Wenzl, Hunter, & Berenson, 1982) and the other is the STABS (Kirmil-Gray et al., 1987). The lack of a significant and meaningful relationship between teacher-rated and self-report Type A appears to be a strong indication that a multiple-measure mode and assessment strategy of Type A behavior is necessary.

The adult Structured Interview (SI) (Rosenman, 1978) is widely considered to be the best single predictor of cardiovascular disease, especially in general population samples (Booth-Kewley & Friedman, 1987; Friedman & Booth-Kewley, 1987b; Matthews & Haynes, 1986). Based on this consideration several structured interviews for adolescents and for children have been developed (Butensky, Faralli, Heebner, & Waldron, 1976; Gerace & Smith, 1985; Kirmil-Gray et al., 1987; Siegel & Leitch, 1981; Smith, Gerace, Christakis, & Kafatos, 1985). For example, the Adolescent Structured Interview (ASI) (Siegel & Leitch, 1981) was adapted from the adult SI. The ASI has been factored into three components (Siegel, Matthews, & Leitch, 1981): Interview Behavior (anger, effort to control), Impatience (time urgency, anger), and Hard-Driving (competitive, effort to control). The total ASI Type A score relates most strongly to the Interview Behavior component (i.e., rated anger and rated efforts to control during the interview). Another behavioral measure adapted from the adult Structured Interview is the Student Structured Interview (SSI) (Kirmil-Gray et al., 1987). The SSI is rated for both Type A content and behavior as well as specific behavior observed during the interview. Use of behavioral measures provide a crucial ingredient in a multimethod assessment of Type A behavior.

A more thorough multimethod assessment of Type A behavior requires at least three kinds of measures: Self-reports, structured behavioral interviews, and teacher, parent, and possibly peer behavior rating scales. Use of such a strategy with an emphasis on extreme composite scores (e.g., upper and lower 20 to 30 percent of a particular age and gender cohort) would relieve the problem of "too many Type A's" (or too heterogeneously defined Type A's) that typically dilutes the predictive and construct validity of the Type A concept. More importantly, if an acceptable standard of assessment could be developed, then progress in scientific understanding concerning Type A behavior in children would be greatly enhanced.

## Descriptive Studies

The history of Type A in adults is intimately tied to its relationship with cardiovascular markers and endpoints, both in a concurrent and a predictive sense. Further, recent findings that reductions in Type A behavior have been directly related to reduced cardiovascular disease morbidity and mortality (Friedman et al., 1986; Nunes et al., 1987) suggest that, if coronary-prone behavior can be identifed in younger people, then primary prevention programs designed to modify that behavior conceivably might reduce cardiovascular disease processes and outcomes over time.

## Physiologic Hyperreactivity

An important modality in the research on Type A behavior in children is the identification of physiological response patterns similar to those found in research with adults. Overall, no consistent differences between Type A and non–Type A children on resting physiological indices have been reported using the STABS/SSI (Eagleston et al., 1986), the HW (Hunter et al., 1982), or the MYTH (Lawler & Allen, 1981). In one study (Siegel et al., 1983), however, the ASI related to resting systolic blood pressure (SBP) and peak SBP. In contrast, when environmental demands have been increased, Type A's have shown more consistent evidence of hyperreactivity (see Lundberg, 1985, in press). For example, ASI Type A ratings were found to relate to increased heart rate under competitive task conditions (Matthews & Jennings, 1984) and the ASI subscales of Impatience and Hard-Driving were also found to relate to self-reports of cardiovascular arousal (Siegel, 1982). Jennings and Matthews (1984) reported that boys high on the MYTH Impatient subscale showed greater heartbeat and beat-by-beat heart rate change. Further, MYTH-rated Type A boys have shown increased systolic blood pressure to a physical challenge (Lundberg, 1983a) and increased heart rate to a timed task, whereas MYTH Type A girls have shown increased systolic blood pressure and heart rate responses to the timed task (Lawler et al., 1981).

These findings suggest that physiological reactivity in Type A's versus non–Type A's is fairly discriminating, reflecting interactions between certain situational factors (e.g., social challenge vs. cognitive task conditions), the particular method of Type A assessment (e.g., self-report vs. structured interview), and the physiological indices targeted (e.g., blood pressure vs. catecholamines). In all,

> "it appears that cardiovascular and endocrine responses of young children assessed according to "Type A-like" behavioral characteristics resemble physiologic responses of Type A and B adults. This suggests that mechanisms hypothesized to predispose to coronary disease might begin to operate in early childhood." (Krantz, Lundberg, & Frankenhaeuser, in press, p. 26)

Further, in a social context, Type A behavior not only may lead to heightened physiologic arousal, but also may be a result of such reactivity (Krantz & Durel, 1982). In order to help better identify and refine the physiological indices of Type A behavior in children and to understand interactions between specific environment, behavior, and physiologic responses, a multiple-method assessment strategy including behavioral observations, teacher ratings, and self-report ratings on the same subject in different situations (i.e., not just at school or in a strange laboratory setting) seems clearly warranted.

## Heritability

Results from the single heritability study to date using the Structured Interview (Rahe, Hervig, & Rosenman, 1978) indicate that the globally assessed Type A is nonheritable. However, subsidiary analyses from the same study also suggest a possible genetic influence for selected behavioral and personality components. For instance, modest but significant heritability estimates of speech characteristics and potential for hostility have been reported for the Structured Interview (Matthews et al., 1983), the JAS Speed and Impatience subscale (Rahe et al., 1978), and the JAS Hard-Driving–Competitiveness subscale (Matthews & Krantz, 1976).

The lack of clarity on this important issue of heritability has two origins. One source of difficulty lies in the assessment of Type A behavior; the other is endemic to the issue of heritability in general. At present, answers to the heritability question are obscured by serious assessment problems. For example, the validity of subscales of the JAS to assess Type A behavior has not been clearly established, yet the only published studies to date showing positive results have relied on this measure of Type A. Coupled with the very modest relationships between self-report and observer ratings of Type A, the resolution of the heritability issue requires a more accurate and discriminating assessment strategy of the Type A behavior pattern, one that will allow a more rigorous examination of specific behavioral components and characteristics. A research strategy using twin studies methodology (MZ vs. DZ twins) and employing multiple assessments is needed to help clarify effects primarily associated with early learning experiences and effects due to genetic influences.

Assessment difficulties are not the only obstacles to understanding the genetic influence on Type A. The complexity of the Type A syndrome quickly dispels any promise of a clear and quick solution to the heritability issue. The enormity of the genetic and extragenetic complexity involved has been clearly acknowledged by human geneticists. Recent work concerning the heritability of neocortical capacities illustrates this complexity. "The human brain probably contains more than $10^{14}$ synapses, and there are simply not enough genes to account for this complexity" (Changeux, cited in Lewin, 1986, p. 155). Further, this synaptic complexity is continuously being rearranged, especially early in development but also in adults, by extragenetic factors such as visual and other sensory experiences. This complexity dilemma has recently been acknowledged in human genetics research where a shift is under way from "simple" genetics to more subtle and complex influences of many genes interacting and being influenced by experience and uncertain regulatory effects. These complex influences stimulating a continuous reorganization of neural (and behavioral) structures lie at the heart of the social constructivist framework. The person constructs and reconstructs reality, emerging as a more complex being (see Ford, 1987; Ford & Ford, 1987; Prigogine & Stengers, 1984). According to Joseph Goldstein: "Now that we are learning about major gene effects at the molecular level we are gaining the tools to begin to open up the black box of the common disease" (cited in Lewin, 1986, p. 156). Goldstein further argues that the more common diseases having subtle, multigene effects may include hypertension, diabetes, and some psychiatric diseases. We strongly suspect that the Type A syndrome may also be associated with such subtle, multigenetic influences.

## Gender

The inconsistencies inherent in study of a complex syndrome like Type A are also present in the reports of gender-related differences. Males have consistently been found to score higher on the teacher-rated MYTH (e.g., Corrigan & Moskowitz, 1983; Lundberg, 1983b; Matthews & Angulo, 1980) than females. These gender differences on the MYTH have generally been attributed to males scoring higher than females on the Impatience–Aggression component. However, no consistent gender differences on ASI Type A rating have been reported; in fact, females have scored higher than males on hostility and impatience dimensions of the ASI (Siegel & Leitch, 1981) and on SSI-Behavior (Kirmil-Gray et al., 1987). At this point we cannot say that anger, for instance, is expressed in the same way for male and female Type A (ASI) children (Siegel, 1984). In addition, generally no consistent gender differences have been found for Hunter-Wolf (HW) rated Type A's (Manning et al., 1987; Weidner et al., 1987; Wolf et al., 1982). One study did report that males rated themselves more Type A (HW) than females. Interestingly, no gender differences within upper-urban and lower-rural SES groups were reported, but both males and females in the upper-urban group had higher HW Type A ratings than males and females in the lower-rural group (Manning et al., 1987). Thus at least for this sample, modest gender differences are suggested within SES groups, but not across groups.

Although numerous other gender-specific differences have been reported on subsidiary analyses, the findings do not form a clear pattern. For example, Bergman and Magnusson (1986) used questionnaire data of 13-year-olds (N = 233) to predict their JAS scores 14 years later. For males, aggressiveness and overambition scales were the best predictors, whereas for females motor hyperactivity was the best predictor for JAS Type A. Female children have been found to be higher in social competence, social networks, perceived as well as self-reported friends, and prosocial skills, and lower in self-esteem than comparable males (Thoresen et al., 1986). Further, females have reported more behavioral symptoms of stress than males (Heft et al., in press).

In sum, the available evidence points to some gender differences in global and component measures of Type A although the general findings have not been consistent. Clearly, additional research specifically designed to focus on gender-related differences among the various facets of Type A in children is needed. Once again, an intensive examination of the Type A construct employing a more rigorous multimodal and multimethod assessment strategy across time and contexts seems necessary before consistent gender-related differences can be adequately identified.

### Ethnicity

Conflicting findings on ethnic differences also have been reported. For example, White children have consistently rated themselves higher on Type

A (Hunter-Wolf) than Black children (Manning et al., 1987; Wolf, 1982; Wolf, Hunter, & Webber, 1979; Wolf, Hunter, Webber, & Berenson, 1981). However, teachers have also consistently rated male and female Black children more often as Type A than White and Hispanic children on the MYTH (Hunter et al., 1985; Murray & Bruhn, 1983). That perceptions and beliefs by teachers, observers, and children about what constitutes socially acceptable behavior differ for White and Black as well as for male and female children may help explain the inconsistent findings. Despite these inconsistencies, the evidence to date supports the existence of Type A in male and female children of different ethnic backgrounds.

## Family Demographics

To date, no association between family demographic variables studied and globally assessed Type A status has been reported. Despite some evidence indicating that Type A in adults is associated with upper socio-economic status levels and family history of coronary heart disease (e.g., Shekelle, Shoenberger, & Stamler, 1976), no association between family income and family history of coronary heart disease for either MYTH-rated Type A children (Matthews, Stoney, Rakaczky, & Jamison, 1986; Murray, Matthews, Blake, Prineas, & Gillum, 1986) or MYTH and STABS/SSI-rated Type A children (Kirmil-Gray, 1987) has been found. However, a recent study (Manning et al., 1987) found a greater prevalence of Type A (HW) in two upper SES groups of children and young adolescents (9-11 and 13-14 yr. olds). In an attempt to estimate the familial aggregation of Type A behavior as assessed by structured interview, Matthews and colleagues (1986) report conducting interviews with all available children over 8 years old and their parents in the study's sample. The efforts of Matthews and colleagues to combine a structured behavioral interview with a teacher rating and a self-report from parents to assess familial aggregation are commendable. More such programs of research using different methods of Type A assessment and studying more heterogeneous populations, including rural and mixed-SES populations, are needed.

## Parent—Child Similarity

Although no strong association between heritability and family demographics and globally defined Type A in children has been reported, Type A ratings between parents and children have shown a degree of similarity. A positive relationship between fathers' and sons' global SI ratings (Bortner, Rosenman, & Friedman, 1970) and a finding that fathers of high Type A boys (STABS/SSI) were significantly more Type A (as measured by Framingham questionnaire and structured interviews) than fathers of low Type A boys (Bracke, 1986) have been reported. Moreover, young Type A (MYTH) boys (but not girls or older boys) were more likely to have Type A (Framingham) mothers and fathers (Matthews et al., 1986). Although a consistent pattern has not emerged, significant gender- and age-specific relationships of components of the children's MYTH and the parents' JAS have been found (e.g., Matthews et al., 1986; Sweda, Sines, Laver, & Clarke, 1986). Again, lack of a more standardized multimethod assessment approach has limited the possibility of finding consistent and meaningful differences.

## Parent and Child Interactions

In addition to the findings of parent–child similarity, research evidence suggests that parents and caregivers may interact with children according to behavior type. In a recent study, fathers of Type A (HW) boys, as compared to fathers of non–Type A boys, reported more often setting high achievement goals for their sons and more often perceived that these goals were not met (Kliewer & Weidner, 1987). Further, non–Type A mothers and female caregivers have been found to "push" Type A (MYTH) children harder and more often than they pressure non–Type A children; by contrast, Type A mothers and caregivers do not interact differently with Type A or non–Type A children. Mothers of Type A children were found to give fewer positive evaluations of the child, to encourage the child to try harder despite successful performances, and to offer the child more rejection. Also in the same type mother–child dyad (e.g., Type A mother–Type A child) the mother was less demanding than in crossed-type dyads (e.g., non– Type A mother–Type A child) (Matthews, 1977; Matthews, Glass, & Richins, 1977). On laboratory tasks, parents of high Type A's (STABS/SSI) were observed to praise and to criticize their child more frequently than parents of low Type A children (Bracke, 1986).

Thus, parents of Type A children seem to encourage their children to try harder and to avoid mistakes more often than parents of non–Type A children. Further, parents of Type A (STABS/SSI) children also appear to be less discriminating about their child's performance, offering more encouragement and more criticism, regardless of how well the child is performing (Bracke, 1986). If this kind of difference is found in other studies, it could help explain the tendency of many Type A's (MYTH, STABS/SSI) to continue making efforts to succeed even though such efforts are often maladaptive (Thoresen et al., 1987).

Although parents of Type A (MYTH, STABS/SSI) children seem to give a greater quantity of evaluative responses to their children's efforts to perform laboratory tasks, those parental evaluations are not necessarily of higher quality (Bracke, 1986). In fact, Matthews (1977) found that mothers of Type A (MYTH) children, particularly non–Type A mothers, gave their children ambiguous standards for evaluating their performance. Thus Matthews and Siegel (1982) hypothesized that as Type A children develop they may be exposed to more situations with less clear performance standards than non–Type A children.

This lack of clarity in external standards may also lead to the development of less clear internal standards and to more excessively competitive and time-urgent behavior. MYTH-rated Type A's do seem to respond to ambiguous situations differently than non–Type A's. For instance, Type A (MYTH) children make greater efforts to excel in an ambiguous condition (Matthews & Volkin, 1981) and respond more vigorously to uncontrollable events (Matthews, 1979) than non–Type A children. Matthews and Siegel (1983) reported that Type A's chose to compare their performance more often against the top-scoring coactor in both clear and ambiguous criteria conditions. In contrast, non–Type A's only compared themselves with the highest scoring coactor in the ambiguous condition. Differences have also been reported in the way extreme MYTH Type A and non–Type A children evaluate themselves and their performances during a cognitively challenging task under ambiguous and clear external standards of performance (Murray et al., 1986). In the clear condition, Type A's reported making more positive self-statements and were more likely to attribute their performance to effort. By contrast, in the ambiguous condition, Type A's gave themselves more negative self-statements, tending to attribute their performance more to luck and task difficulty. In general, Type A's tend to compare their performance to others who have excelled on the task, regardless of whether the basis for evaluation in the task situation is clear or ambiguous (Murray et al., 1986).

Two possible explanations for these differences between MYTH-rated Type A and non–Type A response to clear and ambiguous conditions are suggested. First, Type A's may not have learned to perceive the difference between clear and ambiguous criteria conditions and so chronically push themselves to achieve *and* to avoid failure in ways that their parents have trained them to do. However, the finding that Type A children do make different attributions to the two conditions (e.g., performance due to effort or task difficulty) (Murray, et al., 1985) indicates that at some level they are aware that the task conditions are not identical. Another possible explanation is that, although Type A's may be able to distinguish between conditions, they do not sufficiently trust clearly stated external standards to be valid enough; they must outperform the best coactor as a way of validating their performance. Conjectures about the relative lack of self-esteem and self-worth characteristic of Type A's seem congruent with their tendency to rely more on social comparison to evaluate themselves.

Interesting distinctions have also emerged between parent–child global ratings and behavior observations of on-task interactions. For instance, mothers of high Type A (STABS/SSI) children were not more Type A (as assessed by the Structured Interview and the Framingham Type A Scale [FTAS]) than mothers of low Type A children. However, during laboratory tasks these mothers of high Type A children were observed to behave in a significantly more Type A fashion (Bracke, 1986). Assuming that the mothers' Type A rating was valid, these mothers may have been influenced by both their cognitive expectations of maternal–parental behavior in a challenging task situation and the social behavior of their children in the task situations. Differences in the children's behavior, however, did not explain differences in the mothers' behavior, because high and low Type A children were not observed to act differently, including successfully performing the tasks. This finding of differences in the behavior of mothers during the Structured Interview (as well as on the FTAS) and the laboratory task involving their children (Bracke, 1986) also highlights an assessment issue noted earlier. The context of assessment, especially how challenging or demanding it is perceived to be, can strongly influence the validity of Type A classification.

Parents of high and low Type A (STABS/SSI) children have also been found to differ on characteristics of achievement training, discipline, and modeling of Type A behavior (Bracke, 1986). Parents of high versus low Type A children reported expecting more achievement and independence behavior. In addition, while parents of both high and low Type A children reported rewarding their children's successful performances at a comparable level, the parents of the high Type A children reported that they punished (e.g., criticized) their children more often for unsuccessful performances (Bracke, 1986). This kind of punishing has been related to the development of a high need to avoid failure (McClelland, Atkinson, Clark, & Lowell, 1953; Teevan & McGhee, 1972).

On laboratory tasks parents of high Type A (STABS/SSI) children were observed to be more critical, to praise more, and to exhibit more tension; they were rated by independent observers to be more competitive and more intense, and were more likely to use social comparison data during the task to compare their child's performance to that of other children. When both parents of high Type A children were observed together with their child during performance tasks, the father was observed to model more Type A behavior and the mother was observed to push the child more often to perform better on the task (Bracke, 1986).

High Type A (STABS/SSI) children, especially boys, were also more likely to perceive their parents as using a punishing disciplinary style in response to aggressive behavior by the child (Bracke, 1986). In an earlier retrospective account, Type A (JAS) male students were more likely to recall their fathers as being more physically punishing, and Type A female students recalled their mothers as being more physically punishing than their non–Type A counterparts (Waldron et al., 1980). In Bracke's study (1986), fathers of high Type A (STABS/SSI) boys reported on a questionnaire that they would use more physical and restrictive discipline (i.e., power assertion), while fathers of low Type A males reported that they would more often try to explain the reasons behind the discipline (i.e., induction). Fathers of high Type A males were also rated higher on potential for hostility during the Structured Interview. Further, high Type A males perceived that their fathers would use more physical and punishing discipline (Bracke, 1986). Greater use of parents' power-assertive punishment has been associated with the development of anger and hostility while the use of induction procedures has been related to conscience development (Baumrind, 1971).

## Anger and Hostility

The anger–hostility dimension has recently emerged as possibly the most powerful component of Type A in predicting cardiovascular disease in adults (Booth-Kewley & Friedman, 1987; Matthews & Haynes, 1986; Rosenman, 1985; Spielberger, Johnson, Russell, Crane, & Worden, 1985; Williams, Barefoot, & Shekelle, 1985). Anger has also started to receive more attention in the Type A children literature. For example, Siegel (1984) developed an anger index and examined the relationship between anger and cardiovascular risk in 213 adolescents. The anger index produced two orthogonal factors: frequent anger directed outward and anger-producing situations. Interestingly, the results of this study suggest:

> The adolescent characterized by frequent anger directed outward is anxious, has elevated BP, and is relatively sedentary during leisure time. The adolescent who gets angry in response to a variety of situations is Type A (ASI), overweight, and relatively sedentary at school/on the job. Smoking, the reporting of negative life events, life dissatisfaction, and low self-esteem were associated with both anger scores. (p. 311)

More recently, Thoresen and colleagues (1987) explored anger and hostility in high and low Type A (STABS/SSI) male and female children. Using the Multidimensional Anger Inventory (Siegel, 1986), the high Type A children were found to experience substantially more anger arousal in terms of frequency, intensity, and duration as well as in response to more potential anger-producing situations. Further, high Type A's reported more anger-in and anger-out. By contrast, using the Anger Expression Scale (Spielberger et al., 1985), the high Type A's did not differ in anger expressed outwardly, but were found to express it more inwardly (Thoresen et al., 1987).

These studies strongly suggest that children assessed for Type A by structured interview as well as self-report experience and express more anger than less Type A children. Further, the mode of expression may be less direct and possibly more self-focused. The relationship of different types of anger and hostility constructs, not yet carefully studied in relation to global Type A and children, seems especially worthy of study. A particularily interesting dimension of anger and hostility to explore involves social cognitive processes. Do Type A children, for example, evidence more hostile thoughts in response to situations perceived as socially challenging or personally threatening as adults do (Weinstein, Davision, DeQuattro, & Allen, 1987). Clarification is needed concerning the anger–hostility component of Type A and other measures of anger and hostility.

## Performance and Type A

In an effort to explore possible origins of Type A and what factors might maintain the pattern, several investigators have studied the relationship between Type A and various performance outcomes. If Type A (vs. non–Type A) behavior, or any of its principal components, such as competitiveness, anger–hostility, or impatience, could be shown to relate to enhanced performance outcomes, then a possible reinforcement mechanism might be identified. That is, if Type A behavior directly leads to higher school grades, enhanced athletic proficiency, or increased popularity among peers, then the syndrome might be considered to have positive adaptive value.

Research efforts to examine the relationship between Type A and performance outcomes can be analyzed according to whether the JAS, the FTAS, the MYTH, or the SSI and STABS composite ratings were used to assess Type A. For instance, Waldron and colleagues (1980) found that Type A (JAS) undergraduate students had higher GPAs, took more classes (males only), studied more (females only), and were in class more than non–Type A's. For the female Type A, JAS scores were negatively related to hours per week spent relaxing or sleeping. However, in a study of rural high school students, Fontana and Davidio (1984) reported no differences between JAS Type A and non–Type A students on GPA, sports and extracurricular activities, days absent, and delinquent behavior. In a recent study of college students (Ward & Eisner, 1987), no performance differences were found for Type A and non–Type A (FTAS) groups on a general information test. Interestingly, however, the Type A group showed a greater tendency to unrealistically set high performance standards and to more often fail to reset those standards.

Matthews and Volkin (1981) found that MYTH-rated Type A's (vs. non–Type A's) completed more math problems in an unlimited time condition, but not in a time deadline condition; they also held a weight longer and reported less fatigue relative to the task. Murray and colleagues (1985) found no differences between Type A and non–Type A students on the number of correct or attempted math problems in a challenging cognitive task. Corrigan and Moskowitz (1983) also found no differences between Type A's and non–Type A's on the number of correct choices on a reaction-time task; non–Type A's were significantly slower in reaction time under the no-incentive condition, but not when incentives were involved. Interestingly, Whalen and Henker (1986) reported that higher task performance and perceived competence (e.g., peer ratings of being an athlete and staff ratings of being an athlete, a leader, and being popular) for MYTH-rated Type A's were associated with the MYTH Competitive factor, but not the MYTH Impatience–Aggression factor. The MYTH Competitive subscale was also found by Matthews and colleagues (1986) to relate to higher classroom grades and achievement test scores for both boys and girls. For girls the total MYTH was also related to classroom grades and achievement test scores. Matthews and colleagues (1986) suggested that teachers may have responded more negatively to the impatient and aggressive characteristics in boys than in girls. Generally, evidence for enhanced performance by Type A children appears limited to teacher ratings of competitiveness using the MYTH.

Using SSI and STABS to assess Type A, Arnow and colleagues (1986) found no differences between high and low Type A male and female fifth, seventh, and ninth grade students on classroom grades, standard achievement test scores, athletic success, and participation in sports and other extracurricular activities. Bracke (1986) compared high and low Type A (MYTH and STABS/SSI) male and female sixth grade students and found no differences in performance on two laboratory tasks (block stacking and ring toss). Rodeo and Thoresen (1987) studied more than 100 male and female varsity athletes in various individual and team sports at Stanford. They found that Type A versus non–Type A varsity athletes (assessed by STABS and in a subsample also by the SSI) did not differ in athletic proficiency (performance), athletic potential, or athletic talent as independently rated by their coaches. While male athletes were more Type A than a sample of male nonathlete students (female athletes and nonathletes did not differ), much of this difference was accounted for by higher competition-related scores for the athletes. Further, higher competitiveness in male athletes was limited to the athletic context; no differences were found for greater academic or social competitiveness between athletes and nonathletes.

In sum, Type A typically is not associated with significantly higher classroom grades, achievement test scores, athletic performances, or social competence. Some evidence suggests a positive relationship of the competitive facet of Type A with higher performance. However, much of this evidence is limited to global teacher ratings of competitiveness (MYTH Competitiveness factor). Further, superior performance for Type A children, when reported, is often in terms of the rate or effort of performing (e.g., faster reaction time) rather than the quality or overall correctness of the performance.

An unrecognized performance-related issue involves the possible longer-term effects of Type A on the quality of academic, social, and physical performance in younger people. Unknown at this point are the developmental consequences, in terms of physical, social, and emotional factors, of high and sustained levels of excessively high competitiveness. Answers to questions about enhanced or diminished performance for Type A children, as to quality as well as quantity, require a longer-term perspective that examines more immediate (proximal) *and* more distal performance measures. Of particular concern is the possible performance mix problem for some younger Type A's, involving what some might perceive as superior performance (e.g., completing tasks more quickly) in some areas but leading to inferior performance outcomes in other areas (e.g., more interpersonal problems at school). Essentially, issues of Type A and performance represent a classic problem of process and outcome. That is, various processes working in concert can often produce a contradictory mix of outcomes.

## Summary of Studies

Although children exhibiting Type A have been found to differ significantly from non–Type A's in certain situations, assessment-related problems found in all areas of research limit the consistency and generalizability of results. Overall, no highly consistent physiological differences have been established between Type A and non–Type A children, although the evidence is promising of such differences. Type A children (MYTH), for example, have often but not always shown greater physiologic reactivity to specific situational factors (e.g., social challenge). The few heritability studies to date have not found that globally assessed Type A is a genetically transmitted or determined syndrome. Assessment problems, however, such as only using one measure of Type A on one occasion, have limited definitive answers about physiologic reactivity and heritability. Various gender-related differences on Type A have been reported, but the results have not been consistent. Likewise, ethnic differences have been found, but the results differ according to how Type A has been assessed, SES levels, and gender. Parent–child similarities in the incidence of Type A have been found, especially for fathers and sons. Again, however, clear patterns have not developed, in part because existing measures of Type A for adult females may not be sufficiently sensitive to detect Type A. Thus in many areas including physiologic, genetic, gender, ethnic, and parent–child similarity, differences have been found between Type A and non–Type A children, but confidence in these differences must await more discerning assessment strategies and conceptual frameworks.

Studies of parental behaviors and attitudes as related to Type A children are also limited by the problems just cited. Still, some interesting patterns across assessment methods have recently emerged. Mothers, fathers, and caretakers have been found to interact with children differently, according to the adults' and children's behavior type. Further, parents of Type A children have been found to encourage their children to make greater efforts to succeed and to avoid failure, sometimes regardless of the situation, than parents of non–Type A children. Type A children also seem to respond to ambiguous versus clear task situations differently than non–Type A children—perhaps, in part, due to parental modeling and teaching. Parents of high and low Type A children do not differ in their overall desires for achievement and success of their children, but do differ on the specifics of achievement training, discipline, and modeling of Type A behavior. In one study parents of high Type A's criticized their children more for unsuccessful performances, were rated by observers as more competitive and intense, and more often compared their children's performances to those of other children. Further, high Type A boys perceived that their fathers would use a more physically punishing disciplinary style. The barest outline of a picture is beginning to suggest that a variety of parent–child perceptions and behaviors may be implicated in the development of Type A.

The anger and hostility dimension has been identified as a discriminating and important characteristic of Type A in children. Current research strongly suggests that Type A children experience and express more anger than their non–Type A peers. One of the most deserving areas of further inquiry centers around increasing our understanding of anger and hostility in Type A children and adolescents.

Generally, Type A has not been directly linked to performance superiority. None of the studies using a structured interview and a self-report measure of Type A have found differences between Type A and non–Type A children. Further, some studies have provided evidence that Type A is associated with greater social, emotional, and adverse physiologic symptoms and problems. Future studies may support some performance advantages for Type A children, such as completing tasks more quickly, but these gains may be sharply offset by deficits in other performance areas.

## CONCEPTUAL CONNECTIONS AND CONCERNS

Theory and research concerning Type A, especially in children, need an expanded conceptual frame of reference. Clearly, a more comprehensive multimethod and multimodal assessment approach is overdue. Continuing to assess Type A with a single self-report or adult rating measure will only add to an already confusing collection of findings. By contrast, deriving a composite picture—a multivariate index—of the Type A pattern will permit more sharply focused distinctions between and among children. That picture must include several contextually sensitive portraits composed not only of behavioral reports of others, such as peers and teachers, but also of self-reports, especially ones focused on tapping situational self-perceptions and self-evaluations.

A great deal of conceptual work remains in trying to clarify the boundaries of the Type A construct, including issues of discriminant and convergent validity (Campbell & Fiske, 1959). For example, what is the degree of conceptual and behavioral overlap between children designated as attention deficit disordered ("hyperactive") and Type A children? Is there an appreciable generalized negative affective component in younger Type A children, such that the Type A classification overlaps with chronic depression and generalized lower self-esteem?

Evidence clearly exists that *some* Type A-like characteristics are discernible in children, some as young as 3 years of age (see Lundberg, 1985, in press). Yet the current mechanics of assessing Type A in children and youth suffer from a single and simple trait approach in which individuals are commonly divided, using one measure (e.g., MYTH), into two groups (e.g., A vs. non-A) without reference to other sources of information about the children and without reference to context. Bronfenbrenner's (1979) characterization of most research in child development—the study of strange children in strange places by strangers for the briefest periods of time—seems apt for many studies of Type A and younger people. Generally lacking has been a concern to assess Type A from a more person-centered perspective, one that gathers perceptual- and cognitive-related data about children over time and across specific contexts, along with physiologic, behavioral, and environmental data (see Bem, 1983).

A key obstacle to progress appears to be at the conceptual level. If one construes Type A as an essentially "fixed" or invariant personality trait, one that generalizes across situations and circumstances, then use of a single generalized context-insensitive measure applied on one occasion makes sense. This logic has unfortunately been the rule in prospective studies of Type A in adults where a single self-report measure used on one occasion (e.g., JAS or Framingham Type A Scale) or the Type A Structured Interview has been deemed valid to classify people over several years if not decades (Thoresen & Ohman, 1987). If, however, the Type A construct is instead conceived as a dynamic, predisposing cognitive–behavioral *style*, one sensitive to situations perceived as possibly threatening or challenging, then assessment optimally requires multiple measures employed on more than one occasion that tap perceptual–cognitive, behavioral, and physiologic factors sensitive to particular contexts. By analogy, one typically recognizes the state-specific rather than trait qualities of blood pressure, using at least repeated measures on one occasion and, optimally, obtaining repeated measures in various settings (e.g., home, work, physician's office). At the extreme, some hypertensives may experience markedly elevated blood pressures regardless of the situation, yet most will show considerable variability across time and setting. Type A may also reveal comparable patterns, if adequate assessment procedures are used to examine the possibility.

The focus on assessment in terms of context is also shaped by how Type A is conceptualized. To date, for example, most studies of children using the MYTH on one occasion have, in effect, conceptualized Type A in terms of the classroom teacher's global ratings of a child's school-related competitiveness as well as impatience coupled with social and physical aggressiveness. At issue is the theoretical adequacy of current Type A measures, such as the MYTH, to capture adequately the Type A construct. Recent studies (e.g., Hunter et al., 1985; Murray et al., 1983; Whalen & Henker, 1986) have revealed that the global teacher ratings of Type A often overlap significantly with teacher ratings of hyperactive (i.e., attention deficit disordered) children. In Hunter and colleagues' (1985) study, for example, the best single predictor in multiple regression analyses of teacher-assessed Type A children was the same teachers' ratings of hyperactivity. Yet the Type A construct is not theoretically identical with hyperactivity. The confusion stems in part from method confounding, the shared variance of using global teacher judgments of both constructs. Interestingly, Murray and colleagues (1983) found a modest correlation ($r = .20$) for the MYTH when the same child was rated by the parent and by the teacher using the MYTH. (Note that Kirmil-Gray et al. [1987] found no relationship between a parent-rated behavior checklist of Type A-like actions and the MYTH as well as the structured interview [SSI] and a self-report measure [STABS].) Such a relationship may reflect that the child's rated MYTH characteristics, such as overall competitiveness or impatience, generally differ with the context, that is, the classroom and the home setting. Thus the generalizability of teacher ratings of Type A may be quite weak.

A much larger theoretical question, however, is raised by the studies reviewed here, one that bears on the interpretation of specific findings as well as on the general conclusions about research in this area. The general question concerns the presuppositions or implicit assumptions that seem inherent in any piece of research (Scarr, 1985). Typically, Type A research in children has focused on a few immediate, proximal "objective" variables, such as behavioral or physiologic correlates of children classified as Type A by a single measure on one occasion. These studies have not studied Type A directly; instead, children have been typically classified as Type A or B and then these children have been studied in terms of various physiologic or behavioral correlates. No attention is given to clarifying cognitive, behavioral, or physiologic differences *among* Type A children. Implicit in such studies are premises about relevant variables to examine, in terms of substance (content) as well as method. Stated more simply, it is hard to find out more about something if you're not looking in many different places, some of which will turn out to be the right places.

### Problem Behavior Theory and Drinking: A Conceptual/Empirical Example

Jessor (1984) and his associates, who have studied socially deviant behavior in children and adolescents, offer an excellent example of the type of theoretical framework needed at this point to enhance our understanding of the Type A syndrome in younger people (see also Donovan, Jessor & Jessor, 1983; Jessor, 1982, 1985). The paradigm is briefly presented here to illustrate how research can be productively guided by a theoretical framework that is sufficiently complex.

The conceptual framework used by Jessor is termed problem-behavior theory. It posits two major social–psychological systems—the personality system and the perceived environment system—that determine the behavior system, that is, the various social problem behaviors of young people (e.g., marijuana use, inappropriate sexual intercourse, teenage pregnancies, problem drinking, deviant social behaviors). Examples within the personality system include various values and expectations (e.g., value of academic achievement, value of affection, expectation for independence) along with personal belief structures (e.g., beliefs about social criticism, internal–external locus of control) and personal control structure (e.g., religiosity). The perceived environment system includes views about the more immediate or proximal social environment (e.g., child's view of parent approval of problem behavior) and a friend's modeling of problem behavior along with longer-term, or distal, perceptions of the social environment (e.g., view of parental support, parental controls, compatibility of parents and friends). In addition,

Jessor's conceptual framework includes social demographics (e.g., father's occupation, family structure, and socialization variables such as mother and father's traditional beliefs, mother's tolerance of deviance, parental religiosity, child's involvement with television, and friends' major interests). The model conceives of demographic and socialization structures as antecedent background variables that influence the personality and perceived environment systems, which, in turn, influence social behavior.

Using this framework, Jessor and colleagues have studied the problem of excessive alcohol use, using different research methods ranging from natural case histories to prospective multivariate regression designs using a cohort-sequential protocol (such a design combines cross-sectional and longitudinal data) in examining what covaries with problem drinking among young adolescents up through young adults.

Using problem behavior theory as a framework and a variety of research designs, these investigators have learned a great deal about what factors relate to problem drinking. For example, they learned no one set of data, such as personality or perceived environment variables, adequately predicted or accounted for problem drinking behavior over seven years. Significant correlations between single psychosocial factors and degree of drinking ranged from .20 to .40, a commonly found relationship between personality variables and various outcomes. However, when multiple regression analyses included variables from the entire conceptual framework as suggested by problem behavior theory, the multiple $r$'s for predicting problem drinking status over seven years (from freshman and sophomore high school years to mid- and late twenties) was a robust .79, accounting for about 60 percent of the variance. They also found that the pattern of certain personality variables, such as level of intolerance for socially deviant behavior, markedly changed over the years of adolescence. In this particular case, intolerance of deviant actions diminished over the high school years and then abruptly increased during the early twenties. These data suggest that, as social contexts change, some personality characteristics are also altered.

Another finding made possible by using repeated measures over several years revealed that the probability of being a problem drinker as a young adult was, in part, related to drinking status as a young adolescent. For example, over 50 percent of young adolescent problem drinkers remained so as adults in their late twenties, while young adolescent nondrinkers seldom suffered from a serious drinking problem as adults (less than one in five).

How might researchers studying Type A benefit from the example of Jessor and his colleagues? Some possibilities seem fairly obvious: (1) Use *multiple measures* collected over *repeated occasions*; (2) work within a *conceptual framework* that is sufficiently comprehensive to capture adequately the phenomena of Type A; and (3) employ a *variety* of *research designs*, rather than always using the same design (e.g., only using a pre–post experimental vs. control design), recognizing that any one design at best can only address certain questions. A less obvious implication concerns the marked advantage of a research program approach rather than an ad hoc strategy, one that dictates conducting one or a few studies using the same or highly similar designs.

At present a very promising theoretical framework to study Type A is Bandura's (1986) social cognitive theory. This theory posits that human experience is a function of the reciprocal ("give and take") influences of personal, environmental, and behavioral factors. An expansion of this framework, adding physiologic as another major factor, has been used successfully by Friedman and colleagues (1986) to design and evaluate a treatment program for altering Type A in postcoronary adults as well as an intervention program to reduce Type A in high-level military officers (Gill et al., 1985). Thoresen and his colleagues (e.g., Eagleston et al., 1986; Thoresen et al., 1987) have also employed social cognitive theory to study Type A in children and young adolescents. Other theoretical frameworks such as a social constructivist framework (Ford, 1987; Ford & Ford, 1987) may also provide the needed breadth of focus that can encourage investigators and practitioners to give careful consideration to the reciprocal and dynamic influences of cognitive, behavioral, physiological, and environmental factors in understanding Type A. Such consideration will also reveal, as occurred in Jessor's research program, that specific questions require specific research designs, ranging from well-documented case histories to multivariate longitudinal designs.

## Origins of Insecurity

The central theme of anger and hostility within the Type A construct may have some of its origins in the quality of the parent–child relationship. As discussed earlier, differences have been found in how adult women, including mothers, respond to Type A as compared to non–Type A children. Mothers of Type A (MYTH) children, for example, encourage them to keep trying harder, often despite their successful performance, and also criticize them more often than mothers of non–Type A children (e.g., Matthews et al., 1977). Parents of high Type A (STABS/SSI) children have also been rated as more competitive and more intense in their behavior during situations where their children were performing a challenging task (Bracke, 1986). What might help clarify differences in the ways that Type A children and their parents act and react in certain situations compared to less Type A children and their parents?

One possibility emerges from the literature of child development. Attachment theory, based in part on observational studies of how infants (12 to 18 months old) relate to their mothers, concerns the child's developing sense of personal and social confidence, including self-perceptions of worth, competence (efficacy), and control (see Bretherington & Waters, 1985; Parkes & Stevenson-Hinde, 1982). Theorists concerned with attachment (e.g.,

Bowlby, 1973, 1982) contend that the very young child develops cognitive schemata or mental representations of experience, called *inner working models* of reality. These models strongly influence children's construction of expectations and beliefs about themselves and about others, including relationships between self and others. In contrast to developmental stage theories, attachment researchers believe that "sensitive periods" rather than fixed stages exist for the child, times in which the child is constructing inner working models and is using them to make sense of or give meaning to his or her experience. From this perspective a child's development is viewed as the ongoing interaction of current circumstances and preceding experience, especially the child's cognitive representation of what that past experience means to him or her.

Although the fascinating literature on attachment cannot be thoroughly discussed here, we believe that this perspective on development and behavior may hold promise in helping to clarify why some children manifest Type A-like behavior. Here we discuss briefly some reasons why review of the attachment literature, both empirically and theoretically, seems worthy of attention.

### Getting Attached

Classification of infants as to the quality of their attachment relationship with the parent, usually the mother, yields three major child designations: the securely attached child (Group B), the insecurely attached avoidant child (Group A), and the insecurely attached ambivalent child (Group C). (Different variations of these three major designations will not be presented here.) These designations are typically based on observing the mother and child in a laboratory situation called the Strange Situation (Ainsworth, Bell, & Stayton, 1971; Ainsworth & Wittig, 1969), one in which the mother leaves the child for brief periods of time in a room, some of the times with a stranger involved (e.g., in one sequence the mother leaves the child but the stranger remains in the room). The dependent variable focuses on the observed "reunion" behavior of the child in relation to the mother, that is, how the child behaves when the mother returns to the room after a brief absence.

Attachment researchers believe that the individual differences in behavior observed during such situations represent differences in the way the child creates or constructs what the experience means or represents to him or her, a representation based in part on past experience with the parent. Thus the securely attached child is observed not to be very upset or disrupted by the brief comings and goings of the mother and the stranger, while the insecure–avoidant child tends to act in an angry manner, often physically avoiding the mother, not looking at her directly and acting as if he or she did not care about the mother. In some respects these avoidant reactions appear similar to the anger-in descriptions in older children and adolescents experiencing the emotions of anger, but not expressing the anger in a direct fashion (Spielberger et al., 1985). The insecure–ambivalent child, by contrast, commonly expresses the classic approach–avoidance pattern toward the mother upon her return, with actions that could be labeled as more confused and anxious. As noted earlier, several subclassifications are also used because overlapping behaviors are common between the three basic classifications.

Over the past decade, attachment researchers have studied the stability of these classifications along with various behavioral correlates as these infants have developed and moved into the school years (e.g., Main, Kaplan, & Cassidy, 1982; Sroufe, 1986). These results are of particular interest because the insecurely attached avoidant children have been observed in preschool and elementary school settings to act in ways that appear consistent with some Type A characteristics. For example, Sroufe (1986) reports data, based on observer and classroom teacher ratings, of a 7-year follow-up of infants classified at 12 to 18 months. The avoidant child has been noted, for example, to be more hostile and quick to anger, more socially aggressive during play situations, less positive in expressing feelings toward others, less socially popular, with fewer close peer friendships. Sroufe notes that the quality of the early mother–child attachment is highly predictive of the quality of social relationships that the child has with others in later years.

The more securely attached child, when observed years later, displays more personal and social adaptability, termed *ego resiliency* by Sroufe (1986), acting more flexibly in relations with others as well as with changes in the environment. Such children were observed to display less arousal and upset in stressful situations. Sroufe also reports on the earlier behavior of these children at ages 4 and 5 while they attended nursery school. The results are quite similar. Interestingly, when the children were assessed in their fantasy play, telling a make-believe story about themselves, insecure–avoidant children reported considerably more conflicts and strug- gles with others, including more anger, with few or no other people identified as major people in the story. By contrast, securely attached children reported more positive, cooperative experiences, with greater self-efficacy (perceived competence) and perceived control in terms of successfully taking actions that solved problems leading to pleasant outcomes.

It is interesting to note that Ford and Thompson (1985), in reviewing the attachment literature as well as social cognitive theories of personality development, suggest that perceived competence (e.g., level of self-efficacy) and perceived control (e.g., behavior–outcome expectancies) represent the two major constructs that are central in most developmental theories. These authors suggest that insecurely attached children fall into various combi- nations of perceived competence and control. For example, the Type A child would be primarily classified as suffering from relatively low perceived control of the environment yet adequate perceived competence. Thus the child would be observed to struggle much more than other children in efforts to gain direct control of situations. Further, the child would typically attribute his or her problems to the environment rather than to personal characteristics.

The work of Mary Main and her colleagues (e.g., Main & Weston, 1981, 1982) in many respects confirms these findings. Importantly, Main's work has also focused on the mother's attachment relationship, that is, examining whether the mother herself was securely attached as a child and whether she is at present manifesting behaviors and characteristics associated with insecurely attached relationships. For example, Main and her colleagues (see Main, Kaplan, & Cassidy, 1985) have developed a structured adult attachment interview to gather data on the parent's previous and current relationships. Not surprisingly, they report a significant positive relationship ($r = .62$) between a mother's type of attachment relationship and the child's attachment classification. Such data strongly suggest that the mother's own "working model" of self, in terms of her feeling securely attached, reflects a connection between a child's feelings of security and those of the parent. By contrast, fathers demonstrate a significant but less positive relationship ($r = .37$) between their type of attachment and that of their child.

In a study of 40 parents and their children spanning five years (from age one to six), Main and her colleagues (1985) found that: (1) the relationship of child and mother attachment at one year and six years was quite robust ($r = .76$); (2) the overall social functioning of the 6-year-old child observed during a 20-minute "open-ended" session with the mother significantly correlated ($r = .46$) with the child's earlier attachment classification (i.e., securely attached children displayed more positive social behaviors with mother compared to insecurely attached children); and (3) the securely attached child with the mother present was observed to express greater fluency of speech ($r = .63$), greater "emotional openness" ($r = .68$), and more positive verbal and nonverbal reactions in response to looking at a family photograph ($r = .74$) at age six than did insecurely attached children. Correlations with fathers, however, were dramatically lower, such as an $r = .15$ (instead of the $r = .74$ found for mothers) between attachment classification and positive reactions to viewing the family photograph.

Particularly interesting have been Main and colleagues' (1985) descriptions of insecure–avoidant mothers. Generally, these mothers have demonstrated avoidantlike behaviors toward their children, often warding off intimate physical contact, blocking the children's efforts to approach them, often failing to display physically and verbally affectionate behavior and expressing more anger toward the children. A related finding, noted by Sroufe (1986), was that nursery school teachers displayed much more anger and aggravation with the avoidant child. By contrast, these teachers were observed to display more warmth, acceptance, and confidence toward the secure child and more nurturance and support for the insecurely attached ambivalent child.

These data nicely illustrate the bidirectional nature of social behavior, a sorely neglected perspective in Type A studies of children. That is, Type A behaviors can elicit Type A-like reactions from the social environment.

Further, such data may also bear on the reciprocal nature of social cognitive processes and structures. Perhaps the parent, in effect, "teaches" the child, for example, that one must constantly strive to produce outcomes that are worthy of attention and approval by others, and the child subsequently "teaches" peers, teachers, and others who, in turn, as good learners reciprocate, expecting that the child will constantly strive to produce worthy results. In this way, the child's inner working model of self and of others experiences a great deal of confirmation. As with the inexperienced scientist who unwisely overgeneralizes via inductive inference from seemingly confirmed sample data to the population, the child comes to accept as true his or her beliefs about personal worth and about what others consider good and worthwhile.

How might theory and research in attachment, particularly concerning the insecurely attached avoidant child, relate to Type A? Aside from the more obvious findings in which the avoidant child has been observed and rated as displaying more anger and hostility toward others and perhaps more self-critical appraisal, the development of an anger-oriented appraisal and coping style by the insecure–avoidant child seems especially promising. Conceivably, what might be termed the underlying social cognitive schemata of Type A may emerge in part from the early life experiences of the child who is classified as insecure–avoidant. Further, consideration and study of parent–child interactions and relationships, such as those carried out by attachment researchers, could begin to clarify how the young child begins to adopt at least some of the personal and social perceptions of self and of others, especially those involving perceived worth, competence, and control that have been associated with the Type A syndrome.

## A Narcissistic Reflection

The concept of the narcissistic personality popularized in the past decade (e.g., Lasch, 1978) appears to overlap considerably with the Type A concept. As a construct, narcissism was ascribed with major psychological significance in the early twentieth century by Freud (1914/1925, 1931/1949), who viewed narcissistic tendencies as a universal phase of early child development, following the excessive self-absorption of the child, especially in the autoerotic area, and preceding the establishment of more externally focused object (love) relationships with others. Freud's initial focus was concerned with narcissism not as a personality type disorder—the current perspective—but as a step in the process of psychosexual development. In the 1920s, Wilhelm Reich described the narcissistic character in terms of strong leadership qualities (the "take charge" type), as sometimes arrogant, always energetic, and typically self-assured and self-confident, but in an infantile sense (see Reich, 1949).

In recent years, Kernberg (e.g., 1975, 1976) and Kohut (e.g., 1966, 1971, 1972, 1977) have offered somewhat contrasting psychoanalytic conceptions of the causes of narcissism, but general agreement as to its observable manifestations. Kernberg sees narcissistic people as involved in a great deal of self-referencing in their interaction with others, driven by a pressing need to be loved and admired by others, and seeking a constant stream of "tributes" from others, yet having very little empathy and positive regard for the feelings and concerns of others. Generally unhappy and dissatisfied, the narcissist ceaselessly strives hard to control others, often displaying an engaging yet superficial charm that conceals a personal coldness and a profound distrust and suspiciousness of others.

Kohut's (1971) descriptions of narcissistic personalities highlight their profound angry reactions ("rage") when their self-esteem seems at all threatened or challenged, coupled with a vengeful, hostile attitude, often viewing others as the "enemy." (Note that the word *hostility* comes from the Latin *hostis*, "the enemy.") The narcissistic person holds a grandiose sense of self, one that is strongly associated with serious interpersonal problems, especially at the level of intimate relationships. Perhaps Kernberg (cited in Akhtar & Thomson, 1982) captured much of the essence of the narcissist in observing: "I am grandiose because I feel unlovable and hateful and I fear I cannot be loved unless I am perfect and omnipotent" (p. 15). Such a description closely accommodates clinical observations of some adult Type A's (Friedman & Rosenman, 1974; Price, 1982).

Importantly, almost all scholars who have tried to conceptualize narcissistic behavior and attitudes cite the quality of early childhood experience as a major determinant, primarily a childhood characterized by parents, especially mothers, who were inconsistent in their love and affection, often overly controlling, socially insecure, and out of touch with the child's feelings and fears. Miller's (1981) poignant descriptions of parents of narcissistic children can readily be labeled as Type A; these parents are portrayed as highly competitive and demanding, cynical and distrustful, quick to anger and, crucially, as using the child's performance and achievements as evidence that the parent is worthy of respect and admiration, if not love. Miller argues persuasively that narcissistic parents produce narcissistic children.

Although one can quarrel with the various psychoanalytic rationales offered to explain the narcissistic character (see Millon, 1981), the behavioral and attitudinal descriptions of narcissistic characteristics seem congruent with current descriptions of Type A. For example, the excess of self-referencing speech (*I*, *me*, etc.), the external veneer of being in control with great assurance, the internal structure of genuine self-doubt, profound anger, pervasive distrust, and the problems in establishing and maintaining close, intimate relationships clearly capture major facets of the Type A construct. Further, the parents described by Miller (1981) are strikingly similar to the insecurely attached "avoidant" parents previously noted by attachment researchers (e.g., Main & Weston, 1982). Possibly, some of the wellsprings of what we have termed Type A, especially the underlying pervasive insecurity and self-doubt noted originally by Friedman, Rosenman, and early colleagues, reside in the developmental and experiential strata recognized earlier by psychoanalytic scholars trying to understand excessively self-involved people. The overlapping conceptual fit, however, is probably far from perfect when empirically compared. Unfortunately, scholars of narcissism have not conducted controlled empirical studies, especially those that allow empirical data to challenge and clarify theoretical beliefs. For example, would youngsters labeled as clearly narcissistic be observed to act and react in the same ways as those labeled Type A?

It is tempting to extrapolate from the many clinical descriptions of adults who have been classified as fitting the DSM-III criteria for narcissistic personality disorder (see Akhtar & Thomson, 1982), concluding that the superficially adaptive and seemingly successful behavior of the narcissistic person is indeed the Type A adult in action. It is also tempting to envision narcissistic parents, in how they raise their children, as continually modeling and reinforcing beliefs and behaviors about self and about others that could be described as extremely socially competitive and excessively angry if not hostile. Perhaps the most useful perspective to take at this point is one that acknowledges the possible value of different scholars using various theories and methods arriving at fairly similar conclusions. In that sense one might argue that processes bearing on construct validity are in the making. One can argue, of course, much as in factor-analytic studies, about how best to label the particular construct (e.g., whether we should call it Type A, hostility, narcissistic disorders, etc.). At issue, however, is the need to remain open to at least considering data and concepts gathered in a variety of ways from different sources. In terms of narcissism, for example, the clinical case study descriptions of adults characterized as narcissistic may offer ideas to Type A researchers about better ways to understand and study facets of the Type A syndrome in parents.

## Social Cognitive Processes

One of the most neglected areas of Type A research, yet one that holds promise of the most helpful concepts and data, concerns how Type A's construe and construct everyday reality (Thoresen & Ohman, 1987). Commonly recognized in the field of psychology, often in terms of individual differences, is the established fact that people do not always perceive and believe the same things about the "same" event or situation. Can, for example, the same event, such as filling out a questionnaire or being asked a question in a challenging manner, be considered the same event for all if some people perceive or construe those events as different? Certainly the physical characteristics of a questionnaire can be confirmed as the same across questionnaires. Less certain, however, is that each person processes those questions in the same way. Do all people ascribe the same meaning to each question, do they engage in the same way? Do all people ascribe the same meaning to each question, do they engage in the same "self-talk" while reading questions, and do they hold the same expectations about their ability to answer the question?

Social cognitive processing is a lively topic in many fields (e.g., Cole & Scribner, 1974; Folkman, Lazarus, Gruen, & De Longis, 1986; Gergen, 1985; Rogoff & Lave, 1984; Weiner, 1977), in part because of the growing realization that progess in the social and behavioral sciences, and more recently the biological sciences, requires controlled studies of human cognitive processes. Stated somewhat differently, the argument contends that the complicated workings of the human "black box" cannot solely be inferred by observed behavior or physiologic responses.

Concern by Type A researchers with social and personal cognitions has long existed, and is represented, for example, by the early conjectures of Friedman and Rosenman (e.g., 1974; also see Price, 1982) about negative self-conceptions, inadequate self-esteem, and excessive self-criticalness. Within the literature on Type A children, Matthews (1982) has conjectured that the child's ambiguity about which explicit performance standards to use for self-evaluation may play an important role in encouraging Type A behavior, especially in making more intense effort under ambiguous conditions (Matthews & Volkin, 1981). Considering that much of modern living in complex urban and suburban contexts involves trying to succeed under often ambiguous if not contradictory conditions, the viability of the ambiguous context self-evaluation conjecture about Type A seems highly promising. Add to this ambiguity of standards the need of Type A's for perceived control, along with high levels of self-critical covert talk while performing ambiguous tasks (Murray et al., 1986), and a dynamic social cognitive picture then emerges that appears to be at work in the lives of Type A's. Such social cognitive processes are believed strongly to influence overt behavior, a variety of physiological processes, as well as the social environment (Bandura, 1986).

At present, little is understood about the ways that Type A children perceive reality and construe themselves and others, especially in an ongoing fashion. In what ways do Type A children differ, if at all, from less Type A children in their social perceptions relative to specific situations? Do, for example, Type A children engage in more self-critical and/or socially critical covert talk in general, or is this kind of self-talk limited to situations perceived as highly challenging, competitive, and/or personally threatening? Do Type A children perceive the social behaviors of others as personally challenging or threatening more often? Among Type A children, do some engage in similar levels of self- and socially critical thinking across home, school, and community contexts compared to other Type A children whose critical thoughts are limited to certain contexts? If some children do evidence more generalized "negative" thoughts, how do they differ from other Type A's in terms of physiological and behavioral characteristics?

## The "Take Charge" Perception by Others

Fortunately, a few studies concerned with Type A have been reported that at least help set the stage for inquiry into social cognitive processes in younger people. Strube and his colleagues (e.g., Strube, Lott, Heilizer, & Gregg, 1986), for example, have conducted a series of studies with college students using the JAS to assess Type A. (One can question, however, the validity of using a self-report questionnaire that does not include the anger—hostility factor to assess Type A.) In a recent study (Strube et al., 1986) the perceptions of control and performance were examined, particularly the notion that Type A's are perceived by observers (i.e., the social environment) to exert more control than non–Type A's, regardless of their actual behaviors and the observed performance outcomes. By using a series of computer-mediated symbol tasks in which the actual control of the task by the "actor" (i.e., the student doing the task) was preplanned, these researchers were able to study the self-perceptions of control by the actor as well as by a peer observer across various situations in which actual control by the actor and outcome were systematically varied (from 25 percent to 75 percent control). The results are intriguing in that Type A and non–Type A (JAS) actors did not differ in their own self-perceptions of control. That is, no evidence was found to support the proposition that Type A's in general perceive themselves as having more control. However, under outcome conditions in which the results were positive (i.e., the actor's actions were associated with task success), *observers*, regardless of their own Type A/non–Type A status, consistently rated the Type A actor as having more control than the non–Type A actor, when, in fact, there were no actual outcome differences for the actors. (Under negative outcomes, the observers did not rate Type A's as having more control than non–Type A's.) Further, these investigators found that the perceptions of greater control for Type A's were not due to superior performance (e.g., pressed bar more often, demonstrated more actual control, or were more successful). Impressively, these investigators had the foresight to plan in advance ongoing interviews of the observers about why they judged an actor to have high or low control. While the "objective" performance evidence failed to clarify differences in perceived control, the observer's descriptions of their judgments provided a possible explanation. Typically, observers reported that they rated the Type A actor as having more control (than he actually had) if he moved "decisively," acted "quickly," and seemed to convey a sense that he "knew what he was doing." In sum, JAS Type A's were rated as having more control of the task because they were perceived as more quick, decisive, and competent.

What emerges from this interesting study, primarily from the interview data, is an exciting conjecture about how Type A behavior may influence the social environment that, in turn, may influence the Type A person (Smith & Anderson, 1986). To the extent that a person acts quickly and conveys the impression that he or she is decisive (as in appearing well organized, clearly in charge, and competent), other people, in effect, expect the Type A person to exercise control and authority of situations, even when such control may not be possible. This line of conjecture seems congruent with clinical reports of adult Type A's who often complain that they are frequently expected to perform quick miracles in the face of tremendous odds (Friedman & Rosenman, 1974; Powell & Thoresen, 1987). Such perceived demands or expectations by others could understandably help trigger and maintain the excessive striving and effort that often characterize some Type A's.

These findings may bear on the expectations that parents and teachers have about Type A children. Whalen and Henker (1986), for example, reported that adult observers as well as peers and teachers tended to perceive children who scored high on the Competitive subscale of the MYTH (but not the MYTH Impatience–Aggressiveness subscale) as being good leaders, good athletes, intense, and on task. Data already reviewed on caregivers and mothers interacting with MYTH-rated Type A or non–Type A children also suggested that these adults may hold higher expectations for the Type A children. Parents of high Type A (SSI/STABS) boys and girls in the Bracke (1986) study were also observed to push their children more, perhaps in part because they viewed their children as having or needing to exert more control over situations.

## Perceiving Others as Hostile—and Reacting

Do Type A children help create the kind of social environment that perceives and prompts them to be decisive, to act in a quick, brisk manner, and not to allow others to take control? The work of Dodge and his colleagues (e.g., Dodge & Frame, 1982) may offer some insights. Although Dodge has studied socially aggressive children rather than Type A's, the data and methodology seem highly relevant to the issue of construing social reality in ways that confirm and reinforce Type A–related behavior in children. Commendably, these researchers have used a variety of social task situations (such as open-ended stories, videotaped small-group interaction, and "naturalistic" observations of boys during unstructured play) to explore what may be influencing the social behavior and cognitions of young aggressive boys compared to nonaggressive peers (kindergarten through fifth grade).

In one series of studies (Dodge & Frame, 1982), aggressive boys were found to attribute hostile intentions to others under very ambiguous situations (ones very characteristic of everyday life), especially if the intention of others was perceived as directed at them (actual direction was quite ambiguous) as opposed to being directed at someone else. Thus the aggressive boy was discriminating, only attributing hostility to others *if* he perceived the actions of others as focused on him. This evidence would seem clearly to discredit trait explanations that attribute aggressive or hostile behavior solely to the actor rather than to the interaction of person and particular situations..

This hostile attribution, that is, labeling of the other boy as having hostile intentions, was followed by socially aggressive action by the boy; thus the child's perception of hostility of the other boy prompted overt hostile behavior. One can think of the sequence as a "preemptive strike" strategy, striking the perceived enemy before he can aggress against you. By contrast, non-aggressive boys in the same social situation very seldom construed the ambiguous situation and actions of the other boy as hostile, nor did they promptly respond with socially aggressive behavior.

In another study, socially aggressive boys, in completing a series of stories and then later being asked to recall these stories, remembered significantly more hostile cues and remembered less positive, prosocial cues. In retelling the story, they also fabricated more statements, often negative, made by the story's main character, and consistently construed more ambiguous actions in the story as evidence of hostility. In a third study, the reality of perceived hostility of others was confirmed for aggressive boys. That is, aggressive boys were observed to be the targets of more socially and physically aggressive acts by other boys. Further, aggressive boys initiated 43 percent *more* aggressive acts than they received (presumably in the belief that the best defense is an offense). By contrast, the nonaggressive acts boys in the same situation received 30 percent more aggressive acts than they initiated.

In reflecting on the data, Dodge and Frame (1982) speculated on the possible etiology of the observed tendency of aggressive boys to perceive ambiguous social situations as hostile. In contrast to various social role-taking explanations (i.e., aggressive boys may lack effective social skills) and biased hostile memory explanations, these authors proposed that socially aggressive perceptions and actions may be a function of an inhibition deficit. That is, in fast-moving situations where one has to take prompt action and thus experiences some arousal, the aggressive child may suffer from an inability to inhibit a readily available perception and response, namely, that others probably cannot be trusted and may be hostile and highly competitive. Thus rather than delaying judgment and trying to clarify the situation, the child acts quickly to protect himself or herself and strives by direct action to control the situation. This speculation is an attractive one because it seems to fit various clinical descriptions of adult Type A's (Friedman & Rosenman, 1974; Price, 1982). The impatient, quick, hostilelike judgments often made by adult Type A's are legion.

What emerges from these data is evidence suggesting that Type A children may, in effect, expect or attribute to others (e.g., peers, parents) in many everyday life situations highly competitive, overly critical, and hostile intentions. Such perceptions may understandably encourage these children to think and act in a Type A fashion. Further, in doing so, others—such as peers—may perceive Type A children as fast acting, highly competitive, and socially aggressive with a quickness to criticize and become angry. Hence these shared perceptions may function in concert in the many socially ambiguous situations of everyday life (ambiguous in the sense that the criteria for success remain somewhat unclear as do the "real" intentions of others) to prompt and reinforce Type A behavior.

In terms of parents, Type A children may also construe their parents as highly critical of any shortcoming, such as not displaying maximum effort in every situation and failing to be perfect in performance (Bracke, 1986). Such perceptions, if continually confirmed by experience, could readily encourage the child to work hard and fast, displaying a pronounced competitive drive in the pursuit of exercising command and control of tasks.

## Learning Prototypes

Are these speculations valid? At this point they appear to be at least promising, worthy of controlled study. It is our belief that studies of social cognitive processes and their behavioral, physiologic, and situational correlates could provide a depth and breadth of understanding about Type A in children that is sorely lacking. Such inquiry, however, will require attention to theory and data in the social cognitive arena. Much can be gained by carefully examining the constructs and methods used in several cognitive areas, such as the work of Bower and his colleagues (e.g., Mayer & Bower, 1986) in studying learning and memory in person perception. This research in exploring what is termed schemata learning relative to personality, where schemata are constructs composed of an often incomplete set of features that frequently occur together in a category (such as Type A). Particularly intriguing in this line of inquiry is exploring the processes that people seem to use in creating strong and influential preconceptions about the "types" of people they encounter (e.g., extrovert, shy, friendly). One possible practical implication of this work concerns the Type A construct in that at least some Type A's may suffer from firmly established preconceptions (judgments) about the intentions and attitudes of others in such ways that learning to reconstrue and acquire new ways and patterns of perceiving others is seriously impaired. Conceivably, the acquistion of the social schemata (i.e., personality prototypes) involved may be initiated in childhood. Indeed, the previous discussion of attachment, particularly the notion of the child's inner working model of self and others, could be viewed as schemata.

Another application of studying personal schemata concerns clarification of the Type A construct by researchers. The methodology used to identify specific features of a prototype, such as Type A, can be used to derive a much clearer consensus among experts about what are the specific features of Type A in children (see Thoresen & Ohman, 1987). We have already noted the conceptual confusion and highly related assessment confusion in Type A research on children. Arriving at a consensually validated conceptual model of Type A via a prototype strategy could reduce ambiguity and increase the utility of empirical studies. (see also Cantor & Mischel, 1979; Horowitz, Wright, Lowenstein, & Parad, 1981).

## Type A Coping Processes

Another social cognitive area worthy of comment is the study of cognitive appraisal and coping processes. The work of Richard Lazarus and colleagues seems especially germane because it has focused on trying to understand more specifically the processes involved in how people evaluate and cope with a variety of stressful and demanding life situations (e.g., Cohen & Lazarus, 1979, 1983; Elliott & Eisdorfer, 1982; Lazarus & Folkman, 1984). Coping and appraisal processes are concerned with efforts people make in trying to manage perceived demands, both internal and external demands (Folkman & Lazarus, 1985).

Most investigators currently view coping as a blend of cognitive and behavioral procedures that vary with the particular context (Holahan & Moos, 1986; Lazarus & Folkman, 1984). This blend of coping techniques serves two main functions: Solving problems and regulating emotions. Problem-solving coping is focused on efforts to manage demands that appear to create threat or challenge; regulating emotions concerns efforts to manage the distress that often occurs as a result of the perceived threat or challenge. These two major coping functions (problem solving and emotion control) also show different patterns of variability across different situations. For example, Folkman, Lazarus, Gruen, and DeLongis (1986) found that the uses of the more problem-solving types of coping (e.g., seeks social support, uses planful problem solving) were highly variable for each person over six months across several personally demanding situations. By contrast, some of the more emotion-focused ways of coping, such as positive reappraisal of the situation, showed more stable use across various situations. It is interesting to speculate whether Type A children would demonstrate less flexibility compared to non–Type A's in employing various problem- and emotion-focused coping techniques.

Process-oriented research on the appraisal and coping processes associated with Type A construct could greatly enrich our understanding of this complex syndrome. Studies of children clearly classified as Type A and non–Type A would provide valuable information on similarities and differences in how children think about problem situations—how they appraise them—and what overt and covert actions they take in trying to manage problems and concerns. Of particular interest is how Type A children differ in their primary and secondary appraisal of common events and situations. Do Type A's construe more typical situations as stressful instead of irrelevant, positive, or benign (primary appraisal), and do Type A children evaluate their coping resources differently than less Type A children (secondary appraisal)? Within a coping theory framework (e.g., Folkman, Lazarus,

Dunkol-Schetter, DeLongis, & Gruen, 1986) the Type A construct should reveal major differences between Type A's and non–Type A's in how situations are construed, with Type A's appraising more of them as threatening and challenging.

Research focused on the *patterns* of what might be called Type A coping across time and contexts would go a long way in differentiating among Type A children and adolescents. What might emerge from such studies are different behavioral and physiologic correlates among Type A children who utilize different patterns of coping strategies. Thus some clarification could be gained in how Type A children differ from each other.

## Social Constructivist Perspective

A final observation related to social cognitive processes and structures concerns the need for a dynamic person–environment interaction perspective in theory and research. Intrapsychic-oriented studies that only examine a few cognitive or affective variables typically yield very limited and often invalid information about Type A. Likewise, studies that only assess one or a few brief samples of the person's observable behavior (e.g., a 10-minute sample in the classroom) with little concern for the possible influence of the specific context involved also yield limited information. People as organisms function as open living systems, acting and reacting in often inconsistent ways to life's situations as they are anticipated as well as directly experienced (Cole & Scribner, 1974; Ford, 1987; Ford & Ford, 1987; Vygotsky, 1978). Social constructivist perspectives argue that people must be studied more thoroughly with prime attention to how they go about, over time, constructing and reconstructing their perceptions and beliefs about themselves and their social environment. Within a social constructivist view, particular attention is given to trying to understand the *personal meanings* that people extend to the situations they experience. Much of the work already described about attachment, narcissistic personality, and various social–cognitive processes, such as appraisal and coping strategies, is highly consistent with a social constructivist view.

What deserves brief comment here concerns methodology. While we have repeatedly urged the use of a multimethod and multimodal assessment strategy, the need for richly descriptive controlled empirical case studies, as previously noted, may easily be overlooked. Too often case material has been ignored or denigrated, even though controlled case data have played a vital role in the early stages of developing useful scientific theories concerned with human functioning (Kratochwill, 1978; Mead, 1977; Murphy, 1976; Weimer, 1979). A variety of retrospective and prospective case method strategies are available, such as ethnographic, personal self-monitoring, and social observation techniques. We strongly urge the use of such methods to help fill the blatant data gap that currently exists in the study of Type A and children. Indeed it seems peculiar that the many developmental issues concerning Type A children and their changing contexts have not been addressed in part by gathering the kinds of richly descriptive case material that could illuminate the changing lives and times of these children.

Perhaps researchers have sought too often and too quickly to conduct very time-limited studies that allow statistical confirmation of hypotheses (or more technically, refutation of the statistical null hypothesis) under controlled conditions instead of taking the time to gather systematically a variety of descriptive data that are crucial in the discovery process of science (see Meehl, 1982). From a scientific perspective, maximum progress in an area of inquiry is most likely to occur when a *program* of research is carried out over time, thus affording the needed perspective in designing and conducting a variety of studies (Lakatos & Musgrave, 1970).

## SOME CONCLUDING OBSERVATIONS

Type A-like behaviors and characteristics are observable in children and young adolescents. Some differences exist in Type A across gender, age, ethnicity, and perhaps region, yet these behaviors and characteristics are apparent in a variety of children and adolescents. A major issue, however, concerns how Type A is conceptualized and assessed in younger people. The lack of standardized measures that adequately assess Type A limits understanding of demographics associated with Type A. We suspect that the overall prevalence of Type A, when multiply assessed, is probably not of the same magnitude in the general population as estimates of adult American males (50 to 75 percent), especially white-collar males. A lower rate of prevalence seems highly likely if multiple measures and assessment modes using continuous scoring are used to classify children.

Does Type A in children represent a significant or noteworthy problem—one deserving theoretical, empirical, and clinical concern? We strongly believe that it does. However, long-term studies have not established Type A in children as a significant predictor of cardiovascular disease markers or endpoints or any other chronic disease in adulthood. Further, it is not known whether Type A assessed in childhood represents a highly stable set of behaviors and characteristics into adulthood. One could readily argue that, until prospective studies spanning three or four decades are conducted, the Type A relationship to adult health status will remain unknown and thus does not merit serious concern. That line of reasoning, however, might also negate the value of programs designed to prevent or stop cigarette smoking in youngsters as well as programs designed to treat childhood hypertension, reduce obesity and markedly elevated serum cholesterol levels, as well as promote aerobic conditioning in sedentary children. Available evidence, despite conceptual and assessment issues, is beginning to show that Type A children and young adolescents display some of the same physiologic characteristics as those that are found in adult Type A's.

Although few in number, these studies indicate, for example, that Type A children experience more physiological and behavioral arousal in response to situations perceived as challenging or threatening. Retrospective anecdotal data from postcoronary adults also hint at the relative stability of Type A characteristics; commonly these patients report acting in a Type A fashion for as long as they can remember, often back to their older childhood years.

Clearly, Type A is not an autonomous, isolated pattern that is devoid of relationship with other problems and characteristics. In adult studies such as MRFIT (Shekelle et al., 1985) in which over 200,000 were screened to select 12,000 males who smoked cigarettes and had elevated blood pressure (borderline hypertensives) and higher total serum cholesterol levels (about 250 mg/dl), about three out of four were also classified as Type A (74 percent). In the Recurrent Coronary Prevention Project (Friedman et al., 1986; Thoresen, Friedman, Powell, Gill, and Ulmer, 1985), over 70 percent of the postinfarction patients were smokers, over 40 percent were hypertensives, and their average serum cholesterol level at entry into the study was 260 mg/dl. Studies of children also suggest that some Type A characteristics, such as anger, tend to cluster with other possible risk-related factors, such as smoking, marked physical inactivity (sedentary), elevated systolic blood pressure, negative major life events, and greater life dissatisfaction. Taken together, the evidence so far suggests that children classified as Type A manifest a variety of negative or unhealthy physical symptoms and characteristics that may indeed contribute to a greater predisposition for cardiovascular as well as other chronic diseases (Friedman & Booth-Kewley, 1987a). If this contention eventually proves to be in error, it seems preferable to err in the direction of considering Type A a problem currently needing attention rather than ignoring it because unequivocal hard evidence is lacking.

Understandably, concern with Type A remains primarily focused on cardiovascular-related factors. Generally ignored or unrecognized, however, are data that implicate Type A with various social–emotional and social–cognitive variables, especially those associated with mental health problems. Type A children have significantly less personal and social self-esteem, less social competence, experience more negative life events, and are more socially insecure and socially anxious. In addition, when measured independently of Type A, these children and adolescents clearly convey a great deal of anger. They consistently report experiencing more anger in terms of frequency, intensity, duration, and context. Should research also begin to reveal, as it has with socially aggressive boys, that Type A children more often construe and perceive the intentions and actions of others in many of life's everyday situations as more hostile and competitive, then a troubled social and emotional portrait emerges.

What might be the more immediate as well as longer-term consequences and correlates of the aforementioned social, emotional, and cognitive characteristics? At a global level, one certainly does not sense that consequences will yield positive, happy, joyful experiences, at least in any sustained lasting sense. We suspect that many Type A children may in effect be gradually creating a problematic structure or schemata of self-conception, one in which corresponding social roles are being learned via direct and vicarious social modeling and social contingencies (Hoelter, 1985). Such roles may serve to identify for children how they should think and behave as well as give meaning to their actions in everyday situations. Possibly those meanings are associated with a sense that one must, to succeed and be thought of by others as worthwhile, continually strive and struggle to maintain control and to dominate situations by means of prompt, direct action and often maximum effort. Such a conception, however, may interfere with the ability to consider alternatives, to rethink problems, and to reappraise situations involved with problems (i.e., to take sufficient time to reflect, even relax, in the process of dealing effectively with problems). In effect, Type A in children may be associated with a less flexible coping style, with fewer coping options, in part because these children may not consider themselves capable of taking time to reflect and reappraise, especially if doing so is construed as evidence of a failure to deal promptly and effectively with the situation. While the data on successful performance of various kinds and Type A children are mixed, the evidence at present tentatively supports the general notion that Type A children do not perform better in the academic, social, or athletic areas than their non–Type A peers.

The need for a well-articulated theoretical framework and a multimethod assessment approach has often been cited in this chapter. We believe that investigators in many cases have prematurely settled for rejecting the statistical null hypotheses (at the .05 level) instead of demonstrating how their findings relate directly to theoretically relevant issues or questions. In addition, Type A as a variable has almost always been used as an independent or classification variable, rather than as the primary dependent variable. Experimentally designed studies are needed that alter Type A (or some of its characteristics) and examine the relationship of such changes on selected physiological, behavioral, and/or cognitive variables. For example, is a significant reduction in Type A over several months associated with reductions in physiological symptoms of stress, improved academic performance, increases in social self-esteem, or improved peer or sibling relationships? Good science requires use of a broad array of research designs and methods. Controlled experiments and descriptive studies of Type A are overdue and very much in order.

## REFERENCES

Ainsworth, M. D. S., Bell, S. M., & Stayton, D. J. (1971). Individual differences in strange situation behavior of one-year-olds. In H. R. Schaffer (Ed.), *The origins of human social relations*. London: Academic.

Ainsworth, M. D. S., & Wittig, B. (1969). Attachment and exploratory behavior of one-year-olds in a strange situation. In B. Foss (Ed.), *Determinants of infant behavior* (Vol. 4). London: Methuen.

Akhtar, S., & Thompson, J. A. (1982). Overview: Narcissistic personality disorder. *American Journal of Psychiatry, 139*(1), 12–20.

Arnow, B., Thoresen, C. E., Eagleston, J. R., Kirmil-Gray, K., Bracke, P., & Heft, L. (1986). *Differences in academic and other performance measures for high and low Type A children*. Unpublished manuscript, Stanford University.

Bandura, A. (1986). *Social foundations of thought and action: A social cognitive theory*. Englewood Cliffs, NJ: Prentice-Hall.

Baumrind, D. (1971). Current patterns of parental authority. *Development Psychology Monographs, 4*(2).

Bem, D. J. (1983). Constructing a theory of the triple typology: Second thoughts on nomothetic and idiographic approaches to personality. *Journal of Personality, 51*, 567–577.

Bergman, L. R., & Magnusson, D. (1986). Type A behavior: A longitudinal study from childhood to adulthood. *Psychosomatic Medicine, 48*(1–2), 134–142.

Bishop, E. G., Hailey, B. J., Anderson, H. N. (1987). Assessment of Type A behavior in children: A comparison of two instruments. *Journal of Human Stress, 13*, 121–127.

Booth-Kewley, S., & Friedman, H. S. (1987). Psychological predictors of heart disease: A quantitative review. *Psychological Bulletin, 101*, 343–362.

Bortner, R. W., Rosenman, R. H., & Friedman, M. (1970). Familial similarity in pattern A behavior: Fathers and sons. *Journal of Chronic Diseases, 23*, 3943.

Bowlby, J. (1973). *Attachment and loss: Vol. 2. Separation*. New York: Basic.

Bowlby, J. (1982). *Attachment and loss: Vol. I. Attachment* (2nd ed.). New York: Basic.

Bracke, P. E. (1986). *Parental childrearing practices and the development of Type A behavior in children*. Doctoral dissertation, Stanford University.

Bretherton, I., & Waters, E. (1985). Growing points of attachment theory and research. *Monographs of the Society for Research in Child Development, 50*, (1–2, Serial No. 209).

Bronfenbrenner, U. (1979). *The ecology of human development*. Cambridge, MA: Harvard University Press.

Butensky, A., Faralli, V., Heebner, D., & Waldron, I. (1976). Elements of the coronary-prone behavior pattern in children and teenagers. *Journal of Psychosomatic Research, 20*, 439–444.

Campbell, D. T., & Fiske, D. W. (1959). Convergent and discriminant validation by the multi-trait multi-method matrix. *Psychological Bulletin, 56*, 81–105.

Cantor, N., & Mischel, W. (1979). Prototypicality and personality: Effects of free recall and personality impressions. *Journal of Research in Personality, 13*, 187–205.

Cohen, F., & Lazarus, R. S. (1979). Coping with the stresses of illness. In G. Stone, F. Cohen, & N. E. Adler (Eds.), *Health psychology: A handbook*. San Francisco: Jossey-Bass.

Cohen, F., & Lazarus, R. S. (1983). Coping and adaptation and health and illness. In D. Mechanic (Ed.), *Handbook of health, health care, and the health professions*. New York: Free Press.

Cole, M., & Scribner, S. (1974). *Culture and thought*. New York: Wiley.

Cooper, T., Detre, T., & Weiss, S. M. (1981). Coronary-prone behavior and coronary heart disease. *Circulation, 63*, 1199–1215.

Corrigan, S. A., & Moskowitz, D. S. (1983). Type A behavior in preschool children: Construct validation evidence for the MYTH. *Child Development, 54*, 1513–1521.

Dodge, K. A., & Frame, C. L. (1982). Social cognitive biases and deficits in aggressive boys. *Child Development, 53*, 620–635.

Donovan, J. E., Jessor, R., & Jessor, L. (1983). Problem drinking in adolescence and young adulthood: A follow-up study. *Journal of Studies on Alcoholism, 44,* 109–137.

Eagleston, J. R., Kirmil-Gray, K., Thoresen, C. E., Wiedenfeld, S. A., Bracke, P., Heft, L., & Arnow, B. (1986). Physical health correlates of Type A behavior in children and adolescents. *Journal of Behavioral Medicine, 9,* 341–362.

Elliott, G. R., & Eisdorfer, C. (1982). *Stress and human health.* New York: Springer.

Feurstein, M., Labbe, E. E., & Kuczmierczyk, A. R. (1986). *Health psychology: A psychobiological perspective.* New York: Plenum.

Folkman, S., & Lazarus, R. S. (1985). If it changes it must be a process: A study of emotion and coping during three stages of a college examination. *Journal of Personality & Social Psychology, 48,* 150–170.

Folkman, S., Lazarus, R. S., Dunkol-Schetter, C., DeLongis, A., & Gruen, R. J. (1986). Dynamics of a stressful encounter: Cognitive appraisal, coping, and encounter outcomes. *Journal of Personality & Social Psychology, 50*(5), 992–1003.

Folkman, S., Lazarus, R. S., Gruen, R. J., & DeLongis, A. (1986). Appraisal, coping, health status, and psychological symptoms. *Journal of Personality & Social Psychology, 50*(3), 571–579.

Fontana, A., & Davidio, J. F. (1984). The relationship between stressful life events and school-related performances of Type A and Type B adolescents. *Journal of Human Stress, 10*(1), 50–55.

Ford, D. H. (1987). Humans as self-constructing living systems. Hillsdale, NJ: Erlbaum.

Ford, M. E., & Ford, D. H. (Eds.). (1987). *Humans as self-constructing living systems: Putting the framework to work.* Hillsdale, NJ: Erlbaum.

Ford, M. E., & Thompson, R. A. (1985). Perceptions of personal agency and infant attachment: Toward a life-span perspective on competence development. *International Journal of Behavior Development, 8,* 377–406.

Freud, S. (1925). On narcissism: An introduction. In *Collected papers* (Vol. 4). London: Hogarth. (Original work published 1914).

Freud, S. (1949). Libidinal types. In J. Strachey (Ed. and Trans.), *The standard edition of the complete psychological works of Sigmund Freud* (Vol. 14). London: Hogarth. (Original work published 1931).

Friedman, H. S., & Booth-Kewley, S. (1987a). The "disease-prone personality": A meta-analytic view of the construct. *American Psychologist, 42,* 539–555.

Friedman, H. S., & Booth-Kewley, S. (1987b). Personality, Type A behavior, and coronary heart disease: The role of emotional expression. *Journal of Personality and Social Psychology, 53,* 783–792.

Friedman, M., & Rosenman, R. H. (1974). *Type A behavior and your heart.* New York: Knopf.

Friedman, M., Thoresen, C. E., Gill, J. J., Ulmer, D., Powell, L. H., Price, V. A., Brown, B., Thompson, L., Rubin, D. D., Breall, W. S., Bourg, E., Levy, R., & Dixon, T. (1986). Alteration of Type A behavior and its effect on cardiac recurrences in postmyocardial infarction patients: Summary results of the Recurrent Coronary Prevention Project. *American Heart Journal, 112*(4), 653–665.

Gerace, T. A., & Smith, J. C. (1985). Children's Type A interview: Interrater, test–retest reliability, and interviewer effect. *Journal of Chronic Disease, 38*(9), 781–791.

Gergen, K. J. (1985). The social constructivist movement in modern psychology. *American Psychologist, 40,* 266–275.

Gill, J. J., Price, V. A., Friedman, M., Thoresen, C. E., Powell, L. H., Ulmer, D., Brown, B., & Drews, F. R. (1985). Reduction in Type A behavior in healthy middle-aged American military officers. *American Heart Journal, 110,* 503.

Glueck, C. J. (1986). Pediatric primary prevention of atherosclerosis. *New England Journal of Medicine, 314*(3), 175–177.

Heft, L., Thoresen, C. E., Kirmil-Gray, K., Wiedenfeld, S. A., Eagleston, J. R., Bracke, P., & Arnow, B. (in press). Emotional and temperamental correlates of Type A in children and adolescents. *Journal of Youth & Adolescence.*

Henry, J., & Stephens, P. (1977). *Stress, health and the social environment.* New York: Springer-Verlag.

Hoelter, J. W. (1985). The structure of self-conception: Conceptualization and measurement. *Journal of Personality & Social Psychology, 49,* 1392–1407.

Holahan, C. J., & Moos, R. H. (1986). Personality, coping, and family resources in stress resistance: A longitudinal analysis. *Journal of Personality & Social Psychology, 51,* 389–395.

Horowitz, L M., Wright, J. C., Lowenstein, E., & Parad, H. W. (1981). The prototype as a construct in abnormal psychology: A method for deriving prototypes. *Journal of Abnormal Psychology, 90,* 568–574.

Hunter, S. M., Parker, F. C., Williamson, G. D., Downey, A. M., Webber, L. S., & Berenson, G. S. (1985). Measurement assessment of the Type A coronary prone behavior pattern and hyperactivity/problem behaviors in children: Are they related? The Bogalusa Heart Study. *Journal of Human Stress,* Winter, pp. 177–183.

Hunter, S. M., Wolf, T. M., Sklov, M. C., Webber, L. S., Watson, R. M., & Berenson, G. S. (1982). Type A coronary-prone behavior pattern and cardiovascular risk factor variables in children and adolescents: The Bogalusa Heart Study. *Journal of Chronic Disease, 35*(8), 613–621.

Jackson, C., & Levine, D. W. (1987). Comparison of the MYTH and Hunter-Wolf measures of Type A behavior in children. *Health Psychology, 6,* 255–267.

Jennings, J. R., & Matthews, K. A. (1984). The impatience of youth: Phasic cardiovascular response in Type A and Type B elementary school-age boys. *Psychosomatic Medicine 46*(6), 498–511.

Jessor, R. (1982). Critical issues in research on adolescent health promotion. In T. J. Coates, A. C. Petersen, & C. L. Perry (Eds.), *Promoting adolescent health: A dialog on research and practice.* New York: Academic.

Jessor, R. (1984, November). *Adolescent problem drinking: Psychosocial aspects and developmental outcomes.* Paper presented at the Carnegie Conference on Unhealthful Risk-Taking Behavior Among Adolescents, Stanford, CA.

Jessor, R. (1985). Adolescent development and behavioral health. In J. Matarazzo, S. M. Weiss, J. A. Herd, N. E. Miller, & S. M. Weiss (Eds.), *Behavioral health: A handbook of health enhancement and disease prevention.* New York: Wiley.

Kernberg, O. F. (1975). *Borderline conditions and pathological narcissism.* New York: Jason Aronson.

Kernberg, O. F. (1976). *Object relations theory and clinical psychoanalysis.* New York: Jason Aronson.

Kirmil-Gray, K., Eagleston, J. R., Thoresen, C. E., Heft, L., Arnow, B., & Bracke, P. (in press). Developing measures of Type A behavior in children and adolescents. *Journal of Human Stress.*

Kliewer, W., & Weidner, G. (1987). Type A behavior and aspirations: A study of parents' and children's goal setting. *Developmental Psychology, 23,* 204–209.

Kohut, H. (1966). Forms and transformations of narcissism. *Journal of the American Psychoanalytic Association, 14,* 243–272.

Kohut, H. (1971). *The analysis of the self.* New York: International Universities Press.

Kohut, H. (1972). Thoughts on narcissism and narcissistic rage. *Psychoanalytic Study of the Child, 27,* 360–400.

Kohut, H. (1977). *The restoration of the self.* New York: International Universities Press.

Krantz, D. S., & Durel, L. A. (1983). Psychobiological substrates of the Type A behavior pattern. *Health Psychology, 2,* 393–411.

Krantz, D. S., Lundberg, U., & Frankenhaeuser, M. (1987). Stress and Type A behavior: Interactions between environmental and biologic factors. In A. Baum & J. E. Singer (Eds.), *Handbook of psychology and health: Vol. 5. Stress and coping.* Hillsdale, NJ: Erlbaum.

Kratchowill, T. R. (1978). *Single subject research: Strategies for evaluating change.* New York: Academic.

Lakatos, I., & Musgrave, A. (Eds.) (1970). *Criticism and the growth of knowledge.* Cambridge: Cambridge University Press.

Lasch, C. (1978). *The culture of narcissism.* New York: Norton.

Lawler, K. A., & Allen, M. T. (1981). Risk factors for hypertension in children: Their relationship to psychophysiological responses. *Journal of Psychosomatic Research 25*(3), 199–204.

Lawler, K. A., Allen, M. T., Critcher, E. C., & Standard, B. A. (1981). The relationship of physiological responses to the coronary-prone behavior pattern in children. *Journal of Behavioral Medicine, 4*(2), 203–216.

Lazarus, R. S., & Folkman, S. (1984). *Stress, appraisal, and coping.* New York: Springer Press.

Lerner, R. M., & Busch-Rossnagel, N. A. (Eds.) (1981). *Individuals as producers of their development: A life-span perspective.* New York: Academic.

Lewin, R. (1986). Brain architecture: Beyond genes. *Science, 233,* 155–156.

Lundberg, U. (1983a). Note on Type A behavior and cardiovascular responses to challenge in 3–6 yr. old children. *Journal of Psychosomatic Research, 27*(1), 39–42.

Lundberg, U. (1983b). Sex differences in behavior pattern and catecholamine and cortisol excretion in 3–6 year old day-care children. *Biological Psychology, 16,* 109–117.

Lundberg, U. (1985). Psychobiological stress responses and behavior patterns in preschool children. In J. J. Sanchez-Sosa (Ed.), *Health and clinical psychology* (Vol. 4). New York: Oxford Elsevier (North-Holland).

Lundberg, U. (in press). Stress and Type A behavior in children. *Journal of American Academy of Child Psychiatry.*

Main, M., Kaplan, N., & Cassidy, J. (1985). Security in infancy, childhood, and adulthood: A move to the level of representation. In I. Bretherington & E. Waters (Eds.), *Monographs of the Society for Research in Child Development, 50* (1-2, Serial No. 209), 66–104.

Main, M., & Weston, D. R. (1981). The quality of the toddler's relationship to mother and to father: Related to conflict behavior and the readiness to establish new relationships. *Child Development, 52,* 932–940.

Main, M., & Weston, D. R. (1982). Avoidance of the attachment figure in infancy: Descriptions and interpretations. In C. M. Parkes & J. Stevenson-Hinde (Eds.), *The place of attachment in human behavior.* New York: Basic.

Manning, D. T., Balson, P. M., Hunter, S. M., Berenson, G. S., & Willis, A. S. (1987). Comparison of the prevalence of Type A behavior in boys and girls from two contrasting socio-economic status groups. *Journal of Human Stress, 13,* 116–120.

Margolis, L. H., McLeroy, K. R. Runyan, C. W., & Kaplan, B. H. (1983). Type A behavior: An ecological approach. *Journal of Behavioral Medicine, 6,* 245–258.

Matthews, K. A. (1977). Caregiver–child interactions and the Type A coronary-prone behavior pattern. *Child Development, 48,* 1752–1756.

Matthews, K. A. (1979). Efforts to control by children and adults with the Type A coronary-prone behavior pattern. *Child Development, 50,* 842–847.

Matthews, K. A. (1982). Psychological perspectives on the Type A behavior pattern. *Psychological Bulletin, 91,* 293–323.

Matthews, K. A., & Angulo, J. (1980). Measurement of the Type A behavior pattern in children:

Assessment of children's competitiveness, impatience-anger, and aggression. *Child Development, 51,* 466–475.

Matthews, K. A., & Avis, N. E. (1983). Stability of overt Type A behaviors in children: Results from a one-year longitudinal study. *Child Development, 54*(6), 1507–1512.

Matthews, K. A., Glass, D. C., & Richins, M. (1977). The other-son observation study. In D. C. Glass, *Behavior patterns, stress and coronary disease.* Hillsdale, N.J.: Erlbaum.

Matthews, K. A., & Haynes, S. G. (1986). Type A behavior pattern and coronary disease risk. *American Journal of Epidemiology, 123*(6), 923–959.

Matthews, K. A., & Jennings, J. R. (1984). Cardiovascular responses of boys exhibiting the Type A behavior pattern. *Psychosomatic Medicine, 46,* 484–497.

Matthews, K. A., & Krantz, D. S. (1976). Resemblance of twins and their parents in pattern A behavior. *Psychosomatic Medicine, 28,* 140–144.

Matthews, K. A., Rosenman, R. H., Dembroski, T. M., Harris, E., & MacDougall, J. M. (1983). Familial resemblance in components of the Type A behavior pattern: A reanalysis of the California Twin Study. Unpublished manuscript.

Matthews, K. A., & Siegel, J. M. (1982). The Type A pattern in children and adolescents: Assessment, development, and associated coronary-risk. In A. R. Baum & J. E. Singer (Eds.), *Handbook of psychology and health* (Vol. 2). Hillsdale, NJ: Erlbaum.

Matthews, K. A., & Siegel, J. M. (1983). Type A behaviors for children, social comparison, and standards for self-evaluation. *Developmental Psychology, 19*(1), 135–140.

Matthews, K. A., Stoney, C. M. Rakaczky, C. J., & Jamison, W. (1986). Family characteristics and school achievements of type A children. *Health Psychology, 5*(5), 453–467.

Matthews, K. A., & Volkin, J. I. (1981). Efforts to excel and the Type A behavior pattern in children. *Child Development, 52,* 1283–1289.

Mayer, J. E., & Bower, G. H. (1986). Learning and memory for personality prototypes. *Journal of Personality & Social Psychology, 51,* 473–492.

McClelland, D. C., Atkinson, J., Clark, R. A., & Lowell, E. L. (1953). *The achievement motive.* New York: Appleton-Century-Crofts.

Mead, M. (1976). Towards a human science. *Science, 191,* 903–910.

Meehl, P. E. (1978). Theoretical risks and tabular asterisks: Sir Karl, Sir Ronald, and the slow progress of soft psychology. *Journal of Consulting & Clinical Psychology, 46*(4), 806–834.

Miller, A. (1981). *Prisoners of childhood.* New York: Basic.

Millon, T. (1981). *Disorders of personality: DSM III: Axis II.* New York: Wiley.

Murphy, E. A. (1976). *The logic of medicine.* Baltimore: Johns Hopkins University Press.

Murray, D. M., Blake, S. M., Prineas, R., & Gillum, R. F. (1985). Cardiovascular responses in Type A children during a cognitive challenge. *Journal of Behavioral Medicine, 8,*(4), 377–395.

Murray, D. M., Matthews, K. A., Blake, S. M., Prineas, R. J., & Gillum, R. F. (1986). Type A behavior in children: Demographic, behavioral, and physiological correlates. *Health Psychology, 5*(2), 159–169.

Murray, J. L., & Bruhn, J. (1983). Reliability of the MYTH scale in assessing Type A behavior in preschool children. *Journal of Human Stress, 9,* 25–28.

Murray, J. L., Bruhn, J. G., & Bunce, H. (1983). Assessment of Type A behavior in preschoolers. *Journal of Human Stress, 9*(3), 32–39.

Newman, W. P., Freedman, D. S., Voors, A. W., Gard, P. D., Srinivasan, S. S., Cresanta, J. L., Williamson, G. D., Webber, L. S., & Berenson, G. S. (1986). Relation of lipoprotein levels and systolic blood pressure to early atherosclerosis. *New England Journal of Medicine, 314,* 138–144.

Nunes, E. V., Frank, K. A., & Kornfeld, D. S. (1987). Psychologic treatment for Type A behavior pattern and for coronary heart disease: A meta-analysis of the literature. *Psychosomatic Medicine, 48,* 159–173.

Parker, F. C., Harsha, D. W., Farris, R. P., Webber, L. S., Frank, G. C., & Berenson, G. S. (1986). Reducing the risk of cardiovascular disease in children. In K. Holroyd & T. L. Creer (Eds.), *Self-management of chronic disease.* New York: Academic.

Parkes, C. M., & Stevenson-Hinde, J. (Eds.) (1982). *The place of attachment in human behavior.* New York: Basic.

Powell, L., & Thoresen, C. E. (1987). Modifying the Type A behavior pattern: A small group treatment approach. In J. A. Blumenthal & D. C. McKee (Eds.), *Applications of behavioral medicine and health psychology: A clinician's sourcebook* (Vol. 1). Sarasota, FL: Professional Resource Exchange.

Price, V. A. (1982). *Type A behavior pattern: A model for research and practice.* New York: Academic.

Prigogine, I., & Stengers, I. (1984). *Order out of chaos: Man's new dialogue with nature.* New York: Bantam.

Rahe, R. H., Hervig, L., & Rosenman, R. H. (1978). The heritability of Type A behavior. *Psychosomatic Medicine, 40,* 478–486.

Reich, W. (1949). *Character analysis* (3rd ed.). New York: Farrar, Straus, & Giroux.

Rodeo, S. A., & Thoresen, C. E. (1987). *The Type A behavior pattern and over-use injuries in college athletes.* Manuscript submitted for publication.

Rogoff, B., Gauvain, M., & Ellis, S. (1984). Development viewed in its cultural context. In M. Bornstein & M. E. Lamb (Eds.), *Developmental psychology.* Hillsdale, NJ: Erlbaum.

Rosenman, R. H. (1978). The interview method of assessment of the coronary-prone behavior pattern. In T. M. Dembroski, S. M. Weiss, J. L. Shields, S. G. Haynes, & M. Feinleib (Eds.), *Coronary-prone behavior.* New York: Springer-Verlag.

Rosenman, R. (1985). Health consequences of anger and implications for treatment. In M. A. Chesney & R. H. Rosenman (Eds.), *Anger and hostility in cardiovascular and behavioral disorders.* Washington, DC: Hemisphere.

Roskies, E., Seraganian, P., Oseasohn, R., Hanley, J. A., Collu, R., Martin, N., & Smilga, C. (1986). The Montreal Type A Intervention Project: Major findings. *Health Psychology, 5,* 45–69.

Scarr, S. (1985). Constructing psychology: Making facts and fables for our times. *American Psychologist, 40,* 499–512.

Shekelle, R. B., Hulley, S. B., Neaton, J. D., Billings, J., Borhani, N. O., Gerace, T. A., Jacobs, D., Lasser, N., Mittlemark, M., & Stamler, J. (1985). The MRFIT behavior pattern study: II. Type A behavior and incidence of coronary heart disease. *American Journal of Epidemiology, 122,* 559–570.

Shekelle, R. B., Schoenberger, J. A., & Stamler, J. (1976). Correlates of the JAS Type A behavior pattern score. *Journal of Chronic Diseases, 29,* 381–394.

Siegel, J. M. (1982). Type A behavior and self-reports of cardiovascular arousal in adolescents. *Journal of Human Stress, 8*(3), 24–30.

Siegel, J. M. (1984). Anger and cardiovascular risk in adolescents. *Health Psychology, 3*(4), 293–313.

Siegel, J. M. (1986). The Multidimensional Anger Inventory. *Journal of Personality and Social Psychology, 51*(1), 191–200.

Siegel, J. M., & Leitch, C. J. (1981). Behavioral factors and blood pressure in adolescence: The Tacoma Study. *American Journal of Epidemiology, 113*(2), 171–181.

Siegel, J. M., & Leitch, C. J. (1981). Assessment of the Type A behavior pattern in adolescents. *Psychosomatic Medicine, 43*(1), 45–56.

Siegel, J. M., Matthews, K. A., & Leitch, C. J. (1981). Validation of the Type A interview assessment of adolescents: A multidimensional approach. *Psychosomatic Medicine 43*(4), 311–321.

Siegel, J. M., Matthews, K. A., & Leitch, C. J. (1983). Blood pressure variability and the Type A behavior pattern in adolescence. *Journal of Psychosomatic Research, 27*(4), 265–272.

Smith, T. W., & Anderson, N. B. (1986). Models of personality and disease: An interactional approach to Type A behavior and cardiovascular risk. *Journal of Personality & Social Psychology, 50*(6), 1166–1173.

Smith, J. C., Gerace, T. A., Christakis, G., & Kafatos, A. (1985). Cross-cultural validity of the Miami Structured Interview-1 for Type A in children: The American-Hellenic Heart Study. *Journal of Chronic Diseases, 38*(9), 793–799.

Spielberger, C. D., Johnson, E. H., Russell, S. F., Crane, R., & Worden, T. (1985). The experience and expression of anger. In M. Chesney, W. E. Goldston, & R. H. Rosenman (Eds.), *Anger, hostility, and behavioral medicine*. New York: Hemisphere/McGraw-Hill.

Sroufe, L. A. (1986). *The role of infant–caregiver attachment in development*. Unpublished manuscript, Department of Psychology, University of Minnesota.

Steinberg, L. (1987). Stability (and instability) of Type A behavior from children to young adulthood. *Developmental Psychology, 22*, 393–402.

Strube, M. J., Lott, C. L., Heilizer, R., & Gregg, B. (1986). Type A behavior pattern and the judgment of control. *Journal of Personality & Social Psychology, 50*, 403–412.

Sweda, M. G., Sines, J. O., Laver, R. M., & Clarke, W. R. (1986). Familial aggregation of Type A behavior. *Journal of Behavioral Medicine, 9*(1), 23–32.

Teevan, R., & McGhee, P. (1972). Childhood development of fear and failure motivation. *Journal of Personality & Social Psychology, 21*, 345–348.

Thoresen, C. E., Friedman, M., Powell, L. H., Gill, J. J., & Ulmer, D. (1985). Altering the Type A behavior pattern in postinfarction patients. *Journal of Cardio-pulmonary Rehabilitation, 5*, 258–266.

Thoresen, C. E., & Ohman, A. (1987). The Type A behavior pattern: A person–environment interaction perspective. In D. Magnusson & A. Ohman (Eds.), *Psychopathology: An interaction perspective*. New York: Academic.

Thoresen, C. E., Wiedenfeld, S., Kirmil-Gray, K., Eagleston, J. R., Heft, L., Bracke, P., & Arnow, B. (1987). *Comparison of high and low Type A children on anger and social behaviors*. Unpublished manuscript, Stanford University.

Vygotsky, L. S. (1978). *Mind in society*. Cambridge, MA: Harvard University Press.

Waldron, I., Hickey, A., McPherson, C., Butensky, A., Gruss, L., Overall, K., Schmader, A., & Wohlmuth, D. (1980). Type A behavior pattern: Relationship to variation in blood pressure, parental characteristics, and academic and social activities of students. *Journal of Human Stress, 6*, 16–27.

Ward, C. H., & Eisler, R. M. (1987). Type A behavior achievement striving, and a dysfunctional self-evaluation system. *Journal of Personality and Social Psychology, 53*, 318–326.

Webber, L. S., Cresanta, J. L., Voors, A. W., & Berenson, G. S. (1983). Tracking of cardiovascular disease risk factor variables in school-aged children. *Journal of Chronic Diseases, 36*, 647–660.

Weidner, G., McLellarn, R., Sexton, G., Istvan, J., Connor, S. (1987). Type A behavior and physiologic coronary risk factors in children of the Family Heart Study: Results from a 1-year follow-up. *Psychosomatic Medicine, 48*, 480–488.

Weimer, W. B. (1979). *Notes on the methodology of scientific research*. Hillsdale, NJ: Erlbaum.

Weiner, H. (1977). *Psychobiology and human disease*. New York: Elsevier.

Weinstein, K. A., Davison, G. C., DeQuattro, V., & Allen, J. W. (1987). Type A behavior, hostile cognitions, and early cardiac damage. Unpublished manuscript, University of Southern California.

Whalen, C. K., & Henker, B. (1986). Type A behavior in normal and hyperactive children: Multisource evidence of overlapping constructs. *Child Development, 57,* 688–699.

Williams, R. B., Barefoot, J. C., & Shekelle, R. B. (1985). The health consequences of hostility. In M. Chesney & R. Rosenman (Eds.), *Anger and hostility in cardiovascular and behavioral disorders.* New York: Hemisphere.

Wolf, T., Hunter, S., & Webber, L. (1979). Psychosocial measures of cardiovascular risk factors in children and adolescents. *Journal of Psychology, 101,* 139–146.

Wolf, T. M., Hunter, S. M., Webber, L. S., & Berenson, G. S. (1981). Self-concept, focus of control, goal blockage, and coronary-prone behavior pattern in children and adolescents: Bogalusa Heart Study. *Journal of General Psychology, 105,* 13–26.

Wolf, T. M., Sklov, M. C., Wenzl, P. A., Hunter, S. M., & Berenson, G. S. (1982). Validation of a measure of Type A behavior pattern in children: Bogalusa Heart Study. *Child Development, 53,* 126–135.

# 7

## Self-Reference and Coronary Heart Disease Risk

LARRY SCHERWITZ AND JONATHAN D. CANICK

## INTRODUCTION

Over the last three decades, findings from numerous studies have linked certain psychosocial factors to coronary heart disease (CHD). In the lead is Type A behavior and one of its components, hostility, which have been repeatedly associated with coronary artery disease (CAD) severity (Blumenthal, Williams, & Kong, 1978; Frank, Heller, Kornfeld, Sporn, & Weiss, 1978; Friedman, Rosenman, Straus, Wurm, & Kositchek, 1968; Williams et al., 1980), and CHD mortality and morbidity incidence (Haynes, Feinleib, & Kannel, 1980; Rosenman et al., 1975). In addition, with less

The MRFIT results were developed through direct collaboration with the Minneapolis MRFIT Coordinating Center and the University of Minnesota Department of Biometry, using funds provided by NHLBI Behavioral Medicine grant HL29573 and American Heart Association, California Affiliate grant-in-aid #84-N149. I am grateful to Greg Grandits, of the MRFIT coordinating center, who conducted the statistical analyses, and to the many MRFIT researchers who designed the study and collected the Structured Interview and follow-up data.

systematic support, behavioral scientists have identified a variety of seemingly unconnected elements as possible psychosocial risk factors for CHD, such as the level of social support (Berkman & Syme, 1979; Medalie & Goldbourt, 1976; Ruberman, Weinblatt, Goldberg, & Chaudbury, 1984), the severity of stressful life events (Kits van Heijningen, 1966; Parkes, Benjamin, & Fitzgerald, 1969; Wolf, 1969), and the sense of coherence in life (Antonovsky, 1979).

In this chapter, we describe a series of research studies pertaining to the idea that frequent self-reference in certain kinds of speech is associated with Type A behavior, emotional reactivity, cardiovascular responsivity, and CHD. The empirical findings have led us to seek theoretical explanations that could link speech patterns to psychological, social, and physiological processes. This chapter serves as an introduction and preface to future work. We propose that self-processes (discussed later), reflected in speech, may underlie seemingly disparate psychosocial risk factors.

Currently, the relationship among the various psychosocial risk factors is not clear. It is uncertain whether all of these factors are separate or whether they are different aspects of the same underlying process. What has been lacking is a way to anchor these risk factors in a larger conceptual framework that would explain their foundation and their interrelationships with situational and biological factors. In an attempt to begin the integration of psychosocial factors, we have focused upon self-processes.

## REVIEW OF EMPIRICAL STUDIES

### Self-Reference, Cardiovascular Responsivity, and Emotional Reactivity

The first author's initial encounter with self-reference was serendipitous; it came from an early psychophysiological study of Type A behavior and autonomic reactivity. Because this study was so formative for our later thinking, I will review its salient points. Beginning in 1974, Scherwitz, Berton, and Leventhal (1978) designed an in-depth study of interviewer and subject speech characteristics as well as psychophysiological reactivity in the Structured Interview (SI). In the search for psychophysiological mechanisms mediating Type A and CHD risk, they measured both behavioral and autonomic reactions in 59 male college students who were given a battery of psychophysiological challenges that included mental arithmetic; cold pressor; a psychomotor task; expression of anger, distress, and peaceful experiences; and the SI.

To the researchers' dismay, there was no relationship between either SI- or JAS-defined Type A behavior and any of the autonomic measures including ongoing measures of blood pressure, heart rate, digital vasoconstriction, or skin resistance. In order to explore how Type A behavior was manifested in the SI, we audited the tape-recorded SIs, scoring each for voice emphasis, speed of speaking, latency of answering, and answer content. The results showed no consistent relationship between the separate components and cardiovascular reactivity.

Two clues, however, guided further exploration. As part of the test battery, subjects had been asked to discuss a past incident that had made them very angry and to relate it as if they were telling a sympathetic friend. We reasoned that anger expression would be a good task to assess reactivity, because of the established relationship between clinical impressions of suppressed hostility and hypertension. While Berton was tape-recording the students' anger-inducing incidents and taking their blood pressure from an adjacent room, he observed that some students' blood pressure readings were much higher if they frequently used the self-references *I*, *me*, *my*, and *mine*. The second clue came from the Type A subjects' ratings of how involved they were in the content of the interview. The Type A's who rated themselves as being more involved in the SI had a higher diastolic blood pressure and more digital vasoconstriction.

To pursue the meaning of these correlations and to determine whether Berton's observations of self-references were accurate, we counted all the self-references in these speech episodes of anger-inducing events. We also rated the intensity of verbally expressed anger. The findings showed that the Type A students (N = 23) self-referenced twice as frequently as Type B's (N = 22) and that the self-references of the Type A's were correlated with their (auditor-rated) anger intensity ($r = .45$) as well as their systolic ($r = .54$) and diastolic ($r = .45$) blood pressure.

In looking within the Type A group, it became obvious that Type A behavior corresponded to higher blood pressure levels only if the Type A's were frequent self-referencers. In fact, the Type A subjects who had fewer self-references actually had lower blood pressure readings than the Type B's. For Type B's self-references were not related to either anger intensity or blood pressure. This was the first finding that something about the self as measured by self-reference may interact with Type A behavior and the expression of anger to affect physiological responses.

What actually does self-reference have to do with Type A behavior? To address this question, we correlated the subjects' self-references and the four speech characteristics (i.e., voice emphasis, speed of speaking, latency of answering, and answer content) that we had previously identified and found to be correlated with the interviewer's Type A assessments (Scherwitz, Berton, & Leventhal, 1977). We found that self-references were significantly correlated with voice emphasis ($r = .42$) and with more Type A answer content ($r = .36$). Since voice emphasis is a major criterion for Type A assessment (Blumenthal, O'Toole, & Haney, 1984; Hecker, Chesney, Black, & Rosenman, 1981; Howland & Siegman, 1982; Matthews, Krantz, Dembroski, & MacDougall, 1982; Scherwitz et al., 1977; Schucker & Jacobs, 1977) and answer content is highly correlated with questionnaire measures

(Scherwitz et al., 1977), it is easy to see how high-self-reference individuals would be assessed as Type A.

In other analyses, the high-self-reference subjects, regardless of their behavior type, reported significantly more distress to the cold pressor (hand submerged in water at 4°C for 60 seconds). They also expressed a greater intensity of distress (as rated by our auditors) when asked to discuss a distressing incident than did the low-self-reference subjects.

To summarize the findings from this study (Scherwitz et al., 1978), we found a connection between self-reference and Type A behavior, anger intensity, distress intensity, and vascular reactivity. High-self-reference individuals were more likely to be Type A than Type B, they expressed anger and distress more intensely when discussing a past incident, and the high-self-reference Type A's had much higher blood pressure levels than the low-self-reference Type A's. The study provided the first evidence that self-reference bridged two important processes: emotional reactivity and physiological responsivity.

## Self-Reference, Blood Pressure, and Electrocardiogram Findings

To see whether there was a "bridge" between self-reference and CHD, the next step was to repeat key aspects of the first study using patients with suspected CHD. In an unpublished work by Scherwitz, Ross, Berton, and Leventhal (1979) the SI and blood pressure measurements were repeated with 59 middle-aged men who had been referred by their cardiologists for an exercise stress test. Unknown to the interviewer, half of the subjects had a positive exercise stress test suggestive of CHD.

The results indicated that those with abnormal ECGs were no more likely to be Type A or to self-reference frequently than were those with normal ECGs. This remains puzzling and may reflect a sample selection bias. However, the men with abnormal ECGs showed a strong correlation ($r = .5$ to $.7$) between self-references and blood pressure both at rest and during the SI. By contrast, the men with normal exercise ECGs showed no significant association between self-references and blood pressure. The exercise stress study findings suggested that it was not the frequency of self-references per se, but the association of self-references with blood pressure that may distinguish men with CHD. This suggested that self-reference was not necessarily tapping into a separate risk component, but was measuring a phenomenon underlying other risk factors.

## Self-Reference and Coronary Artery Disease Severity

To determine whether self-reference was related to more certain measures of CHD, we repeated the SI with a much larger sample of 150 male patients who were hospitalized to undergo a coronary angiogram (Scherwitz et al., 1983). Before angiography was performed, each of the 150 patients received the Type A SI along with other psychosocial and medical tests. We found that self-reference frequency correlated with the history of previous myocardial infarction (MI) ($r = .19$; $p = .02$), the index of disease severity ($r = .22$; $p = .008$), time on the treadmill ($r = -.30$; $p = .05$), percentage of maximum heart rate attained ($r = -.30$; $p = .08$), angiographically determined ejection fraction ($r = -.25$; $p = .008$), and number of occluded arteries (> 50 percent) ($r = .20$; $p = .01$). The relationship between self-reference frequency and number of occluded arteries remained significant after being statistically adjusted for Type A behavior, smoking, cholesterol, and blood pressure.

At the time, these findings provided the best evidence to date that self-reference was associated with CHD. While it remained possible that patients would self-reference more after developing heart disease (and not the other way around), further analyses suggested that this was not the case. The link between self-reference and CAD severity was strongest ($r = .50$) among those patients who had not had angina or an MI.

However, not all of the results from self-reference studies have been positive. An unpublished study by Krantz (1984) found a significant negative correlation between self-reference and CAD severity; another unpublished report by Dembroski (personal communication, March 15, 1985) found no relationship between self-reference and CAD severity (although self-reference was correlated, $r = .37$, with his measure of potential for hostility). Because the data analyses have never been published, it is difficult to compare the results to our own, but we think these results seriously question the hypothesis that self-references in the SI are always associated with CHD.

## Prospective Studies of Self-Reference and CHD

**Self-Involvement and Recurrent CHD.**   As part of the Recurrent Coronary Prevention Project, Powell and Thoresen (1985) analyzed 49 speech characteristics from videotaped SIs of individuals who had sustained their first MI. The subjects were 118 nonsmoking men; 44 sustained a recurrent coronary heart disease (RCHD) event after the interview and 74 (randomly chosen controls) remained free of RCHD during the 2-year follow-up. Powell audited the videotapes of the SIs for each subject and conducted a comprehensive analysis of verbal and nonverbal behaviors, many of which have been used to characterize Type A behavior.

The results showed that 15 of 49 characteristics were statistically related to RCHD in univariate analyses. However, in a multivariate analysis including six physiological factors (e.g., Peel index, systolic and diastolic blood pressure, body mass, cholesterol, age), only four variables independently predicted heart attack recurrence. Comparing the standardized regression coefficients, the strongest predictor was the Peel index ($r = .63$), which is composed of age, number of previous infarctions, shock, heart failure, and conduction or rhythm abnormalities. The second strongest predictor of recurrent CHD was intensity ($r = .57$; $p < .001$), which is a summary measure of strength of emotional response to the interview, including positive emotion (e.g., enthusiasm) and negative emotion (e.g., irritation) on a 5-point scale with the anchors: detached-intense. Self-reference density to the question "About what do you feel insecure?" was the third most predictive ($r = .54$; $p < .001$), followed by periorbital pigmentation ($r = .37$; $p < .05$). Self-references to two other SI questions did not predict a second heart attack.

Powell (1981) conducted analyses to explore whether certain interactions of Type A components would predict RCHD better than each component separately. She found that the combination of intensity (described earlier) and self-reference was a better predictor of RCHD than either factor alone. This finding echoes a theme of other studies (Scherwitz et al., 1978; Scherwitz, Graham, Grandits, Buehler, & Billings, 1986) and supports our hypothesis that something measured by self-references may underlie the riskiness of other psychosocial factors.

**Ancillary Study Using the MRFIT SIs.**    The research at this point had been with people who either had already developed heart disease or were not at risk. For the next study, to determine whether self-reference would be associated with future CHD (Scherwitz, Graham, Grandits, Buehler, & Billings, 1986), we used material from a long-term CHD risk reduction program, the Multiple Risk Factor Intervention Trial (MRFIT) with 12,866 male subjects (MRFIT Group, 1982). The MRFIT had tested whether men who were taught ways to reduce cholesterol, hypertension, and cigarette smoking would have less heart disease 6 to 8 years later compared to a control group who were not taught to reduce their CHD risk. All MRFIT participants were considered at high risk for heart attack, based upon serum cholesterol levels, blood pressure, and smoking. But at the start of the program none had yet experienced any sign of heart disease.

The MRFIT also tested the prospective relationship between Type A behavior and heart disease by measuring Type A behavior in a subgroup of 3110 participants before the program began. Fortunately, these baseline Type A SIs were tape-recorded, and we used this data as the raw material for our study of self-reference in the MRFIT.

Eight years after the MRFIT project began, 193 individuals from the 3110 interviewed had shown some clinical signs of heart disease. We matched this group with 384 MRFIT men who had remained free of any coronary problems during follow-up. We predicted that, after the role of other heart disease risk factors had been statistically adjusted, self-reference would be correlated with CHD morbidity and mortality.

To test these hypotheses, we reviewed the audiotapes of baseline SIs for all 577 participants and counted all spoken *I*'s, *me*'s, and *my*'s; *mine* occurred too infrequently to be included in the analysis. As in previous studies, we counted all spoken clauses to measure speech quantity. This yielded two crude measures of self-reference: (1) total number of self-references (frequency) and (2) self-references per clause (density, a control for speech quantity). In multivariate analyses, we then used statistical methods to adjust for age, diastolic blood pressure, cholesterol, cigarette smoking, and Type A behavior.

The multivariate results partially supported the predictions. As anticipated, the participants who later developed all forms of CHD had a few more self-references (75.1) than their controls (71.7) ($p = .017$). Those who had angina had slightly more self-references (77.0) than their controls (72.8) ($p = .06$). Most salient was the much greater self-reference frequency and density in those who died from heart disease (77.6 frequency and .76 density) compared with their matched controls (69.2 frequency and .71 density) ($p = .06$, $p = .01$, respectively).

However, contrary to predictions, those who survived a heart attack had fewer self-references (64.1) than those who remained free of CHD (72.8) ($p = .75$). This was puzzling, and we did not have an explanation for it until we assessed which risk factors could best distinguish those who died from those who survived a heart attack. In this analysis those who had a heart attack were divided into two groups according to whether they died or survived. Using a discriminant function analysis with the other risk factors entered as predictors, we found self-reference frequency to be the only significant predictor (due to the small sample) of CHD death ($p = .025$; relative risk [$RR$] of 2.0). In a similar analysis, self-reference density did not reach statistical significance ($p = .09$; $RR = 1.87$). Thus self-reference was more strongly associated with survival from an MI than with its occurrence.

What about self-references and Type A behavior? Do they interact to predict CHD? To answer this question, we conducted three analyses for Type A by dividing the sample in two different ways: A's versus B's, and A1's versus everybody else. Within these categories, we split the sample at the median into high and low self-reference frequency and density, and calculated the $RR$ ratios using the Type B-like group as the comparison. For the A versus B comparison there were no differences, but for the A1's versus A2's and B's comparison the self-involved Type A1's had over twice the risk of incurring all-cause CHD ($RR = 2.2$). The results are consistent with the explanation that self-reference was interacting with extreme Type A behavior to increase CHD risk.

What about Type A components? Do they interact with self-references to predict CHD incidence? To answer this question, we scored four speech characteristics (SCs) from the 577 case-control MRFIT SIs: voice emphasis, speed of answering, speed of speaking, and Type A answer content (Scherwitz, Graham, Grandits, & Billings, 1986). These four characteristics have all been correlated with global assessments in previous studies (Scherwitz et al., 1977). We wanted to see whether their predictiveness for CHD incidence differed by level of self-reference, so we divided each of the four SCs into three levels: high, medium, and low. Within each level, we calculated $RR$ ratios comparing high and low self-reference frequency and density (median split).

The results showed no interaction between speed of answering or answer content and self-references, but there was an interaction for voice emphasis and speed of speaking. Previously, we found that voice emphasis was the strongest predictor of CHD incidence among the Type A components measured, with a *RR* ratio of 1.3 (Scherwitz, Graham, Grandits, & Billings, 1986). However, when we contrasted the high and low self-reference measures, the results clearly showed that the predictiveness of voice emphasis was dependent upon the level of self-reference frequency. Among those who were most emphatic, the group with high self-reference frequency had a 1.8 times greater risk of CHD than the high-emphatic, low-self-reference group. The same trend is evident, even stronger, for speed of speaking. The group that spoke most quickly with high self-reference density had a 3.0 times greater risk of CHD than the group that spoke most quickly with low self-reference density. The results clearly show that predictiveness of both speed of answering and voice emphasis, two key Type A indicators, is dependent upon level of self-referencing. Put another way, the predictiveness of self-reference is dependent upon the level of speed and emphasis in the voice.

Consistent with previous studies (Powell & Thoresen, 1985; Scherwitz et al., 1978; Scherwitz et al., 1983), the MRFIT results lend further credibility to the hypothesis that self-reference is related to CHD risk. First, the prospective design rules out the possibility that individuals who first develop heart disease later self-reference more frequently because none of the subjects had CHD when the SIs were conducted. Second, the study was done with a large sample from five geographic areas, thereby increasing the generalizability of the findings. Third, the relationship between self-reference and coronary heart disease remained statistically significant when adjusted for other risk factors.

The results showing self-reference to be the best predictor of death from heart attack are intriguing. We suspect from previous research (Scherwitz et al., 1978) that emotional and blood pressure reactivity are higher in individuals who self-reference frequently. Perhaps a chronic tendency toward hyperreactivity and a lack of physiological modulation prove lethal.

The most interesting MRFIT finding is that extreme Type A behavior, voice emphasis, and speed of speaking all appear to interact with self-reference in predicting CHD incidence. This adds further support to previous studies (Powell & Thoresen, 1985; Scherwitz et al., 1978) showing that self-reference acts differently from the other psychosocial risk factors in that it performs in interactions with other factors to predict CHD better than it performs alone.

## Summary of Empirical Work Relating Self-References to CHD

The results from our early study (Scherwitz et al., 1978) found self-references to correlate with anger intensity, distress, and Type A behavior.

The high-self-reference individuals were more psychologically reactive; they expressed more Type A content, more intensity of anger and distress, and they were more autonomically reactive. These results suggested the possibility that, at least with those assessed as Type A, self-processes may underlie or serve as the context for behavioral, autonomic, and emotional reactivity.

At this point we turned our attention to exploring the link between self-reference and CHD. The next study (Scherwitz et al., 1979) found self-reference to be highly correlated with blood pressure in individuals with abnormal exercise ECGs; and in a study of angiography patients (Scherwitz et al., 1983), self-reference was positively correlated with previous MIs, treadmill performance, ejection fraction, as well as coronary atherosclerosis. This provided evidence, albeit retrospectively, that self-reference was associated with CHD.

The MRFIT results provided the strongest evidence that self-reference is associated with CHD, particularly CHD mortality. The prospective design, the large sample, and the control for other risk factors increased our confidence that self-reference measures something that reflects part of the psychosocial risk process. And as just reviewed, we found that self-reference interacted with extreme Type A1 behavior, speed of speaking, and voice emphasis in predicting CHD incidence. What is most interesting about the findings is that we and other investigators have made empirical links, sometimes tenuous, between an objectively scorable speech measure and emotions, two Type A components, physiological reactivity, CHD morbidity, RCHD, and CHD incidence.

But not all studies have found self-reference to be associated with CHD. Krantz (1984) and his colleagues found self-reference to correlate negatively with angiographically determined CAD severity. And most convincingly, in preliminary results that will be reported in more detail in a research paper in preparation, we did not find self-reference to be associated with CHD incidence in the Western Collaborative Group Study (WCGS). While we are not certain why the results of these two studies were negative, it is clear that we need a better understanding of what self-reference measures, how structural, situational, and interpersonal factors affect these measures, and just how whatever self-reference does measure is interacting with other psychosocial risk factors.

## STUDIES RELATING SELF-REFERENCE TO PSYCHOLOGICAL PROCESSES

The second author has brought a clinical and psychological perspective to the study of self-referencing, and he has contributed to much of the thinking in the remaining sections. Clinical psychologists and psychiatrists have linked objective counts of self-references to emotions and psychopathology, and we will now review some of the most relevant studies. In the most systematic clinical study of self-reference, Weintraub (1981) counted *I*, *me*, and *we* references in several studies. Weintraub's method was to ask subjects to talk into a tape recorder about anything they chose for 10 minutes. He used this method to study the differences between normal and neurotic groups. He found that, relative to a group of normals, self-references were more frequent for impulsives, depressives, binge eaters, compulsives, and alcoholics. Relative to all other groups, the depressives had the greatest frequency of *I* and *me* references, which Weintraub noted as being consistent with the observation of Freud (1914/1957) that the "trait of insistent talking about himself and pleasure in the consequent exposure of himself predominates in the melancholiac" (p. 94). It essentially suggests that excessive self-referencing is a way of experiencing pleasure through exhibition; it is the melancholic's compromise formation (neurotic conflict) to both draw much attention to self while at the same time belittling this attention by reporting only depressive content. Our thinking is that excessive self-referencing serves two purposes: reassurance and amending self and a request for other's attention and support; both are a linguistic form of rallying around the flag. In depression, self-reference is the action of a beleaguered self rather than a pleasure-seeking self. The melancholic is lacking in the beliefs and feelings of self-esteem, confidence, self-sustenance, and ability to synthesize, ergo excessive self-referencing.

Weintraub's findings are consistent with previous research by Ruesch and Prestwood (1949) and Lorenz and Cobb (1953) that found that anxious individuals self-referenced more than nonanxious individuals. Gottschalk, Gleser, and Hambidge (1957) found proportionately greater self-references in hospitalized psychotics than controls. A person feels anxious and tense as part of the fight-or-flight reaction to threat; the *I*, *me*, or *my* is perceived to be under attack. They can react in several ways: (1) They can act through confidence in their ability to master the challenge; (2) they can become explosive, hostile, and aggressive toward the perceived threat; or (3) they can fold into themselves, becoming implosive, depressed, and melancholic.

In general, Weintraub sees excessive self-references as reflecting a lack of separation and objectivity. Psychologically and behaviorally, we theorize that either (1) people who self-reference continuously may be doing so because they do not experience a consolidated identity or a sense of equilibrium; or (2) their identity is too rigidly constructed. We theorize that individuals without a consolidated identity use self-references to attempt to define who they are, and individuals with too rigid an identity use self-references to maintain this identity in the face of changing circumstances. In stressful circumstances those without a consolidated identity are overwhelmed, as their interpretations of identity are too field dependent and therefore unstable. Individuals who have too rigid an identity struggle to control the circumstances' effects upon their identity.

Because psychotherapy deals very much with the client's self-concept, individuals with unstable or rigid identities probably have more difficulty benefiting from psychotherapy. This is consistent with Natale, Dahlberg, and Jaffe's (1978) findings that there is a negative association between the use of self-references and improvement in psychotherapy, and it is consistent with Friedman and colleagues' (1984) observation that egocentric Type A's have the most difficulty reducing their Type A behavior.

Supporting Weintraub in linking self-reference to psychopathology are the research findings by Exner (1973), who used a written measure of self-focus based upon sentence completions. Exner developed the Self Focus Sentence Completion questionnaire, an instrument consisting of 30 sentence stems, for example, "I wish . . . ," "My mother . . . ," 25 of which contain self-references (*I, me, my*, etc.). The subjects' completions to these partial sentences are categorized into positive, negative, or ambivalent self-focus.

In a study of 19 job interviewees for a semiskilled factory position, Exner found that those subjects using frequent self-references had a preponderance of self-focus versus external focus on the sentence completion test. Exner is suggesting that there is an overlap between the measures of written sentence completions and spoken self-references.

Comparing sentence completion scores of nonpsychiatric groups with those of psychiatric groups, Exner found that individuals diagnosed as psychopaths and reactive schizophrenics had a much higher self-focus than normals. However, individuals who were severely depressed, particularly those who were suicidal, had less self-focus than external world focus. Exner's findings conflict with Weintraub's findings just reported that depressives and melancholiacs had higher self-referencing. While it is not clear or certain which clinical populations self-reference more, excessive self-referencing consistently indicates a lack of balance in a person's sense of self and identity. Equilibrium and balance play critical roles in health and illness. In regard to this, Exner developed the idea of egocentric balance; a state of health requires a balance between self and external concerns rather than a preoccupation with one or the other. According to Exner, extreme concern with either self or external world signifies or results in pathology. There is considerable consensus that there should be a balance between self and other. Freud's (1957) concept of narcissism, Kohut's (1966) narcissistic balance, Piaget's (1954) interaction phenomena, and Kegan's (1982) self–other balance all imply that at the core of adjustment problems is a lack of balance.

## THEORETICAL SECTION

### Definitions

If self-reference is associated with CHD, then what are self-references? What do they measure? And how could they reflect a psychosocial risk process? In this section we speculate in answering these questions. We need a working definition of self to theorize about the nature of self-reference. *Self is a psychosocial construct that serves to make meaning in and of the world.* The construction of identity is a cognitive process that provides an operational definition of Who am I?, What is mine?, and What is the difference between you and me? Defining what identity is and how it works is a challenge. Identity is not a set of concrete meanings, but a set of patterns for the organization and the articulation of meaning.

## Self-References, Pronouns, and Psychological Roles

But how do we use language to express the mental operations of self? The first place to look is at pronouns. We have operationally defined self-reference by the use of pronouns *I*, *me*, *my*, *myself*, and *mine* in speech. This grammar of self is not only structural, but functional as well. In language personal pronouns do a majority of the work in referring to people, so they occur very frequently in speech. These self-pronouns along with the more other-oriented self pronouns, for example, *we*, *our*, and *us*, and the third-person pronouns, for example, *he*, *she*, and *they*, function in speech to distinguish the *who* in thought and conversation. First-person pronouns are the only verbal way of referring to ourselves and our possessions, other than using a name or a third-person reference (which is rare in dialogue).

Personal pronouns differ grammatically by case: in English the nominative, objective, and possessive cases distinguish roles pronouns play in speech. Each of the first-person pronouns has a unique grammatical role, and we think they also have corresponding psychological roles as actor, object, and possessor.

The pronoun *I* is used overwhelmingly as the subject of a clause in the SI; the *I* is the agent doing the action of the connected predicate or verb phrase. Psychologically, *I* takes the perspective, representing the speaker's experience. In the SI, *I*'s comprise 85 percent of all self-references, a finding we can attribute in part to the typical "Do you . . . ?" question form of the SI, which naturally elicits a "Yes, I . . . " or "No, I . . ." response. In the MRFIT study (Scherwitz, Graham, Grandits, Buehler, & Billings, 1986), *I* frequency alone was associated with CHD incidence.

In a completely different role, the self-reference *me* functions as a direct object, an indirect object, or object of preposition. As a direct or indirect object, *me* receives the action of the predicate. It is the *what* or *who* that the subject focuses upon with the predicate. As an object of a preposition, the *me* is the receiver of the preposition's direction, for example, "He did this to me." *Me* occurs with the second most frequency in the SI at 9 percent, but is weakly or not at all linked to heart disease (Scherwitz, Graham, Grandits, Buehler, & Billings, 1986).

The third self-reference, *my*, is used in English as a possessive adjective; it modifies the object of possession, laying claim to it, for example, "my car." *My* functions to extend the boundaries of the self internally, externally, or socially. It is with *my* that we possess, own, and control. Though it occurs least often, 6 percent, it has been found to be the strongest correlate of CHD incidence in the MRFIT and in a recent study of angiography patients (Canick, 1986).

*Mine* is used in English also as a possessive predicate adjective, for example, "That is mine." With *mine*, the speaker owns the subject through the linking verb *to be*. Because the questions of the SI were not about ownership, *mine* did not occur with sufficient frequency to be used in our analysis. Also not occurring in sufficient frequency for analysis was the word *myself*, which is used as a reflexive pronoun.

## Major Assumptions of Theoretical Approach

1. The psychosocial risk for CHD is more than a stress-producing situation, a behavior pattern, a degree of social support, and a pattern of hostile feelings. Rather than segmented components operating in isolation, these components are themselves manifestations of an underlying process of self and identity. The risk for CHD stems from an misalignment of self and context. This misalignment is reflected in language.

2. Language is a primary vehicle for acculturation; it evolved culturally and interpersonally to serve thinking and communication and it reflects much about these social processes. In this role language helps define an individual's identity in terms of the cultural milieu—family, school, country, and so on. Names and personal pronouns play a large part, in terms of both the structure of the language and how individuals construct identity.

## Theoretical Speculations

But what do we mean by identity? Identity represents a psychic cohesiveness, creating a feeling that we are the same person we were a year ago even though much may have changed. Identity provides a focus, a point of reference, to perceive others as well as ourselves. And we think that the normal process of identity maintenance changes throughout the life span, thus providing the basis of cognitive and moral development.

The need to maintain an identity is fundamental to the existence of an organism. Lichtenstein (1961) suggests:

> The capacity to maintain or hold onto an identity is a fundamental characteristic of all living organisms, one to which we refer when we think of self-preservation and self-reproduction. Animals and children deprived of identity maintenance simply die. (pp. 246–247)

We agree with Erikson (1956, 1968) that the coherence of identity is an important consideration. There is a considerable clinical literature that maintains that narcissistic behavior results from an individual's struggle to construct and maintain a coherent identity. For example, Fairbanks (1944) proposed that pronouns are used in an attempt to strengthen ego boundaries; this is consistent with Kernberg's (1976) view of narcissism as an attempt to protect an extremely fragile sense of identity.

We theorize that a fragile or overly vulnerable identity constantly perceives and experiences threat to either the agent (*I*) or the agency (*my*). Constant maintenance of identity without achieving equilibrium becomes wearing and draining. Perhaps this is why so many Type A persons describe their heart attack as a relief from the constant struggles and tensions they experience. Despite accomplishments, Type A persons are driven by concerns of failure and competition. They lack a developed or maintained self-esteem. Self-esteem is important nurturance to a fully functioning and healthy individual. Feeling constantly beleaguered adds not to a sense of control and mastery but to a sense of failure.

The paradigms a person uses to construct and organize himself or herself (i.e., his or her identity) and the world have multiple consequences for cognitive and physiological functioning. Self-referencing serves linguistically to cement and patch identity while simultaneously signifying what is not identity. Yet these paradigms are not just "things" that are isolated in the psychosocial realm; they are also embodied. Such organic representations of brain and identity are commonly evident in the body's autoimmune systems, which must consistently differentiate self from not self.

Our research and study suggest that self and identity provide sequelae to cardiovascular and physiological functioning as well. Identity is organismic; it is at once biological, psychological, and social. Self-referential activity occurs on many levels of human organismic functioning to create and maintain self in both symbolic and concrete forms. Self-referential activity follows a logic that is construed through identity.

## Self-Involvement and Other Psychosocial Risk Factors

In the following sections, we present a conceptual analysis that maintains that self-involvement contributes to underlying psychosocial risk. While the research findings are not always consistent, it is reasonable to conclude that aspects of hostility, Type A behavior, and social isolation increase the risk of CHD. From our theoretical perspective there are no discrete boundaries between these different psychosocial factors so that they should be studied simultaneously.

**Self-Involvement and Type A Behavior.**   The two pioneers who originated the concept of Type A behavior, Meyer Friedman and Ray Rosenman, recognized the connection between self-reference and Type A behavior more than 10 years ago. In their lay publication *Type A Behavior and Your Heart* they characterized Type A's as egocentric:

> You possess Type A behavior pattern . . . if you find it *always* difficult to refrain from talking about or bringing the theme of any conversation around to those subjects which especially interest and intrigue you, and when unable to accomplish this maneuver, you pretend to listen but really remain preoccupied with your own thoughts. (Friedman & Rosenman, 1974, p. 101)

The clinical insight from Friedman and Rosenman appears to be valid. In analyzing speech from the SI, we and other researchers have repeatedly found self-references to be much higher in Type A than Type B individuals (Lovallo & Pishkin, 1980; Scherwitz et al., 1978; Scherwitz et al., 1983). Also, careful detailed analyses by Scherwitz and colleagues (1978) have shown that high-self-reference individuals speak more emphatically and report that they are more Type A in their answers than do low-self-reference individuals. Because these are the primary criteria for assessing someone as Type A by the SI or by questionnaires (Scherwitz et al., 1977), it is easy to see why high-self-reference individuals could be assessed as Type A.

Based upon our earlier work, Hecker and colleagues (1981) devised a measure of self-involvement they called aggrandizement. The self-aggrandizement scale was developed to detect an inflated self-image, and we think it is strongly, but not necessarily, related to self-reference. As Hecker and colleagues measured it, self-aggrandizing behaviors included the following kinds of statements in the SI: (1) calling attention to one's superior position (e.g., "I send my secretary to the post office"); (2) exaggerating one's own importance (e.g., "I have rescued more projects than I care to remember"); and (3) making an arrogant statement. They rated SI answers to questions using a 4-point scale from low to high aggrandizement. In a sample of tape-recorded SIs of 75 middle-aged aerospace employees, they scored self-aggrandizement and 19 other speech characteristics. In the analysis that intercorrelated these 20 speech characteristics, four of the five correlations that exceeded $r = .50$ included self-aggrandizement. Self-aggrandizement was the strongest correlate of hostility ($r = .64$), exactingness ($r = .65$), and competitiveness ($r = .51$), and the fourth strongest correlate of global Type A ratings ($r = .42$). More than any other component, self-aggrandizement was a central correlate of the other Type A components.

Although similar in some respects, Type A behavior and self-reference are not the same thing, depending of course on how interviewers or auditors make their ratings. Only half of the Type A's in our first study were more self-involved than Type B's. And in our MRFIT study as well as our earlier work we found that high-self-involved individuals either spoke more slowly or answered more slowly than low-self-involved individuals. It is important to point out that answering slowly does not fit with the clinical description of Type A or how it was assessed. Rather, the high-self-reference individuals seemed more involved in the content of the questions and therefore took longer to answer. We think this represents a willingness to reflect upon their personal experiences.

There are interesting parallels among self-reference, Type A characteristics, and clinical descriptions of narcissism. Kernberg (1975) describes the narcissist as presenting an unusual degree of self-reference in his or her interactions. Schwartz-Salant (1982) notes that extreme self-reference is dominant in the narcissistic character, so that someone else's words are immediately transformed into a story or fantasy about oneself. Kohut (1966) has made the same point and aptly described this phenomenon as the mirror transference.

Schwartz-Salant's (1982) book characterizes the narcissist as having: (1) an inner world that is full or rage, hate, envy, and emptiness; (2) chronic incessant doing, which, stated positively, means relatively active consistent work in some areas that permits the narcissist partially to fulfill his or her ambitions of greatness and obtain admiration from others; (3) often a sense of powerlessness and lack of effectiveness, though he or she may be seen by others as confident and powerful; (4) low empathetic ability and high hostility; (5) low ability to tolerate criticism; and (6) pride in having no needs. These descriptions bear strong similarity to Friedman and colleagues' (1982) descriptions of Type A's as being egocentric, Glass's (1977) theory that coronary proneness derives from needs for control, Wolf's (1969) Sisyphus complex, and Dembroski and MacDougall's (1978) findings that Type A's would rather work alone.

Using the self-construct, we can also draw upon developmental theories that might shed further light upon Type A behavior. For example, we draw upon Kegan's (1982) theory of self-development, which proposes that there are five qualitative stages of self-identity. Of most interest for our discussion is the institutional self, which appears to develop most typically during late adolescence. Kegan characterizes the institutional self as embedded in personal autonomy where self-authorship is primary as in work or love. As such this self-identity has the capacity for independence, the assumption for authority, and exercises personal enhancement or achievements.

The institutional self is useful in the adolescent in developing independence from parents and skill mastery to take on adult roles. "If the strength of the institutional balance is its autonomy, it would be as true to say that its weakness lies in its embeddedness in this autonomy" (p. 223). For, being embedded in autonomy, we see others as separate and this makes it much easier to be competitive, hostile, and alienated.

According to Kegan, this institutional self identity gradually wears thin sometime in middle age and the individual becomes most uncomfortable in transition from one stage to the next. Kegan's description of individuals in this transition period has some similarities to characterizations of coronary-prone behaviors. He says that the individual "may experience the fear of losing one's balance, which consists of feelings of negative self-evaluation, feelings that one's personal organization is threatened or about to collapse, fears about losing one's control and one's precious sense of being distinct" (p. 223).

Perhaps, if we can safely use Kegan's stage framework, coronary proneness represents a stage of arrested identity development. At any rate, there is little evidence that most coronary patients have reached Kegan's last stage of development, the interindividual stage, where the self-identity is embedded in the interpenetration of social systems. Individuals in this stage cultivate the capacity for interdependence, self-surrender, and intimacy.

**Self-Involvement and Hostility.**   Hostility is currently the most popular candidate in the search for the psychogenic Type A components (Barefoot, Dahlstrom, & Williams, 1983; Dembroski, MacDougall, Williams, Haney, & Blumenthal, 1985; Williams et al., 1980). Hostility has been linked with blood pressure reactivity (Dembroski, MacDougall, Shields, Petitto, & Lushene, 1978), CAD severity (Dembroski et al., 1985; Williams et al., 1980), and death from all causes including CHD (Barefoot et al., 1983). Most recently, hostility, scored from the SI, has been linked with CHD incidence in the WCGS, the epidemiological study that best established Type A behavior as a risk factor (Hecker et al., 1985).

The few studies that have examined the connection between self-reference and hostility have found a link. Dembroski and his colleagues (Dembroski, personal communication, March 15, 1985) found potential for hostility to correlate with self-reference ($r = .37$) in the SI. In addition, Canick (1986) found both self-reference frequency and density positively and highly correlated with potential for hostility. In another study, Hecker and colleagues (1981) found in an analysis of 75 SIs of middle-aged males that self-aggrandizement—defined as behavior that either called attention to the speaker's status or exaggerated the speaker's importance—correlated more strongly with hostility ($r = .64$) than any other measure. These results are consistent with the role of self-processes in the development and expression of anger and hostility.

Self-involvement may underlie hostility in several ways. We speculate that the predisposition for hostility relates to how threatened we perceive our identity to be, both as subject and object, and depends on how we cope with these perceived threats. For example, if we think of ourselves as necessarily the smartest, the strongest, the most powerful, or the most attractive, then we are vulnerable to anyone who confronts such claims or compares favorably. This presents a threat to our self-image. Hostility may be a frequently employed strategy for warding off such threats.

Hostility that is reflected by the possessive self references *my* and *mine* is concerned with threats to or regaining possession of its objects, attributes, thoughts, or feelings. As we have mentioned, the self-reference that best predicted CHD in the MRFIT study was *my*. Why is this? Psychologically, *my* acts to extend the self outward toward possessions, reflecting our attachment to various aspects of our environment. When a person uses many *my*'s in speech, this may reflect a self-concept that is overextended or over controlled. The more we possess the more there is to protect and control, thereby increasing our sense of vulnerability, which may be a major antecedent to hostility.

**Self-Involvement and Social Support.**   We theorize that identity is formed and maintained by a collaboration of self and others through biological, psychological and social modes. An *I* not only distinguishes itself from others (not *I*'s), but requires others in order to distinguish itself. The interaction between self and other is relevant to the understanding, assessment, and treatment of the Type A person who is typically physiologically reactive. A major aspect of this interaction is expressed in an individual's engagement–involvement with another, which Singer (1974) theorizes to be a central psychophysiological mechanism as well. Singer and her coworkers' studies laid the groundwork for the assumption that the transactional qualities between the subject and examiner are influential in determining the patterns of psychological and physiological responses during laboratory experiments. The most crucial aspect of this transaction is whether the subject becomes involved with the examiner.

Singer defined engagement–involvement as a transactional phenomenon, reflected by the degree to which an individual actually locks into and invests in an interpersonal transaction. It includes features of attention, alerting, arousal, affect, and affection, but it refers to more than these alone. Singer felt the concept would be useful in psychophysiology as it provides a way to attempt to characterize the effort one notes in a person's transacting. Each person has his or her own characteristic level of engagement, which is in part determined and conditioned by physiological reactions.

We think there is an intimate connection between self-involvement and social support, based upon Singer and colleagues' work. We theorize that self-involvement can adversely affect social support and can also result from adverse experiences with social support. If as a child one did not receive attention to needs, support, and ability to depend, one would be forced into a more self-involved position (Lewis, Brooks-Gunn, & Jaskir, 1986). Similarly, the more we are preoccupied by our own thoughts, feelings, and behaviors, the less we will be able to focus on others' experiences and needs. As a result, others will find it difficult to communicate with self-involved individuals, and self-involved individuals will find it difficult to trust and depend on others to listen, attend, and respond.

This is not to say that self-involved individuals are hermits. They need other people, for it is often through others that they achieve what they want or get the adoration they need. While using someone else as an object to achieve one's own aims characterizes part of human relations, the nature of that relationship is qualitatively different from a relationship where individuals experience one another as unique subjects.

## SUMMARY: RELEVANCE OF SELF-PROCESSES AND TYPE A BEHAVIOR

The concept of self, self-involvement, and the measure of self and other references in speech provide the potential for a better understanding of psychosocial risk for CHD. For example, the above mentioned work on self-references in the SI provides evidence of how emotional and autonomic responses are linked, and thus adds connective tissue to the link between Type A behavior and CHD. In the study of social support, the use of self and other pronouns from speech can provide a dialectic one can use to study the interactions (both symbolic and real) of self and other. Similarly, for hostility one can use the self versus other and source versus target distinctions to differentiate forms of hostility. The underlying construct of identity is important because how an individual is defined may well determine the use of hostility as a coping mechanism, and it may also determine the capacity for intimacy as a necessary predisposition for giving and receiving social support. Another important consideration is that by using the construct of self and identity one can tap into the rich and varied ideas, methods, and findings on self-processes from developmental psychology, social psychology, and psychoanalysis in order to address the questions of how the psychosocial risk factors evolved in a individual, what functions they serve, how they are connected to one another, and how they might best be treated.

## REFERENCES

Antonovsky, A. (1979). *Health stress and coping*. San Francisco: Jossey-Bass.

Barefoot, J. C., Dahlstrom, G., & Williams, R. B. (1983). Hostility, CHD incidence, and total mortality: A 25-year follow-up study of 255 physicians. *Psychosomatic Medicine, 45,* 59–64.

Berkman, L. F., & Syme, S. L. (1979). Social networks, host resistance, and mortality: A nine-year follow-up study of Alameda County residents. *American Journal of Epidemiology, 109,* 186–204.

Blumenthal, J. A., O'Toole, L. C., & Haney, T. H. (1984). Behavioral assessment of the Type A behavior pattern. *Psychosomatic Medicine, 46,* 415–423.

Blumenthal, J. A., Williams, R. B., & Kong, Y. (1978). Type A behavior pattern and coronary atherosclerosis. *Circulation, 58,* 634–639.

Canick, J. (1986). *Self-involvement, hostility, and severity of coronary artery disease.* Unpublished doctoral dissertation, California School of Professional Psychology, Berkeley.

Dembroski, T. M., & MacDougall, J. M. (1978). Stress effects on affiliation preferences among subjects possessing the Type A coronary-prone behavior pattern. *Journal of Personality & Social Psychology, 36,* 23–33.

Dembroski, T. M., MacDougall, J. M., Shields, J. L., Petitto, J., & Lushene, R. (1978). Components of the type A coronary behavior pattern and cardiovascular response to psychomotor performance challenge. *Journal of Behavioral Medicine, 1,* 159–176.

Dembroski, T. M., MacDougall, J. M., Williams, R. B., Haney, T. L., & Blumenthal, J. A.

(1985). Components of Type A, hostility, and anger-in: Relationship to angiographic findings. *Psychosomatic Medicine, 47,* 219–233.

Erikson, E. (1956). The problem of ego identity. *Journal of the American Psychoanalytic Association, 4,* 56–121.

Erikson, E. (1968). *Identity: Youth and crisis.* New York: Norton.

Exner, J. (1973). The Self Focus Sentence Completion: A study of egocentricity. *Journal of Personality Assessment, 37,* 437–455.

Fairbanks, H. (1944). Quantitative differentiation of spoken language. *Psychological Monographs, 56,* 19–38.

Frank, K. A., Heller, S. S., Kornfeld, D. S., Sporn, A. A., & Weiss, M. B. (1978). Type A behavior pattern and coronary angiographic findings. *Journal of the American Medical Association, 240,* 761–763.

Freud, S. (1957). On narcissism. In J. Strachey (Ed. & Trans.), *The standard edition of the complete psychological works of Sigmund Freud* (Vol. 14). London: Hogarth. (Original work published 1914)

Friedman, M., & Rosenman, R. (1974). *Type A behavior and your heart.* New York: Faucet Crest.

Friedman, M., Rosenman, R. H., Straus, R., Wurm, M., & Kositchek, R. (1968). The relationship of behavior pattern A to the state of the coronary vasculature: A study of 51 autopsied subjects. *American Journal of Medicine, 44,* 525–537.

Friedman, M., Thoresen, C. E., Gill, J. J., Powell, L. H., Ulmer, D., Thompson, L., Price, V., Rabin, D., Breall, W. S., Dixon, T., Levy, R., & Bourg, E. (1984). Alteration of Type A behavior and reduction in cardiac recurrences in postmyocardial infarction patients. *American Heart Journal, 108,* 237–248.

Friedman, M., Thoresen, C., Gill, J., Ulmer, D., Thompson, L., Powell, L., Price, V., Elek, S., Rabin, D., Breall, W., Piaget, G., Dixon, T., Bourg, E., Levy, R., & Tasto, D. (1982). Feasibility of altering Type A behavior pattern after myocardial infarction. Recurrent Coronary Prevention Project Study: Methods, baseline results and preliminary findings. *Circulation, 66,* 83–92.

Glass, D. C. (1977). *Behavior patterns, stress, and coronary disease.* Hillsdale, NJ: Erlbaum.

Gottschalk, L. A., Gleser, G. C., & Hambidge, G. J. (1957). Verbal behavior analysis, some content and form variables in speech relevant to personality adjustment. *Archives of Neurology & Psychiatry, 77,* 300–311.

Haynes, S. G., Feinleib, M., & Kannel, W. B. (1980). The relationship of psychosocial factors to coronary heart disease in the Framingham study: III. Eight-year incidence of coronary heart disease. *American Journal of Epidemiology, 111,* 37–58.

Hecker, M., Chesney, M., Black, G., & Rosenman, R. (1981). Speech analysis of Type A behavior. In J. K. Darby (Ed.), *Speech evaluation in medicine.* New York: Grune & Stratton.

Hecker, M., Frautschi, N., Chesney, M., Black, G., & Rosenman, R. (1985, March). *Components of the Type A behavior and coronary heart disease.* Paper presented at the meeting of the Society of Behavioral Medicine, New Orleans.

Howland, E. W., & Siegman, A. W. (1982). Toward the automated measurement of the Type-A behavior pattern. *Journal of Behavioral Medicine, 5,* 37–54.

Kegan, R. (1982). *The evolving self.* Cambridge: Harvard University Press.

Kernberg, O. (1975). *Borderline conditions and pathological narcissism.* New York: Jason Aronson.

Kernberg, O. (1976). *Object relationships theory and clinical psychoanalysis.* New York: Jason Aronson.

Kits van Heijningen, H. (1966). Psychodynamic factors in acute myocardial infarction. *International Journal of Psychoanalysis, 47,* 370–374.

Kohut, H. (1966). Forms and transformations of narcissism. *Journal of the American Psychoanalytic Association, 14,* 243–272.

Krantz, D. (1984). [letter to the editor]. *Psychosomatic Medicine, 46*, 67–68.

Lewis, M., Brooks-Gunn, J., & Jaskir, J. (1985). Individual differences in visual self-recognition as a function of mother–infant attachment relationship. *Developmental Psychology, 21*, 1181–1187.

Lichtenstein, H. (1961). Identity and sexuality: A study of their interrelationship in man. *Journal of the American Psychoanalytic Association, 9*, 179–260.

Lorenz, M., & Cobb, S. (1953). Language behavior in psychoneurotic patients. *Archives of Neurology & Psychiatry, 69*, 684–693.

Lovallo, W. R., & Pishkin, V. (1980). A psychophysiological comparison of Type A and B men exposed to failure and uncontrollable noise. *Psychophysiology, 17*, 29–36.

Matthews, K. A., Krantz, D. S., Dembroski, T. M., & MacDougall, J. M. (1982). Unique and common variance in Structured Interview and Jenkins Activity Survey measures of the Type A behavior pattern. *Journal of Personality & Social Psychology, 42*, 303–313.

Medalie, J., & Goldbourt, V. (1976). Angina pectoris among 10,000 men: II. Psychosocial and other risk factors as evidenced by a multivariate analysis of a five year incidence study. *American Journal of Medicine, 60*, 910–921.

The MRFIT Group. (1982). The Multiple Risk Factor Intervention Trial: Risk factor changes and mortality results. *Journal of the American Medical Association, 248*, 1465–1477.

Natale, M., Dahlberg, C. C., & Jaffe, J. (1978). The relationship of defensive language behavior in patient monologues to the course of psychoanalysis. *Journal of Clinical Psychology, 34*, 466–470.

Parkes, C. M., Benjamin, B., & Fitzgerald, R. G. (1969). Broken heart: A statistical study of increased mortality among widowers. *British Medical Journal, 1*, 740–743.

Piaget, J. (1954). *The construction of reality in the child* (1937). New York: Basic.

Powell, L. (1981). *Indicators of the Type A behavior pattern and recurrent coronary heart disease.* Unpublished doctoral dissertation, Stanford University.

Powell, L., & Thoresen, C. (1985). Behavioral and physiologic determinants of long-term prognosis after myocardial infarction. *Journal of Chronic Disability, 38*, 253–263.

Rosenman, R. H., Brand, R. J., Jenkins, C. D., Friedman, M., Straus, R., & Wurm, M. (1975). Coronary heart disease in the Western Collaborative Group Study: Final follow-up experience of 8 ½ years. *Journal of the American Medical Association, 233*, 872–877.

Ruberman, W., Weinblatt, E., Goldberg, J. D., & Chaudbury, B. (1984). Psychosocial influence on mortality after myocardial infarction. *New England Journal of Medicine, 311*, 552–559.

Ruesch, J., & Prestwood, A. R. (1949). Anxiety: Its initiation, communication and interpersonal management. *Archives of Neurology & Psychiatry, 62*, 527–550.

Scherwitz, L., Berton, K., & Leventhal, H. (1977). Type A assessment and interaction in the behavior pattern interview. *Psychosomatic Medicine, 39*, 229–240.

Scherwitz, L., Berton, K., & Leventhal, H. (1978). Type A behavior, self-involvement, and cardiovascular response. *Psychosomatic Medicine, 40*, 593–609.

Scherwitz, L., Graham, L. E., Grandits, G., & Billings, J. (1986). *Speech characteristics and coronary heart disease incidence in the MRFIT.* Unpublished manuscript.

Scherwitz, L., Graham, L., Grandits, G., Buehler, J., & Billings, J. (1986). Self-involvement and coronary heart disease incidence in the Multiple Risk Factor Intervention Trial. *Psychosomatic Medicine, 48*, 187–199.

Scherwitz, L., McKelvain, R., Laman, C., Patterson, J., Dutton, L., Yusim, S., Lester, J., Kraft, I., Rochelle, D., & Leachman, R. (1983). Type A behavior, self-involvement, and coronary atherosclerosis. *Psychosomatic Medicine, 45*, 47–57.

Scherwitz, L., Ross, M., Berton, K., & Leventhal, H. (1979). *Self-involvement and blood pressure reactivity in individuals with ischemic heart disease.* Unpublished manuscript.

Schucker, B., & Jacobs, D. R. (1977). Assessment of behavioral risk for coronary disease by voice characteristics. *Psychosomatic Medicine, 39,* 219–228.

Schwartz-Salant, N. (1982). *Narcissism and character transformation.* Toronto: Inner City Books.

Singer, M. T. (1974). Presidential address—Engagement-involvement: A central phenomenon in psychophysiological research. *Psychosomatic Medicine, 36,* 1–17.

Weintraub, W. (1981). *Verbal Behavior: Adaptation and Psychopathology.* New York: Springer.

Williams, R. B., Haney, T., Lee, K. L., Kong, Y., Blumenthal, J., & Whalen, R. E. (1980). Type A behavior, hostility, and coronary atherosclerosis. *Psychosomatic Medicine, 42,* 539–549.

Wolf, S. (1969). Psychosocial forces in myocardial infarction and sudden death. *Circulation, 39,* 40 (Suppl. IV), 74–83.

# 8

# Coronary-Prone Components of Type A Behavior in the WCGS: A New Methodology

MARGARET A. CHESNEY, MICHAEL H. L. HECKER, AND GEORGE W. BLACK

The Type A behavior pattern was described by Rosenman and Friedman as an action–emotion complex that is

> exhibited by an individual who is engaged in a relatively chronic and excessive struggle . . . to obtain a usually unlimited number of things from the environment in the shortest period of time and/or against the opposing efforts of other persons or things. (Rosenman, 1978, p. xv)

As discussed in other chapters in this volume, an impressive body of epidemiologic evidence has implicated Type A behavior in the severity of coronary atherosclerosis, in the prevalence and incidence of coronary heart disease (CHD), and in the severity of coronary atherosclerosis (for reviews see Matthews & Haynes, 1986; Review Panel on Coronary-Prone Behavior and Coronary Heart Disease, 1981; Rosenman & Chesney, 1985).

The first of the prospective studies to examine a causal relationship between Type A behavior and heart disease was the Western Collaborative Group Study (WCGS) (Rosenman et al., 1964). This 8.5-year investigation revealed that men assessed as Type A by means of a Structured Interview (SI) administered at intake had approximately twice as much risk of developing CHD over the follow-up period as their Type B counterparts had (Rosenman et al., 1975). This risk persisted after adjustment for other CHD risk factors (Rosenman, Brand, Sholtz, & Friedman, 1976). Since the WCGS, the Framingham Heart Study (Haynes, Feinleib, & Kannel, 1980) and the French-Belgian Collaborative Study (French-Belgian Collaborative Group, 1982) have provided additional evidence that Type A behavior is a risk factor for CHD. Angiographic (Blumenthal, Williams, Kong, Schanberg, & Thompson, 1978; Frank, Heller, Kornfeld, Sporn, & Weiss, 1978; Zyzanski, Jenkins, Ryan, Flessas, & Everist, 1976) and autopsy (Friedman et al., 1973) studies have further contributed to the evidence that Type A behavior is associated with coronary atherosclerosis, the process underlying CHD.

Recently, the pattern of studies confirming a significant association between Type A behavior and CHD was broken. Several prospective studies of persons at high risk for CHD, including the Multiple Risk Factor Intervention Trial (MRFIT) (Shekelle et al., 1985), the Multicenter Post-Infarction Program (Case, Heller, Case, Moss, & the Multicenter Post-Infarction Research Group, 1985), and the Aspirin Myocardial Infarction Study (Shekelle, Gale, & Norusis, in press), failed to support the role of Type A behavior as an independent CHD risk factor. Similarly, a number of studies of patients referred for angiographic evaluation of coronary atherosclerosis have failed to find a relationship between Type A behavior and severity of coronary artery disease (Bass & Wade, 1982; Dimsdale, Hackett, Black, & Hutter, 1978; Dimsdale, Hackett, & Hutter, 1979; Kornitzer et al., 1982; Krantz et al., 1981; Scherwitz et al., 1983). The lack of evidence associating Type A behavior with disease in these studies has led some investigators to question the association between the global Type A behavior pattern and CHD and has led to confusion in the medical community.

There are several possible explanations for the inconsistencies observed in the Type A literature. One is that the risk associated with Type A behavior is less prominent in subjects at high risk because of the other risk factors or existing disease. In each of the trials and in the angiographic studies that found no association with Type A behavior the patients comprising the sample were at high risk, whereas the subjects followed in the WCGS and the French-Belgian Collaborative Study exhibited averaged normal levels of the risk factors. A second explanation is that the subjective nature of the SI produces a measurement of the Type A behavior pattern that is vulnerable to subjective bias and drift over time. A third possibility is that certain components of the multidimensional Type A behavior pattern are more directly related than others to CHD endpoints. This chapter is intended to review and provide new information relevant to this third explanation. In the first section, the original clinical definition of, and assessment procedure for, the Type A behavior pattern will be described. Research efforts to examine the separate components of the behavior pattern will be reviewed in the second section. The third section will present the initial results from a recent study of the relationship between Type A components and CHD incidence in the WCGS. Future directions for research on Type A components and coronary-prone behaviors will be outlined in the fourth and final section.

## THE CLINICAL DEFINITION OF TYPE A BEHAVIOR

Originally, Rosenman and Friedman (1959) developed the concept of the coronary-prone Type A behavior pattern from clinical observations of their patients with CHD. Its originators noted that earlier clinical portrayals of CHD patients (Dunbar, 1943; Gertler & White, 1954; Kemple, 1945; Menninger & Menninger, 1936; Osler, 1892) were consistent with their new conceptualization. Given the clinical origins of the definition of the Type A behavior pattern, it is not surprising that the first procedure for assessing Type A behavior was the Structured Interview (Rosenman et al., 1964). This interview was designed to examine a subject's responses to questions about everyday activities and potentially challenging situations. Tape-recorded interviews were assessed by judges who were clinically trained to attend to the various facets of the behavior pattern in arriving at a global rating. The Structured Interview was first used to separate subjects in the WCGS into four groups: Type A1, Type A2, Type B3, and Type B4. Those subjects who displayed the Type A behavior pattern in the interview (Type A1 or Type A2) were classified as Type A and those who did not (Type B3 or Type B4) were classified as Type B. Since then, the Structured Interview has continued to be the Type A assessment of choice because it outperforms pencil-and-paper methods in predicting clinically relevant endpoints (Chesney, Eagleston, & Rosenman, 1980) and best fits the Type A construct (Byrne, Rosenman, Schiller, & Chesney, 1985). The relative strength of the interview can be attributed to the fact that it provides an opportunity for direct assessment of behavior, not unlike the clinical observations originally made by Rosenman and Friedman. However, maintaining the reliability of behavior pattern assessment and the limited specificity afforded by the dichotomous nature of the Type A–Type B distinction have proved to be problematic. In an attempt to address these problems, efforts to explicate further the various facets or components of the Type A behavior pattern were undertaken.

## PREVIOUS RESEARCH ON TYPE A COMPONENTS

### Type A Components and CHD

The first effort to study the relationship between components of the Type A behavior pattern and CHD used data from the WCGS. The original sample and methodology followed in the WCGS are described in detail in previous reports (Rosenman et al., 1964; Rosenman et al., 1976). In this study, a comprehensive examination, including assessment of cardiovascular risk factors and Type A behavior, was given to 3524 male subjects between the ages of 39 and 59. At the intake examination, a number of subjects were found to exhibit electrographic patterns of previous myocardial infarction (MI). Of these subjects, 25 men were not aware of their condition and were thus classified as having had a "silent" myocardial infarction. Component ratings of the interviews of these subjects and 75 matched controls were made based on the content and style of interview responses. Among the components studied, the group with silent MI showed significantly more manifest hostility and reported significantly higher past achievements than control subjects (Jenkins, Rosenman, & Friedman, 1966).

Of the entire cohort of 3524 WCGS subjects, 3154 were determined to be free of CHD at the comprehensive examination at intake. These subjects were reexamined annually for 8.5 years to document the incidence of CHD. Interim data on CHD incidence at the 4.5-year follow-up (Rosenman et al., 1970) were used to select the sample for a component analysis of Type A behavior. By this interim follow-up, 133 men had developed CHD. The design of this component study was to select, for each of these 133 cases, two CHD-free control subjects matched for company of employment and age. Independent raters were to have scored the audiotaped intake Type A Structured Interviews for specific components of the behavior pattern. For convenience, the sample of cases and matched control subjects was split by age. Sixty-three cases were between the ages of 39 and 49, and 70 cases were between the ages of 50 and 59. Unfortunately, the component analysis was performed only on the younger cohort. Of the 63 cases in this age group, interview data for 1 subject were lost. Therefore, a sample of 62 cases and 124 matched controls was studied. Figure 8.1 illustrates the derivation of this sample from the WCGS cohort.

The component scoring in this study was performed by Dr. Ray Bortner, who was unaware of the subjects' behavior pattern rating or heart disease status. Each subject's responses to the 37 interview questions were coded for evidence of Type A behavior. In addition, clinical judgments were made on the basis of the subjects' speech stylistics and related behaviors exhibited across the interview. These stylistics included interruptions, sighing, explosive voice modulation, vigorous responses, evidence of tight self-control, and potential for hostility. Unfortunately, the specific criteria on which the

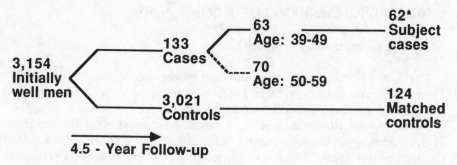

*Interview not available on 1 subject

**FIGURE 8.1.**   Source of case-control sample for the study of Type A components and CHD incidence during the first 4.5 years of the WCGS follow-up.

ratings of these characteristics were based were not documented before Dr. Bortner's death.

Analysis of the component data scored by Dr. Bortner provided the first indication that some dimensions of the behavior pattern were more predictive of CHD than others. In particular, the most significant differences between cases and control subjects were found on the clinical judgment of potential for hostility ($p < .01$), the subjects' responses regarding anger expression ($p < .01$), the subjects' reporting competitive behavior ($p < .01$), the subjects' responses regarding anger frequency ($p = .02$), irritation at waiting in lines ($p < .05$), and clinical judgments of explosive ($p < .05$) and vigorous ($p = .02$) speech stylistics.

Since the WCGS, the relationship between components of Type A behavior and CHD incidence has been examined in two prospective studies. One of these was the MRFIT, in which, as noted above, global ratings of Type A behavior were not found to be related to clinical CHD endpoints. Encouraged by evidence that self-involvement (i.e., a focus on the self) is associated with CHD risk and morbidity, Scherwitz and his colleagues (Scherwitz, Graham, Grandits, Buehler, & Billings, 1986) scored the self-references made in the SI administered at intake into MRFIT to 193 individuals who manifested their first CHD event and 384 individuals who remained free of CHD during the 7-year follow-up. Neither the total number of self-references nor self-reference density was predictive of nonfatal myocardial infarction or angina. However, for those patients who suffered a fatal myocardial infarction, self-referencing was the strongest predictor of mortality among all of the standard risk factors. This research is discussed in detail in Chapter 7 by Scherwitz in this volume.

The second study since the WCGS examining the relationship between Type A behavior and CHD endpoints was conducted as part of the Recurrent

Coronary Prevention Project (RCPP) (Powell & Thoresen, 1985). In this study, SI responses given by a sample of 118 nonsmoking, postcoronary male subjects were scored for 49 components and possibly related signs and symptoms of the Type A behavior pattern. Of these, 15 showed univariate relationships to recurrent cardiac events. It is of interest that, among the 15, nine involve some form of hostility, irritation, annoyance, or anger (e.g., self-report of anger arousal while driving, anger provoked by waiting). Using a multivariate analysis, four of the 15 variables remained significant: intensity (i.e., strength of positive [enthusiasm] or negative [irritation] responses), self-involvement, periorbital pigmentation, and anger arousal while driving.

## Type A Components and Severity of Coronary Atherosclerosis

The relationship of Type A components to the severity of coronary artery disease (CAD) has been examined in two studies (Dembroski, MacDougall, Williams, Haney, & Blumenthal, 1985; MacDougall, Dembroski, Dimsdale, & Hackett, 1985). As noted previously, Type A behavior was found to be associated with angiographically documented severity of coronary atherosclerosis in some but not all studies. In both of these component studies, global ratings of Type A behavior did not show a significant relationship to disease severity. However, the component rating of potential for hostility and subjects' self-reports of holding anger in when provoked were significantly related to severity of coronary atherosclerosis. One of these investigations (MacDougall et al., 1985) constituted in part a reanalysis of the Structured Interviews that had been previously reported to show no association with disease severity. These two studies indicate that the hostility component of the Type A behavior pattern is associated with clinical CAD even when global ratings of the behavior pattern are not. Taken together, these findings and those from the studies of the WCGS and RCPP sample suggest that hostility is coronary prone while other facets of the behavior pattern such as loudness, explosive speech stylistics, and job involvement may not be.

Further evidence implicating hostility in the incidence of CAD is provided by studies that have used Cook and Medley's Hostility scale (Cook & Medley, 1954), an MMPI-derived scale to assess hostility. As discussed in more detail in Chapter 9 by Williams and Barefoot in this volume, high scores on this scale have been found to be associated with CHD incidence and all-cause mortality in two prospective studies (Barefoot, Dahlstrom, & Williams, 1983; Shekelle, Gale, Ostfeld, & Paul, 1983) and with severity of CAD in a study of patients undergoing angiography (Williams et al., 1980). These findings, however, were not confirmed by a prospective study (McCranie, Watkins, Brandsma, & Sisson, 1986) in which the MMPI was given as part of an evaluation for medical school admission—a condition that may have influenced self-report of hostility. This study and other researchers (Megargee, 1985; Rosenman, Swan, & Carmelli, Chapter 2 this volume), have raised questions about the construct validity of this scale as a measure of hostility.

## Type A Components and Reactivity

Another line of research examining components of the Type A behavior pattern has focused on the relationship of component behaviors to physiological hyperreactivity to stress. The investigations of hyperreactivity are of interest because excessive adrenergically mediated physiological arousal in response to stress is the leading explanation of the mechanism by which Type A behavior may lead to coronary atherosclerosis and increased risk for CHD (see Houston, Chapter 10, this volume). Some studies have suggested that the same components that have been found to predict disease endpoints, particularly hostility, are more highly correlated than others with excessive cardiovascular response to mild and moderate laboratory stressors (Allen, Lawler, Matthews, & Rakaczy, 1984; Dembroski, Mac-Dougall, Shields, Petitto, & Lushene, 1978; Dembroski, MacDougall, & Lushene, 1979). Specifically, these studies showed that the hostility component was consistently the strongest correlate of hyperreactivity among the components studied (including loud and explosive voice, response latency, rapid and accelerated speech, and competitiveness). In some studies, competition for control of the interview also showed a significant relationship to reactivity (Allen et al., 1984).

Not all studies have confirmed an association between hostility and reactivity. In one investigation (Glass, Lake, Contrada, Kehoe, & Erlanger, 1983), while no evidence of an association between global Type A behavior and reactivity was found, an inverse relationship between the hostility component and blood pressure reactivity was reported. Anderson, Williams, Lane, and Monon (1984) reported that changes in cardiovascular responses to a laboratory task presented under a challenging condition were not related to subjects' scores on Cook and Medley's Hostility scale, or measures of anger expression and Type A behavior.

## Type A Components and Global Type A Behavior

Much of the early research on Type A components focused on examining the extent to which specific components of the behavior pattern correlated with global Type A ratings. These studies, while not identifying coronary-prone behavior, helped elucidate the facets within the global behavior pattern and provided a foundation and methodology that were used in subsequent studies with clinical CHD endpoints (Jacobs & Schucker, 1981). In independent studies, Scherwitz, Berton, and Leventhal (1977) and Schucker and Jacobs (1977) showed that numerous dimensions of speed and volume of speaking distinguished Type A from Type B individuals. In fact, among the numerous speech characteristics studied, four (speed, volume, explosive words, and a short response latency) that were significantly related to global Type A ratings, when considered together, showed a correlation of $r = .71$ with global ratings of the behavior pattern. Pursuing these findings, Feldstein and his associates (Feldstein, Siegman, Barkley, Simpson, & Kobren, 1984) have attempted to develop automated systems to score or rate the more quantitative Type A speech characteristics, such as interruptions and speed of speaking. The importance of this trend toward more reproducible and reliable assessments of Type A components is emphasized by the evidence discussed in this chapter, which points to the need to move beyond global ratings of the multidimensional Type A behavior pattern and to focus on ratings of specific Type A components. The next section will report on the development of such an operationally defined system and present data on its application to the WCGS.

## A REEXAMINATION OF TYPE A COMPONENTS IN THE WCGS

### The Type A Component Scoring System

An operational assessment procedure was developed to define and assess specific dimensions of the Type A behavior pattern.[*] This procedure involves the division of the recorded Type A Structured Interview into 20 segments. Each segment begins with one of the key questions of the interview and includes the subject's response and all subsequent dialogue until the next key question is asked. The 20 key questions of the interview are presented in Table 8.1. The behaviors exhibited by the subject during each of the 20 segments are scored in terms of 14 operationally defined components, which are defined to represent previously described facets of the Type A behavior pattern (Rosenman et al., 1964) and other variables thought to be related to CHD risk. Summary definitions of these components are presented in Table 8.2. A comprehensive protocol specifies and illustrates detailed scoring criteria for each component. This protocol, which consists of a code book and a library of reference tapes, was designed to minimize the need for raters to make subjective judgments. In the code book, different behaviors relating to the same component are identified and assigned numerical scores. The reference tapes are used to define and quantify several speech characteristics, such as Loudness of Voice and Speaking Rate. Examples of the scoring criteria for each of the components are shown in Table 8.3. The score sheet used for coding the SI is a cell matrix of 20 columns (representing the segments of the interview) and 14 rows (representing the components to be scored). Each cell is given a score from a 5-point scale

---

[*] A preliminary version of this assessment procedure is described in Hecker, Chesney, Black, and Rosenman (1981).

**TABLE 8.1. KEY QUESTIONS IN THE WCGS TYPE A STRUCTURED INTERVIEW**

1. Does your job carry heavy responsibility?
2. Were you on any athletic teams in high school or college?
3. Did you attend night school or take correspondence courses to advance your career?
4. Are you satisfied with your present job?
5. Do you think of yourself as hard-driving and ambitious, or as relaxed and easy-going?
6. When you play competitive games with children, do you purposely let them win?
7. In games with contemporaries, do you play to win or for the fun of it?
8. Is there any competition in your job?
9. Do you have another job or participate in civic activities?
10. When you take snapshots, do you develop your own films?
11. When you have an appointment to meet your wife or a friend, will you be there on time?
12. What are your major hobbies?
13. Do you get impatient when you are watching a slow worker?
14. Do you often do two things at the same time, like reading while eating?
15. Do you walk fast?
16. Are you irritated if you have to wait for a table in a restaurant?
17. When someone is talking to you, do you often find yourself thinking about other things?
18. Do you feel that time is passing too quickly each day to get everything done?
19. Are you irritated if you are caught behind a slow automobile and cannot pass?
20. How frequently do you get angry or upset?

(ranging from 0 to 4), depending on the level or intensity of the corresponding behavior exhibited during a given interview segment. The score sheet is presented in Figure 8.2.

To score a Structured Interview, the rater plays back the interview three times. These repeated playbacks are necessary because data have shown that raters cannot simultaneously attend to all the behaviors that may occur during a single segment. By playing the interview back multiple times, the rater is able to concentrate on a small group of components that require a similar mode of assessment. During Playback I, Immediateness, Type A Content, Anger In, and Anger Out are scored. Except for Immediateness (the inverse of response latency), these components require listening only to what the subject is saying, not to the way it is being said. During Playback II, Competitiveness, Hostility, Self-Aggrandizement (similar to self-involvement), Exactingness, and Despondency are scored. These components require evaluation of both the verbal content and the emotional tone of the subject's speech. Finally, during Playback III, Loudness of Voice, Syllabic Emphasis, Speaking Rate, Acceleration, and Hard Voice are scored. These speech

**TABLE 8.2.    SUMMARY DEFINITIONS OF COMPONENTS**

| Component | Definition |
|---|---|
| Immediateness | Quickness with which the subject responds to the key questions. The inverse of response latency. |
| Type A Content | Content of the subject's responses indicative of Type A behavior (e.g., report of heavy job responsibility in response to the first key question). |
| Anger In, Anger Out | Content of the subject's response to specific questions in the SI about the suppression or expression of anger. |
| Competitiveness | Competitive behavior exhibited during the interview (e.g., interrupting the interviewer, asking irrelevant questions, or requesting unnecessary clarification). |
| Hostility | Reports of anger or irritation involving others or unpleasant situations, and hostility expressed toward the interviewer (e.g., complaints about others, depreciation of interviewer). |
| Self-Aggrandizement | Claims of superiority relative to others (e.g., conceit, pompous statements, boasting). |
| Exactingness | Excessive and unnecessary attention to detail, both in interpreting questions and providing answers (e.g., volunteering numerical information, requesting additional information before responding to questions). |
| Despondency | Depressed viewpoint or mood evidenced in content or tone of responses (e.g., statements of loss, pessimism, sadness, and withdrawal as a coping style). |
| Loudness of Voice | Loudness of voice during responses. |
| Syllabic Emphasis | Sudden increases in loudness that emphasize particular syllables, that is, explosive speech. |
| Speaking Rate | Speed of speaking in passages that are free of thought pauses and emotional interruptions. |
| Acceleration | Temporary increases in speaking rate, usually at the end of sentences. |
| Hard Voice | Speech that reflects excessive muscular tension in the laryngeal structures. |

characteristics are scored independently of the verbal content of the subject's answers. For each component included in the first and second playbacks, each of the 20 interview segments is given a score that indicates the extent to which relevant behaviors are evident during that segment. For the third playback, raters integrate their assessment of the speech characteristics over five consecutive interview segments at a time and then use a 5-point scale to rate these characteristics. Thus for the 20 segments of the interview, raters provide four ratings of each speech characteristic.

**TABLE 8.3. SCORING CRITERIA FOR TYPE A COMPONENTS**

| Component | Criteria | Score |
|---|---|---|
| Immediateness | Latency between question and response > 0.5 seconds | 0 |
| | Latency approximately 0.5 seconds | 1 |
| | No latency | 2 |
| | End of question "cut off" | 3 |
| | Most of question "cut off" | 4 |
| Type A Content | Protocol gives specific criteria for each question for scoring content of self-reported Type A behavior | |
| | Response characteristic of marked Type B behavior | 0 |
| | Response characteristic of predominantly Type B behavior | 1 |
| | Response characteristic of mixed Type A and Type B behaviors | 2 |
| | Response characteristic of predominantly Type A behavior | 3 |
| | Response characteristic of marked Type A behavior | 4 |
| Anger In | Protocol gives specific criteria for each applicable question for scoring reports of suppressed anger | |
| | Very high level of anger | 4 |
| | High level of anger | 3 |
| | Moderate level of anger | 2 |
| | Low level of anger | 1 |
| | No anger | 0 |
| Anger Out | Protocol gives specific criteria for each applicable question for scoring reports of expressed anger | |
| | Very high level of anger | 4 |
| | High level of anger | 3 |
| | Moderate level of anger | 2 |
| | Low level of anger | 1 |
| | No anger | 0 |
| Competitiveness[a] | Interrupts interviewer | |
| | Once during segment | 2 |
| | More than once during segment | 3 |
| | Asks an irrelevant question | 2 |
| | Attempts to reverse roles with interviewer | 3 |
| Hostility[a] | Withholds answer | 1 |
| | Depreciates interviewer | |
| | Indirectly | 3 |
| | Directly | 4 |
| | Voice has hostile tone | 2 |

**TABLE 8.3.** (*Continued*)

| Component | Criteria | Score |
|---|---|---|
| Self-Aggrandizement[a] | Focuses on job responsibility, personal accomplishments, social position, etc. | |
| | Mild degree | 1 |
| | Moderate degree | 2 |
| | Marked degree | 3 |
| | Makes an unqualified pronouncement | 2 |
| Exactingness[a] | Response is unnecessarily detailed | |
| | Mild degree | 1 |
| | Moderate degree | 2 |
| | Marked degree | 3 |
| | Asks a question to provide more structure | 2 |
| Despondency[a] | Mentions a personal limitation or disability | |
| | Mild degree | 1 |
| | Moderate degree | 2 |
| | Marked degree | 3 |
| | Voice has despondent tone | 2 |
| Loudness of Voice[b] | Very soft voice, barely above a whisper | 0 |
| | Soft voice, suggests weakness and fatigue | 1 |
| | Voice of average loudness | 2 |
| | Loud voice, suggests strength and vitality | 3 |
| | Very loud voice, audible strain and discomfort | 4 |
| Syllabic Emphasis[b] | Speech is dynamically flat | 0 |
| | Weak syllabic emphasis | 1 |
| | Average syllabic emphasis | 2 |
| | Strong syllabic emphasis | 3 |
| | Speech is very explosive | 4 |
| Speaking Rate[b] | Very low speaking rate | 0 |
| | Low speaking rate | 1 |
| | Average speaking rate | 2 |
| | High speaking rate | 3 |
| | Very high speaking rate | 4 |
| Acceleration[b] | Almost no acceleration | 0 |
| | Average acceleration | 1 |
| | Moderate acceleration | 2 |
| | Considerable acceleration | 3 |
| | Extreme acceleration | 4 |
| Hard Voice[b] | Has very soft, warm, and melodious voice | 0 |
| | Has soft or warm voice | 1 |
| | Has neutral voice | 2 |
| | Has hard or cold voice | 3 |
| | Has very hard, cold, and monotonous voice | 4 |

[a] For these components, the score is the sum of points (not exceeding 4) assigned to different types and degrees of behaviors occurring in each segment.
[b] Each of these components is associated with specific perceptual criteria that are defined in terms of expert ratings of reference interviews.

WCGS Subject: _____

Rating Date: _____

Rater Number: _____

Column headers (diagonal):

A. Heavy job responsibility
B. High school activities
C. Further education
D. Job level satisfaction
E. Self/spousal assessment
F. Games with children
G. Games with peers
H. Competition at work
I. Other jobs/civic activ.
J. Develop own firms
K. punctuality/waiting
L. Hobbies
M. Slow worker
N. Simultaneous tasks
O. Rapid activities
P. Waiting in restaurant
Q. Thinking while listening
R. Time passing too quickly
S. Slow driver
T. Frequency of anger

| Component | Columns |
|---|---|
| 1. Immediateness | ( 1-20) |
| 2. Type A Content | (21-40) |
| 3. Anger In | (41) |
| 4. Anger Out | (42) 02 |
| 5. Competitiveness | ( 1-20) |
| 6. Hostility | (21-40) |
| 7. Self-Aggrandizement | (41-60) 03 |
| 8. Exactingness | ( 1-20) |
| 9. Despondency | (21-40) |
| 10. Loudness of Voice | (41-44) |
| 11. Syllabic Emphasis | (45-48) |
| 12. Speaking Rate | (49-52) |
| 13. Acceleration | (53-56) |
| 14. Hard Voice | (57-60) 04 |

FIGURE 8.2. Form used for rating Type A components in the Structured Interview, showing matrix of 14 components and 20 interview segments.

## Coronary-Prone Components in the WCGS

The WCGS provided the basis for an investigation of coronary-prone components of the Type A behavior pattern using the component scoring system described in the foregoing paragraphs. As noted previously, an examination of the relationship between Type A components and CHD incidence over the first 4.5 years of the WCGS follow-up was reported on by Matthews, Glass, Rosenman, and Bortner (1977). The original follow-up of the WCGS cohort continued for 8.5 years, and during this time additional subjects developed CHD. The original cohort consisted of 3154 male subjects between 39 and 59 years of age. These subjects were free of CHD at intake in 1960–1961 and were followed prospectively for an average of 8.5 years. The subjects were employed by 10 companies in the state of California and were involved primarily in white-collar occupations. The Structured Interview was administered to the entire sample at intake for assessment of Type A behavior. Global ratings of the behavior pattern were made at intake and yielded approximately equal numbers of Type A and Type B subjects. By 1969, at the end of the 8.5-year follow-up period, 257 subjects had developed clinical manifestations of CHD (i.e., coronary death, electrocardiographically confirmed nonfatal myocardial infarction, or angina pectoris).

The component scoring system described earlier was used to score the Structured Interviews of the men who developed CHD over the 8.5-year follow-up period and a sample of matched controls who did not develop CHD during this period. Of the 257 men developing CHD, recorded interviews for seven subjects were either inaudible or lost, reducing the sample of CHD cases to 250. Each of the 250 cases was matched with two controls selected from the 2897 other original participants in the WCGS. Each matched control was required to have been employed at the same company and have been of the same age as the CHD case at entry. In those rare occurrences where a match of the same age was impossible, a control was chosen who was 1 year younger or older than the case. When more than one subject met these criteria, the two matched controls were selected on the basis of having subject identification numbers numerically closest to the subject number of the case. Thus in summary, 500 control subjects were matched with cases on the basis of company of employment, age, and time of entry into the study. The combined mean age at intake for CHD cases and controls was 48.5. Figure 8.3 illustrates the derivation of this sample from the WCGS cohort. This study of coronary-prone components of the Type A behavior pattern differs from the earlier analysis by Matthews and colleagues (1977) in two ways. First, the sample studied in the current investigation is larger and has a wider age range. Second, the component scoring system developed for this study relies on operationally defined components, whereas the scoring procedure used by Bortner for the earlier study was not documented.

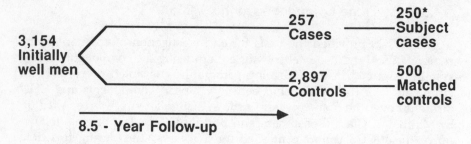

8.5 - Year Follow-up

*Interviews not available on 7 subjects

**FIGURE 8.3.** Source of case-control sample for the study of Type A components and CHD incidence during the 8.5 years of the WCGS follow-up.

Two experienced raters used the component scoring system to evaluate the 750 case and control interviews. The raters had no knowledge of either the identities of CHD cases and controls or the previously determined global rating of the behavior pattern. To minimize possible effects of rater differences and temporal shifts in applying scoring criteria, the three related interviews (one CHD case and two matched controls) were always assigned to the same rater for evaluation during the same week.

A risk analysis using a logistic model was employed to examine the relationship between each of the components and CHD incidence. The results of this analysis are presented in Table 8.4 in terms of relative risks.* The relative risk (*RR*) represents the ratio of CHD incidence for an individual at one standard deviation above the mean value of the component to the incidence of an individual at one standard deviation below the mean. The univariate analysis showed that five components were significantly related to CHD incidence: Hostility (*RR* = 1.92, $p < .001$); Speaking Rate (*RR* = 1.66, $p = .003$); Immediateness (*RR* = 1.62, $p = .009$); Competitiveness (*RR* = 1.5, $p = .013$); and Type A Content (*RR* = 1.38, $p = .045$). These findings indicate that not all of the Type A components, as assessed by the component scoring system, are related to disease. The components found to be related to CHD incidence fall into three groups: a posture toward others that is characterized by hostility and competitiveness, time urgency–impatience, and self-report of Type A behaviors. When the strength of the association between the Type A components and disease incidence was examined, it was evident that the strongest univariate predictor of

---

*Results for Anger In and Anger Out were not included in this analysis. The WCGS data set represents the first systematic application of the Structured Interview, and as such provided only one question directly dealing with anger. Other potentially useful questions did not include sufficient follow-up for assessment of anger expression.

**TABLE 8.4. UNIVARIATE FINDINGS OF THE LOGISTIC ANALYSIS OF BEHAVIORAL COMPONENTS AND CHD INCIDENCE IN THE WESTERN COLLABORATIVE GROUP STUDY**

| Component | Standardized Logistic Coefficient | Standardized Relative Risk | | p Value |
|---|---|---|---|---|
| | | Value | 95% Confidence Interval | |
| Immediateness | .4806 | 1.62 | 1.13–2.32 | .009 |
| Type A Content | .3221 | 1.38 | 1.01–1.89 | .045 |
| Competitiveness | .4039 | 1.50 | 1.09–2.06 | .013 |
| Hostility | .6509 | 1.92 | 1.39–2.65 | <.001 |
| Self-Aggrandizement | .0298 | 1.03 | .74–1.44 | .862 |
| Exactingness | .1870 | 1.21 | .88–1.64 | .237 |
| Despondency | −.2599 | .77 | .55–1.08 | .131 |
| Loudness | .2599 | 1.30 | .94–1.79 | .111 |
| Syllabic Emphasis | .1720 | 1.19 | .83–1.69 | .342 |
| Speaking Rate | .5050 | 1.66 | 1.19–2.30 | .003 |
| Acceleration | −.1099 | .90 | .65–1.23 | .502 |
| Hard Voice | .2438 | 1.28 | .94–1.74 | .121 |

CHD endpoints in the WCGS was hostility, a finding consistent with the previous work associating Type A components with CHD incidence, severity of coronary atherosclerosis, and hyperreactivity.

The relationship between the components and global Type A ratings was also examined. As shown in Table 8.5, all of the components were significantly related to global ratings; however, there were differences in

**TABLE 8.5. SPEARMAN CORRELATION COEFFICIENTS FOR ASSOCIATION OF TYPE A COMPONENTS AND GLOBAL TYPE A RATINGS IN THE WCGS**

| Component | Spearman r | p Value |
|---|---|---|
| Immediateness | .188 | <.001 |
| Type A Content | .323 | <.001 |
| Competitiveness | .230 | <.001 |
| Hostility | .175 | <.001 |
| Self-Aggrandizement | .249 | <.001 |
| Exactingness | .128 | .001 |
| Despondency | −.065 | .077 |
| Loudness of Voice | .317 | <.001 |
| Syllabic Emphasis | .222 | <.001 |
| Speaking Rate | .207 | <.001 |
| Acceleration | .100 | .006 |
| Hard Voice | .202 | <.001 |

the magnitudes of the associations. The largest correlations were Content and Loudness of Voice; the smallest correlations were Despondency and Acceleration. It is of interest that Hostility (with $r = .175$) was not one of the larger correlations. This indicates that the original global Type A ratings in the WCGS did not incorporate the same elements of hostility as does the hostility component in the scoring system used in this reexamination of the WCGS. A modest correlation between component ratings of hostility and global Type A behavior was also observed in two angiography studies (Dembroski et al., 1985; MacDougall et al., 1985); ratings of hostility in the Structured Interview were related to disease severity, while global ratings of Type A behavior were not. In the component scoring system used here, the conceptualization of hostility is similar to that used by Dembroski and colleagues (1985). Specifically, hostility is viewed as a predisposition to respond directly and indirectly to challenge with various kinds and intensities of anger and related mood states, including irritation and annoyance, disgust, resentment, and frustration.

## CURRENT STATUS AND FUTURE DIRECTIONS

The present findings build on the growing evidence in the literature that the Type A behavior pattern consists of coronary-prone components, such as hostility, and more benign components, such as loud and explosive speech. To identify target behaviors for intervention or to interpret findings from Type A research, and to resolve inconsistencies in the literature with regard to the relationship between Type A behavior and disease, it is essential that the benign and coronary-prone components of Type A behavior be differentiated and evaluated separately.

The Type A behavior pattern is a complex syndrome consisting of components that can be differentiated and examined statistically for their independent relationships to CHD. Among these components, hostility has emerged as having the strongest relationship to coronary heart disease endpoints in a number of studies and is receiving considerable attention. In some arenas, it appears that hostility is being promoted as the *only* coronary-prone characteristic of interest. In this regard, it is important to note that another component of Type A behavior—competitiveness—appears across the research to be of significance. Moreover, in the most recent analysis of the WCGS case-control data set, two measures related to time urgency (speaking rate and immediateness) also predicted endpoints. Further research is needed to evaluate the potential interactions among these coronary-prone components. For example, it may be that the potential for hostility is expressed in the presence of time urgency. This association is consistent with the common description of the context in which hostility is experienced. Specifically, it is common for the Type A individual who scores high on measures of the hostility component to report that his experience of anger, irritation, or annoyance "depends on the situation" and, in particular, that it depends on whether or not he is in a hurry.

Another important area for future research involves examining components of Type A behavior, particularly hostility and competitiveness, in groups other than White males. With few exceptions, the research reported on in this chapter has focused exclusively on men. The extent to which the relationships observed between hostility and CHD endpoints will be found in females, minority groups, and blue-collar working males is not established. The angiographic studies at Duke University (Blumenthal et al., 1978; Williams et al., 1980) included women and showed a similar relationship to that observed in males, suggesting that, like Type A behavior, these coronary-prone behaviors are relevant for males and females. However, specific information about the expression of coronary-prone behavior in women is lacking. This information definitely is needed, given that heart disease is the leading cause of death for adult females, as it is for adult males.

Yet another important area for future research focuses directly on hostility. The problems that have existed in the Type A literature and that were discussed previously in this chapter involved the need for objective measurement strategies and conceptual disentangling of the multidimensional nature of Type A behavior. Unfortunately, the construct of hostility presents many of the same problems. It is a vaguely defined construct that lacks a consensual definition. It can be referred to as a personality trait or as a predisposition to respond to challenge with anger. Measurement of hostility and its related constructs needs to distinguish between anger and hostility as moods or behaviors, and between the experience of anger and hostility and the expression and intensity of these feelings. Fortunately, what we have learned in developing operational definitions to examine components of Type A behavior may be beneficial as we grapple with the new coronary-prone behavior of hostility and its possible correlates, competitiveness and time urgency.

## REFERENCES

Allen, T. A., Lawler, K. A., Matthews, K. A., & Rakaczky, C. J. (1984). Speech stylistic components of the Structured Interview and cardiovascular reactivity in college males. *Psychophysiology, 21*, 567.

Anderson, N. B., Williams, R. B., Jr., Lane, J. D., & Monou, H. (1984). The relationship between hostility and cardiovascular reactivity following a mild harassment intervention. *Psychophysiology, 21*, 568.

Barefoot, J. C., Dahlstrom, W. G., & Williams, R. B. (1983). Hostility, CHD incidence, and total mortality: A 25-year follow-up study of 255 physicians. *Psychosomatic Medicine, 45*, 59–63.

Bass, C., & Wade, C. (1982). Type A behavior: Not specifically pathogenic? *Lancet, 2*, 1147– 1150.

Blumenthal, J. A., Williams, R., Kong, Y., Schanberg, S. M., & Thompson, L. W. (1978). Type A behavior and angiographically documented coronary disease. *Circulation, 58,* 634–639.

Byrne, D. G., Rosenman, R. H., Schiller, E., & Chesney, M. A. (1985). Consistency and variation among instruments purporting to measure the Type A behavior pattern. *Psychosomatic Medicine, 47,* 242–261.

Case, R. B., Heller, S. S., Case, N. B., Moss, A. J., & the Multicenter Post-Infarction Research Group (1985). Type A behavior and survival after acute myocardial infarction. *The New England Journal of Medicine, 312,* 737–741.

Chesney, M. A., Eagleston, J. E., & Rosenman, R. H. (1980). The Type A Structured Interview: A behavioral assessment in the rough. *Journal of Behavioral Medicine, 2,* 255–272.

Cook, W. W., & Medley, D. M. (1954). Proposed hostility and pharisaic-virtue scales for the MMPI. *Journal of Applied Psychology, 38,* 414–418.

Dembroski, T. M., MacDougall, J. M., & Lushene, R. (1979). Interpersonal interaction and cardiovascular responses in Type A subjects and coronary patients. *Journal of Human Stress, 5,* 28–36.

Dembroski, T. M., MacDougall, J. M., Shields, J. L., Petitto, J., & Lushene, R. (1978). Components of the Type A coronary-prone behavior pattern and cardiovascular responses to psychomotor performance challenge. *Journal of Behavioral Medicine, 1,* 159–176.

Dembroski, T. M., MacDougall, J. M., Williams, R. B., Haney, T., & Blumenthal, J. A. (1985). Components of Type A, hostility, and anger-in: Relationship to angiographic findings. *Psychosomatic Medicine, 47,* 219–233.

Dimsdale, J. E., Hackett, T. P., Block, P. C., & Hutter, A. M. (1978). Type A personality and extent of coronary atherosclerosis. *American Journal of Cardiology, 42,* 583–586.

Dimsdale, J. E., Hackett, T. P., & Hutter, A. M. (1979). Type A behavior and angiographic findings. *Journal of Psychosomatic Research, 23,* 273–276.

Dunbar, H. F. (1943). *Psychosomatic diagnosis.* New York: Hoeber.

Feldstein, S., Siegman, A. W., Barkley, S. E., Simpson, S., & Kobren, R. (1984). Judged and actual speech rates as indices of coronary prone behavior. *Behavioral Medicine Update, 6,* 29.

Frank, K. A., Heller, S. S., Kornfeld, D. S., Sporn, A. A., & Weiss, M. B. (1978). Type A behavior pattern and coronary angiographic findings. *Journal of the American Medical Association, 240,* 761–763.

French-Belgian Collaborative Group (1982). Ischemic heart disease and psychological patterns. *Advances in Cardiology, 29,* 25–31.

Friedman, M., Manwaring, J. H., Rosenman, R. H., Donlon, G., Ortega, P., & Grube, S. M. (1973). Instantaneous and sudden deaths: Clinical and pathological differentiation in coronary artery disease. *Journal of the American Medical Association, 225,* 1319–1328.

Gertler, M. M., & White, P. D. (1954). *Coronary heart disease in young adults.* Cambridge, MA: Harvard University Press.

Glass, D. C., Lake, C. R., Contrada, R. J., Kehoe, K., & Erlanger, L. R. (1983). Stability of individual differences in physiological responses to stress. *Health Psychology, 2,* 317–341.

Haynes, S. G., Feinleib, M., & Kannel, W. B. (1980). The relationship of psychosocial factors to coronary heart disease in the Framingham Study: III. Eight-year incidence of coronary heart disease. *American Journal of Epidemiology, 111,* 37–58.

Hecker, M. H. L., Chesney, M. A., Black, G. W., & Rosenman, R. H. (1981). Speech analysis of Type A behavior. In J. K. Darby (Ed.), *Speech evaluation in medicine.* New York: Grune & Stratton.

Jacobs, D. R. Jr., & Schucker, B. (1981). Type A behavior pattern, speech, and coronary heart disease. In J. K. Darby (Ed.), *Speech evaluation in medicine.* New York: Grune & Stratton.

Jenkins, C. D., Rosenman, R. H., & Friedman, M. (1966). Components of the Type A behavior pattern: Their relation to silent myocardial infarction and blood lipids. *Journal of Chronic Diseases, 19,* 599–609.

Kemple, C. (1945). Rorschach method and psychosomatic diagnosis: Personality traits of patients with rheumatic disease, hypertension, cardiovascular disease, coronary occlusion and fracture. *Psychosomatic Medicine, 7,* 85–89.

Kornitzer, M., Magotteau, V., Degre, C., Kittel, F., Struyven, J., & van Thiel, E. (1982). Angiographic findings and the Type A pattern assessed by means of the Bortner scale. *Journal of Behavioral Medicine, 5,* 313–320.

Krantz, D. S., Schaeffler, M. A., Davia, J. E., Dembroski, T. M., MacDougall, J. M., & Schaffer, R. T. (1981). Extent of coronary atherosclerosis, Type A behavior, and cardiovascular response to social interaction. *Psychophysiology, 18,* 654–664.

MacDougall, J. M., Dembroski, T. M., Dimsdale, J. E., & Hackett, T. P. (1985). Components of Type A, hostility, and anger-in: Further relationships to angiographic findings. *Health Psychology, 4,* 137–152.

Matthews, K. A., Glass, D. C., Rosenman, R. H., & Bortner, R. W. (1977). Competitive drive, Pattern A, and coronary heart disease: A further analysis of some data from the Western Collaborative Group Study. *Journal of Chronic Diseases, 30,* 489–498.

Matthews, K. A., & Haynes, S. G. (1986). Type A behavior pattern and coronary risk: Update and critical evaluation. *American Journal of Epidemiology, 123,* 923–960.

McCranie, D. W., Watkins, L. O., Brandsma, J. M., & Sisson, B. D. (1986). Hostility, coronary heart disease (CHD) incidence, and total mortality: Lack of association in a 25-year follow-up study of 478 physicians. *Journal of Behavioral Medicine, 9,* 119–125.

Megargee, E. I. (1985). The dynamics of aggression and their application to cardiovascular disorders. In M. A. Chesney & R. H. Rosenman (Eds.), *Anger and hostility in cardiovascular and behavioral disorders.* New York: Hemisphere.

Menninger, K. A., & Menninger, W. C. (1936). Psychoanalytic observations in cardiac disorders. *American Heart Journal, 11,* 10.

Osler, W. (1892). *Lectures on angina pectoris and allied states.* New York: Appleton.

Powell, L. H., & Thoresen, C. E. (1985). Behavioral and physiologic determinants of long-term prognosis after myocardial infarction. *Journal of Chronic Diseases, 38,* 253–263.

Review Panel on Coronary-Prone Behavior and Coronary Heart Disease (1981). Coronary-prone behavior and coronary heart disease: A critical review. *Circulation, 63,* 1199–1215.

Rosenman, R. H. (1978). The interview method of assessment of the coronary-prone behavior pattern. In T. M. Dembroski, S. M. Weiss, J. L. Shields, S. G. Haynes, & M. Feinleib (Eds.), *Coronary-prone behavior.* New York: Springer-Verlag.

Rosenman, R. H., Brand, R. J., Jenkins, D., Friedman, M., Straus, R., & Wurm, M. (1975). Coronary heart disease in the Western Collaborative Group Study: Final follow-up experience of 8½ years. *Journal of the American Medical Association, 233,* 872–877.

Rosenman, R. H., Brand, R. J., Sholtz, R. I., & Friedman, M. (1976). Multivariate prediction of coronary heart disease during 8.5 year follow-up in the Western Collaborative Group Study. *American Journal of Cardiology, 37,* 903–910.

Rosenman, R. H., & Chesney, M. A. (1985). Type A behavior pattern: Its relationship to coronary heart disease and its modification by behavioral and pharmacological approaches. In M. R. Zales (Ed.), *Stress in health and disease.* New York: Brunner/Mazel.

Rosenman, R. H., & Friedman, M. (1959). The possible relationship of the emotions to clinical coronary heart disease. In G. Pincus (Ed.), *Hormones and atherosclerosis.* New York: Academic.

Rosenman, R. H., Friedman, M., Straus, R., Jenkins, C. D., Zyzanski, S. J., & Wurm, M. (1970). Coronary heart disease in the Western Collaborative Group Study: A follow-up experience of 4½ years. *Journal of Chronic Diseases, 23,* 173–190.

Rosenman, R. H., Friedman, M., Straus, R., Wurm, M., Kositchek, R., Hahn, W., & Werthessen, N. T. (1964). A predictive study of coronary heart disease: The Western Collaborative Group Study. *Journal of the American Medical Association, 189,* 113–120.

Scherwitz, L., Berton, K., & Leventhal, H. (1977). Type A assessment and interaction in the behavior pattern interview. *Psychosomatic Medicine, 39,* 229–240.

Scherwitz, L., Graham, L. E., Grandits, G., Buehler, J., & Billings, J. (1986). Self-involvement and coronary heart disease incidence in the Multiple Risk Factor Intervention Trial. *Psychosomatic Medicine, 48,* 187–199.

Scherwitz, L., McKelvain, R., Laman, C., Patterson, J., Dutton, L., Yusim, S., Lester, J., Kraft, I., Rochelle, D., & Leachman, R. (1983). Type A behavior, self-involvement, and coronary atherosclerosis. *Psychosomatic Medicine, 45,* 47–57.

Schucker, B., & Jacobs, D. R., Jr. (1977). Assessment of behavioral risk for coronary disease by voice characteristics. *Psychosomatic Medicine, 39,* 219–228.

Shekelle, R. B., Gale, M., & Norusis, M. (in press). Type A score (Jenkins Activity Survey) and risk of recurrent coronary heart disease in the Aspirin Myocardial Infarction Study. *American Journal of Cardiology.*

Shekelle, R. B., Gale, M., Ostfeld, A. M., & Paul, O. (1983). Hostility, risk of coronary heart disease, and mortality. *Psychosomatic Medicine, 45,* 109–114.

Shekelle, R. B., Hulley, S. B., Neaton, J. D., Billings, J. H., Borhani, N. O., Gerace, T. A., Jacobs, D. R., Lasser, N. L., Mittlemark, M. B., & Stamler, J., for the Multiple Risk Factor Intervention Trial Research Group (1985). The MRFIT behavior pattern study, Type A behavior and incidence of coronary heart disease. *American Journal of Epidemiology, 122,* 559–570.

Williams, R. B., Haney, T. L., Lee, K. L., Kong, Y., Blumenthal, J. A., & Whalen, R. E. (1980). Type A behavior, hostility, and coronary atherosclerosis. *Psychosomatic Medicine, 42,* 539–549.

Zyzanski, S. J., Jenkins, C. D., Ryan, T. J., Flessas, A., & Everist, M. (1976). Psychological correlates of coronary angiographic findings. *Archives of Internal Medicine, 136,* 1234–1237.

# 9

## Coronary-Prone Behavior: The Emerging Role of the Hostility Complex

REDFORD B. WILLIAMS, JR. AND JOHN C. BAREFOOT

## INTRODUCTION

The notion that states of mind might contribute to afflictions of the heart is by no means a modern conception. Throughout recorded history careful observers have noted that various behaviors, emotions, and personality attributes appear to be associated with alterations in cardiovascular function as well as with manifestations of coronary heart disease (CHD). In 1628 William Harvey observed, "A mental disturbance provoking pain, excessive joy, hope or anxiety extends to the heart, where it affects its temper, and rate, impairing general nutrition and vigor" (1628/1928, p.

Preparation of this paper was supported in part by grants from the National Heart, Lung, and Blood Institute (HL-18589, HL-22740, and HL-36587), the National Institute of Mental Health (MH-70482), and the John D. and Catherine T. MacArthur Foundation

106). The eminent eighteenth century physician John Hunter asserted, "My life is in the hands of any rascal who chooses to annoy or tease me" (Stephen & Lee, 1975, p. 290). And it was, because he died suddenly after a heated argument at a hospital board meeting! In an oft-quoted passage, Sir William Osler described the typical coronary patient as "not the delicate, neurotic person . . . but the robust, the vigorous in mind and body, the keen and ambitious man, the indicator of whose engine is always at 'full speed ahead' " (1910, p. 839).

Such observations as these have led naturally to the impression that psychological and behavioral factors play a causal role in the pathogenesis of CHD. This was the state of affairs when, spurred by their own clinical experience and the realization that the traditional "physical" risk factors (e.g., smoking, hypertension, and hyperlipidemia) predict fewer than half the new cases of CHD, Meyer Friedman and Ray Rosenman coined the term *Type A behavior pattern* (TABP) to denote a constellation of behaviors that characterized most of their patients with CHD (Friedman & Rosenman, 1974). Persons displaying the fully developed TABP were characterized by high levels of competitive achievement striving, incessant time-urgent behavior that led to persistent acceleration of physical or mental activity, and high levels of free-floating hostility.

Friedman and Rosenman knew it unlikely the medical community would accept their hypothesized involvement of TABP in the pathogenesis of CHD solely on the basis of their clinical impressions. To make their case, they undertook a prospective epidemiologic study, the Western Collaborative Group Study (WCGS), of more than 3000 middle-aged men who were healthy at intake into the study. To provide a valid and reliable means of assessing TABP, they developed the Structured Interview (SI), which relies more on the presence of emphatic and vigorous voice stylistics than it does on the content of responses as the major criteria in TABP designation (Dembroski & MacDougall, 1985; Friedman, Brown, & Rosenman, 1969; Schucker & Jacobs, 1977).

About one-half of the WCGS subjects were classified as Type A at intake; the remainder, who did not display the constellation of behaviors making up the TABP, were classified as Type B. After following up the WCGS men for 8.5 years, Rosenman and colleagues (1975) reported that the Type A subjects were about twice as likely as the Type B's to show clinical manifestations of CHD. This increased CHD risk among the Type A men remained significant after multivariate statistical adjustment for the traditional risk factors.

The WCGS results constituted the first solid epidemiologic evidence that TABP is an independent CHD risk factor. Subsequent research found increased coronary atherosclerosis (CAD) among Type A subjects, whether verified by autopsy in the WCGS (Friedman, Rosenman, Straus, Wurm, & Kositchek, 1968) or by coronary angiography by independent research groups (Blumenthal, Williams, Kong, Schanberg, & Thompson, 1978; Frank,

Heller, Kornfeld, Sporn, & Weiss, 1978; Zyzanski, Jenkins, Ryan, Flessas, & Everist, 1975). This body of research findings led an independent group of scientists convened by the NHLBI (Review Panel on Coronary-Prone Behavior, 1981) to conclude that TABP was associated with increased risk for CHD over and above that conferred by the traditional physical risk factors. The panel further concluded that the increased CHD risk attributable to TABP is of "the same order of magnitude as the relative risk associated with any of these [traditional risk] factors" (p. 1199).

At this point it appeared that the medical community had for the first time acknowledged a psychosocial factor as a bona fide CHD risk factor. Almost immediately, however, negative findings began to emerge from a series of studies, causing many to question whether the panel's conclusions may not have been premature. As a result, the current state of affairs with respect to research on coronary-prone behavior may best be described as one of confusion. The TABP hypothesis appears less robust now than it did at the time of the panel's meeting in 1978 (Shekelle, Hulley, et al., 1985).

To bring some order to this confusion, as well as to provide some indication of where research on coronary-prone behavior is heading, the remainder of this chapter will address the following issues: (1) implications of the negative TABP studies; (2) the emergence of the hostility complex* as the sole "toxic" aspect of the globally defined TABP; and (3) recent evidence regarding biological mechanisms whereby coronary-prone behavior is translated into disease.

## NEGATIVE STUDIES: WHITHER THE TABP HYPOTHESIS?

Recent studies that have failed to find significant associations between TABP and various indices of CHD fall into two general categories: prospective epidemiological studies and cross-sectional studies of patients undergoing coronary angiography.

---

*At the present time there is probably no single term that adequately describes all the aspects of hostility and related constructs that appear relevant to coronary-prone behavior. As review in this chapter will make clearer, important aspects include a cynical mistrust of others, a contemptuous dislike of others, and a tendency to express these negative feelings overtly. Rather than risking premature closure as to which aspects of hostility should be included in the construct of coronary-prone behavior, we have chosen to use the term *hostility complex* to denote a set of related constructs that appear to be important aspects of coronary-prone behavior, much as the term *Type A* was originally used to describe a constellation of related behavioral tendencies. Just as recent research shows that the hostility complex is a more specific descriptor of coronary-prone behavior than Type A behavior, it is likely that future research will produce findings that indicate which aspects of the hostility complex are most relevant, thus leading eventually to the most specific and sensitive descriptive term for coronary-prone behavior.

With only a few exceptions (see Matthews & Haynes, 1986, for a review), TABP whether assessed by the SI or the Jenkins Activity Survey (JAS; Jenkins, 1967), has failed to predict new or recurrent CHD events in prospective epidemiological studies, particularly in samples that, for one reason or another, are at increased risk of developing CHD. Neither SI nor JAS assessments predicted CHD events or mortality among CHD-free subjects with multiple risk factors in the large-scale and carefully executed MRFIT study (Shekelle, Hulley, et al., 1985). JAS-assessed TABP also failed to predict recurrent CHD events in post-MI patients in two studies (Case, Heller, Case, & Moss, 1985; Shekelle, Gale & Norusis, 1985). While these populations differ from the original WCGS sample in being at higher risk of CHD at intake, they do raise serious doubts that Type A behavior is the best we can do in defining coronary-prone behavior.

Turning to studies of angiographic patient samples, the picture has been equally bleak since the original positive findings. Of 10 subsequent studies, only a single study (Williams et al., 1980), using the SI to assess TABP, found an unequivocal positive relationship between TABP and CAD severity. The remaining 9 studies (see Matthews & Haynes, 1986, for a detailed review of these studies) failed to find a significant TABP–CAD association.

Possible reasons for this paucity of positive findings in post-1978 angiographic studies are suggested by the results of a recent, comprehensive multivariate analysis of data on 2289 angiographic patients who were evaluated at Duke University Medical Center (Williams et al., 1986). JAS-assessed TABP was unrelated to CAD severity in this sample. On the other hand, when the SI assessment was used, significant positive TABP–CAD association was found, but only among the younger patients. Among patients older than 55, there was a reversal of this association, with Type B patients having significantly more severe CAD. This reversal is interpreted as reflecting a survival effect: Among the older patients, there may be fewer Type A's with severe CAD due to development of disease among Type A's at an earlier age, leading them to be no longer available for study. The presence of a positive Type A effect only among the younger patients was paralleled by a similar diminution in effect size for both smoking and hyperlipidemia in the older patients of this study. As we shall describe, similar survival effects have been invoked to explain age differentials in risk factor effects in prospective epidemiological studies.

These findings help to explain why so many of the angiographic studies just referred to have been negative. First, none took age into account. Thus the reversal of the TABP–CAD relationship among older patients could well have obscured a positive finding among younger patients. Second, even in the younger patients in the large Duke sample of over 2000 patients, the size of the TABP–CAD association was small, far smaller, in fact, than the smoking or hyperlipidemia effects. A power analysis based on the TABP effect size in the Duke sample showed that, even if the negative studies had been limited to younger patients, the 7 negative studies with sample sizes of 150 or less would have had a statistical power of only 17 percent to detect a real TABP–CAD relationship. Finally, the 2 remaining negative angiographic studies with larger sample sizes both used questionnaire-based methods to assess TABP. As noted earlier, even in the large Duke sample, the most highly regarded questionnaire method, the JAS, failed to correlate with CAD severity.

Taken altogether, the considerations just listed indicate that the negative angiographic studies cannot be accepted as adequate tests of the null hypothesis that TABP is not related to angiographically documented CAD severity. Nevertheless, the fact remains that even in the large Duke sample the size of the TABP effect is relatively small. Even though TABP does appear associated with more severe CAD among younger angiographic patients, the size of this association is so small that its clinical significance might be questioned.

From this review of the recent negative evidence, it appears reasonable to conclude that we can probably do better than the globally defined TABP in arriving at a definition of coronary-prone behavior. This conclusion is strengthened considerably if one considers that there may be an important distinction between the concepts of TABP and coronary-prone behavior. Thus not all aspects of the multifaceted TABP may be coronary prone, just as not all components of the total serum cholesterol confer increased CHD risk. If only certain aspects of the multidimensional TABP are "toxic," then assessment of the global TABP will provide a measure that contains a considerable amount of "noise" in addition to the coronary-prone "signal." A growing body of recent research in which different aspects of the global TABP have been assessed using various methods and related to CHD endpoints suggests specific improvements in the working definition of coronary-prone behavior.

## THE EMERGENCE OF THE HOSTILITY COMPLEX

The first clue that some aspects of the global TABP are more coronary prone than others came when 62 new CHD cases in the WCGS were compared with 124 symptom-free men using a components rating system for the SI developed by Dr. Ray Bortner (Matthews, Glass, Rosenman, & Bortner, 1977). The best discriminator between cases and controls was the SI-defined potential for hostility, followed by anger directed outward, competitiveness, experience of anger more than once per week, vigorous answers, irritation at waiting in lines, and explosive voice modulation. Most of these attributes are probably significantly intercorrelated and appear to represent aspects of the hostility complex. Multivariate analyses were not performed on these data, however, so it is impossible to say now whether the hostility–anger measures were accounting for all the significant variance in behavioral differences between cases and controls.

Based on Matthews and colleagues' (1977) findings, the long-standing interest in hostility and anger expression in the pathogenesis of CHD (Diamond, 1982), and the repeated conceptual emphasis Friedman and Rosenman (1974) have placed on hostility aspects of the TABP, there has been increased research focused in the past several years on hostility and related aspects of the TABP, which for descriptive purposes are herein termed the hostility complex. This research, which we shall describe, provides strong support for the hypothesis that the hostility complex reflects the major and probably the only aspect of the global TABP that is coronary prone.

The research linking aspects of the hostility complex with various CHD endpoints can be grouped into two categories, based on the assessment approaches used: (1) questionnaire-based approaches, especially those using the Cook and Medley (1954) Hostility (Ho) scale from the MMPI; and (2) SI-based approaches to the measurement of potential for hostility (PoHo), components of hostility, and anger-coping styles. As will become evident, the findings from these two lines of research are complementary and, taken together, lead to a much clearer definition of at least one aspect of coronary-prone behavior, namely, the hostility complex.

## EVIDENCE OBTAINED USING THE COOK-MEDLEY HO SCALE

More than 10 years ago, the Duke research group began to collect, in addition to the SI- and JAS-based TABP measures, MMPI and other psychosocial data on nearly all patients referred for diagnostic coronary angiography. Guided by the considerations reviewed earlier in this chapter, as well as by preliminary indications (Blumenthal & Williams, unpublished data) that Ho scores are positively correlated with CAD severity, they evaluated the relationship between CAD severity and both SI-based assessment of TABP and MMPI-based Ho scores (Williams et al., 1980). Both TABP and Ho scores were found to be significantly related to CAD severity in a sample of 424 male and female patients. The effect size was larger, however, for Ho scores. While Type A patients were 1.27 times more likely than non-A's to have a clinically significant arterial occlusion, those patients with high Ho scores were 1.46 times more likely to have significant disease than patients with low Ho scores. Multivariate analyses showed that, when gender and TABP were controlled, the significance of the Ho–CAD association became stronger, while control for Ho scores and gender resulted in a weakening of the significance of the TABP–CAD association.

These findings have several implications regarding which aspects of TABP are coronary prone. Recall that evidence reviewed earlier in this chapter clearly indicated that questionnaire-based measures of the *global TABP* are inferior to the SI-based assessment in correlating with any indices of CHD. Yet the questionnaire-based Ho measure shows a stronger effect size in relating to CAD than the SI-based TABP categorization in Williams and colleagues' (1980) study. It seems unlikely that any questionnaire could assess as well as direct observation during the SI the emotional overtones, exaggerated psychomotor mannerisms, and vigorous voice stylistics considered essential features of the TABP (Rosenman, in press). Therefore, the finding of a stronger effect size for Ho scores suggests that these motor behaviors may not be crucial aspects of the TABP with respect to coronary proneness. Moreover, if even a questionnaire-based measure of the hostility complex correlates more strongly with CAD than the SI-based assessment of the global TABP, it would indicate that the hostility complex reflects the only aspect of the global TABP that is coronary prone.

It is important to note here that the Ho scale should not be viewed as a measure of the global TABP. It does not necessarily bear any direct relationship to the time urgency and competitive achievement striving aspects of the TABP. Rather, it reflects only that aspect of the TABP related to the hostility complex. It is not surprising, therefore, that Ho scores have been found to be only weakly, albeit significantly, correlated with SI assessments of the global TABP (Williams, Barefoot, & Shekelle, 1985). Ho scores are more strongly correlated, however, with SI-based assessments of potential for hostility (Dembroski, MacDougall, Williams, Haney, & Blumenthal, 1985).

Further evidence that the Ho scale is measuring an aspect of the hostility complex that is coronary prone is provided by findings from two prospective epidemiological studies that were stimulated by Williams and colleagues' (1980) finding of a Ho–CAD association. Shekelle, Gale, Ostfeld, and Paul (1983) reported a significant prediction of increased 10-year CHD event rates as a function of higher Ho scores among the 1877 middle-aged (mean age = 45) males who originally completed the MMPI in the Western Electric Study more than 20 years ago. Barefoot, Dahlstrom, and Williams (1983) found a four-to-five-fold higher CHD event rate over a 25-year follow-up period in those with higher Ho scores among 255 physicians who had completed the MMPI during a medical school clerkship 25 years previously (when their mean age was 25).

Thus higher Ho scores were not only found to be correlated with more severe CAD in a cross-sectional study, but were also predictive of increased CHD rates in both young and middle-aged men over follow-up periods of 10 to 25 years. The effect size for CHD events' prediction by Ho scores was larger in the physician study than among the Western Electric Study participants, suggesting action of survival effects. If those with high Ho scores are dying or developing chronic disease at a younger age, then men with high Ho scores who survive to middle age likely represent a biologically hardier group than a sample of young men with high Ho scores, who have not yet been affected by survival effects. Even more strongly indicative of such survival effects, the effect size for prediction of all-cause mortality by higher Ho scores was also larger in the physician study.

Additional evidence of the action of such survival effects with respect to behavior–disease relationships comes from a recently reported analysis of long-term outcome data from the WCGS (Ragland, Brand, & Rosenman,

1986). In contrast to the significant prediction of CHD events by TABP during the initial 8.5 years of follow-up in the WCGS, during the years subsequent to that period TABP did not predict CHD events. More detailed analyses showed that the size of the TABP effect diminished across the later years of follow-up. This diminution in effect size is again suggestive of a survival effect: Surviving Type A men are biologically hardier due to dropout of more biologically vulnerable Type A men during the earlier years of follow-up. Similar explanations have been advanced to explain the diminution of the smoking–CHD relationship among older groups (Dawber, 1980), and it should surprise no one to find similar survival effects occurring with respect to TABP– and Ho–CHD relationships.

In both the Western Electric and physician studies, the relationship of Ho scores to both CHD and mortality outcomes appeared nonlinear, with no further increase in risk once an apparent "threshold" Ho score was exceeded. However, in a prospective study of 118 lawyers followed up 25 years after completing the MMPI while in law school, a significant *linear* relationship has been found between Ho scores and all-cause mortality (Barefoot, Williams, Dahlstrom, & Dodge, 1987). Interestingly, the all-cause mortality risk ratio in this much smaller sample was comparable (five-fold higher mortality rate in high vs. low Ho scorers) to that observed earlier in the physician study. While the apparent absence of a dose–response relationship between Ho scores and health outcomes in all but one study may be of some concern, it is important to recall that SI-defined TABP did not show a dose–response effect in the WCGS.

Before concluding this section on the Ho scale, it is important to note that one study, comparable in most respects to Barefoot, Dahlstrom, and Williams's (1983) study, has failed to find Ho scores predicting adverse health outcomes. This study involved a sample of 478 physicians followed up 25 years after they completed the MMPI while visiting the Medical College of Georgia (MCG) for their admission interviews (McCranie, Watkins, Brandsma, & Sisson, 1986). In Barefoot and colleagues' (1983) study, the students completed the MMPI as a class exercise during their psychiatry clerkships and were told that the results would not affect their grades, but would be used for research purposes only. In contrast, the MCG physicians completed the MMPI as part of the application process during a visit for interviews that would play a key role in determining whether they were admitted to medical school. Not surprisingly, Ho scores were unusually low in the MCG sample, which is consistent with the idea that evaluation apprehensiveness in the MCG sample stimulated the subjects to give more socially desirable responses on the MMPI. Thus the validity of the MCG MMPI data must be questioned, and the failure to replicate the earlier Ho results cannot be accepted as a valid test of the null hypothesis with respect to Ho–disease effects.

McCranie and colleagues' (1986) study does serve the useful purpose, however, of documenting how the conditions under which any assessment tool is administered can exert a profound influence upon that tool's validity. Thus when evaluation apprehensiveness is aroused by the test conditions, responses on a self-report instrument can be so affected as to render them useless in measuring the construct the tool was designed to assess. It might also be surmised that, had the MCG subjects been evaluated using the SI under the same conditions, even their "overt" behavioral responses would likely have been more guarded. It is important to note, however, that this problem is not unique to psychobehavioral assessment tools. A glucose tolerance test or a lipid panel obtained after the ingestion of a large fatty meal would be a no more valid measure of carbohydrate or lipid metabolism than the MMPI is of psychological traits when given to medical school applicants.

What is the nature of the psychological characteristic(s) measured by the Ho scale? First of all, it appears to be a very stable trait, with test–retest correlations of .84, and .85 in Shekelle and colleagues' (1983) and Barefoot and colleagues' (1983) studies, respectively. A growing body of research suggests that many of the Ho scale items might be more accurately described as indicants of cynicism, since they reflect a general distrust of human nature and motives. This description is supported by the emergence of a major Cynicism factor from factor analyses of the Ho scale (Costa, Zonderman, McCrae, & Williams, 1986), as well as of the entire MMPI item set (Costa, Zonderman, McCrae, & Williams, 1985; Johnson, Butcher, Null, & Johnson, 1984). In a large-scale study of the construct validity of the Ho scale, Smith and Frohm (1985) conclude that "the scale primarily assesses suspiciousness, resentment, frequent anger and cynical distrust of others rather than overtly aggressive behavior or general emotional distress" (p. 503). They also found that persons with high Ho scores report more anger, less hardiness, more frequent and severe hassles, and fewer and less satisfactory social supports. Thus the terms *cynical mistrust* (Costa et al., 1986) and *cynical hostility* (Smith & Frohm, 1985) have been proposed as more accurate descriptors than *hostility* of the psychological characteristic measured by the Ho scale.

Very recent research by Barefoot and colleagues (1987) suggests that a subset of Ho scale items reflecting cynical mistrust of people in general and the tendency to respond to frustration with increased experience and expression of anger is a stronger predictor of all-cause mortality than the entire 50-item Ho score. In contrast, items reflecting the attitude that others' bad behavior is directed personally toward the respondent were not predictive. These results suggest that, just as the components scoring approach to TABP using the SI has uncovered more specific correlates of CHD severity, it is likely that further attempts to refine self-report measures of the hostility complex will lead to better measures of coronary-prone behavior.

Taken together, the findings obtained using the Ho scale appear quite consistent and suggest that it is measuring a trait that has "a broad effect on survival" (Shekelle et al., 1983, p. 114). Its consistent correlation with

CAD and prediction of increased CHD risk are strong indications that the Ho scale is measuring an important aspect of coronary-prone behavior. At the same time, Ho scores have been even stronger predictors of mortality due to any cause. A task for future research will be to determine whether some subset of Ho items (e.g., as in Barefoot et al., 1987) or some combination of Ho scores with other measures (e.g., as in Albright, King, Taylor, Haskell, & DeBusk, 1986; or Weidner, Sexton, McLellarn, Matarazzo, & Conner, 1986) will produce a more specific index of coronary-prone behavior. If not, then we will be left with the conclusion that the trait measured by the Ho scale is a general risk factor for a wide variety of adverse health outcomes, the precise natures of which are likely to be due to underlying biological predispositions in each individual. If such turns out to be the case, it should not come as any great surprise, nor should it be too disturbing to anyone, because both smoking and hyperlipidemia are also "nonspecific" risk factors—both predict increased risk of CHD and cancer in most populations studied to date.

Whatever the outcome of future research, the prediction of adverse health outcomes, including CHD, by the Ho scale has now been firmly established in several prospective studies, and its effect size (four- to five-fold higher risk of CHD events and six-fold higher risk of dying, with an absolute mortality rate of 14 percent, in young physicians with high Ho scores; and a similar effect size in young lawyers) is comparable to that associated with the presence of all three "physical" risk factors combined (Aravanis, 1983; Blackburn, 1983; Keys, 1970; Pooling Project Research Group, 1978). Thus the Ho scale must be considered a robust indicator of coronary-prone as well as of "mortality-prone" behavior. Further research to uncover the psychological and physiological mechanisms underlying the Ho scale's predictive capacity will likely prove useful in efforts to understand better the nature of coronary-prone behavior and, ultimately, to devise effective measures for prevention and treatment.

## EVIDENCE OBTAINED USING SI-BASED ASSESSMENTS OF HOSTILITY

Another useful approach in refining our understanding of coronary-prone aspects of the global TABP has been to use the SI as a means of assessing separately the various attributes contained in both the conceptual and operational definitions of the TABP. Derived from the original components scoring approach developed by Bortner and applied in Matthews and colleagues' (1977) study, this scoring system has been developed further by Dembroski and coworkers (see Dembroski, 1978; Dembroski & Mac-Dougall, 1983, 1985) and provides for ratings of speech stylistics including loudness, explosiveness, rapid–accelerated speech, and response latency. Another important measure of the hostility complex is provided by this assessment system: Potential for Hostility (PoHo), which is conceptualized as the relatively stable tendency to react to a broad range of frustration-inducing events with psychological and/or behavioral responses indicative of anger, irritation, disgust, contempt, resentment, and the like (Dembroski et al., 1985). Another important aspect of the hostility complex that is assessed using this scoring system is anger-coping style, or anger-in, which is indexed by content responses indicative of an inability or unwillingness to confront the source of a frustration.

In contrast to the self-report measure of the hostility complex that is provided by the Ho scale, the PoHo conceptualization is primarily based on overt behavioral responses. It is distinct from anger, which is considered a primary emotional state as such. PoHo is also distinct from the more attitudinal trait measured by the Ho scale, though persons characterized by a cynical mistrust of people in general would be expected to react to frustration-inducing events in the manner just described for persons high on PoHo. The correlation between PoHo and Ho is significant, but modest ($r = .37$, $p < .01$; Dembroski et al., 1985), suggesting that, while related, these two measures of the hostility complex dimension are not simple proxies for one another. Research currently in progress will evaluate the relationship between recently derived subcomponents of the Ho scale (Barefoot et al., 1987) and PoHo and its subcomponents.

A major contribution of the SI-based components scoring technique toward the definition of coronary-prone behavior has come from two recent studies in which components of the hostility–anger dimension were found correlated with CAD severity in angiographic samples. In a reanalysis of 131 taped SIs from the Duke sample, Dembroski and colleagues (1985) found that both PoHo and anger-in were significantly and positively correlated with CAD severity, even after statistical adjustment for age, sex, and the traditional risk factors. Another intriguing finding was that, although insignificantly and *positively* correlated with CAD severity in univariate analyses, a measure of Type A speech stylistics, namely, explosiveness, became significantly and *negatively* correlated with CAD in a multivariate analysis controlling for PoHo and anger-in.

In a similar reanalysis of SI data from a sample of patients originally studied at Massachusetts General Hospital (MGH) (Dimsdale, Hackett, Hutter, Block, & Catanzano, 1979), MacDougall, Dembroski, Dimsdale, and Hackett (1985) also found both PoHo and anger-in to be significantly and positively correlated with CAD severity. In this sample, explosive speech also became negatively correlated, although with marginal significance ($r = -.14$; $p = .10$), with CAD severity after statistical adjustment for PoHo and anger-in. Another component reflecting the time urgency aspects of the TABP—time pressure—was also significantly *negatively* correlated with CAD severity in this study.

As with the studies using the Ho measure, these studies using the SI-based assessment of the hostility complex also make important contributions toward clarifying the nature of coronary-prone behavior. First, in both the

Duke and MGH samples, globally defined TABP was not significantly related to CAD severity, though in the Duke sample there was a marginally significant positive relationship when only the extreme TABP groups were examined. In light of the small effect size for TABP noted earlier (Williams et al., 1986), this failure to detect a TABP effect in these small samples, both including fewer than 150 patients, is not surprising. The fact that in both studies measures of the hostility complex related significantly to CAD severity, despite small sample sizes, provides convincing evidence that this dimension is far more strongly related to CAD severity—and hence is a better index of coronary-prone behavior—than the global TABP itself.

Another potentially important finding in both studies is the negative associations between CAD severity and other (i.e., apart from those related to the hostility complex) aspects of the TABP that emerge with statistical adjustment for PoHo and anger coping style. The negative correlations of both explosiveness and time pressure with CAD severity suggest that, when measures of the hostility complex are controlled for, other aspects of the TABP may be not only uncorrelated with CHD risk, but, rather, may actually represent protective factors. It is tempting to speculate that, just as some components of the total serum cholesterol are toxic (LDL fraction) and some protective (HDL fraction), so may it be with TABP. That is, the hostility complex may be toxic, while "enthusiastic" speech and speed in accomplishing goals may be protective. If so, the inclusion of people in whom these protective effects are operating among groups designated as Type A, for instance, in the MRFIT study, may cancel out the toxic effects of hostility complex factors and thus account for the failure of global TABP to predict CHD events.

The significant positive association between anger-in and CAD severity in Dembroski and colleagues' (1985) and MacDougall and colleagues' (1985) studies appears at first glance to contradict the earlier report of Matthews and colleagues (1977) that SI ratings of potential for hostility and anger-*out* predict incident CHD cases in the WCGS. This apparent contradiction may be explained by the effect of more severe CAD, with its attendant increase in symptoms of chest pain, to *cause* patients to learn to inhibit the expression of anger, as would also the common admonition to CHD patients to "avoid emotional upsets." At the same time it is less easy to see how the presence of more severe disease would result in increased cynical mistrust and irritation toward others.

To ascertain the correctness of these interpretations, it will be necessary to evaluate the prediction of CHD events in a prospective study of persons free of any signs or symptoms of CHD. If they are correct, then PoHo should predict increased CHD risk, while anger-in should not. Chesney (Chapter 8, this volume) reports that anger-in did not differentiate cases from controls in the WCGS. Work currently in progress by Dembroski (personal communication, March 21, 1987) to evaluate the prediction of CHD events in the MRFIT study by PoHo and other SI-based measures of TABP components will also help to clarify these issues.

In another study employing components scoring techniques with SI data, Hecker, Frautschi, Chesney, Black, and Rosenman (1985; also see Chesney, Hecker, & Black, Chapter 8, this volume) compared component scores of all available CHD cases (N = 250) in the WCGS with those of 500 matched controls free of CHD during the initial 8.5 year follow-up. Again, a measure of potential for hostility emerged as the best significant discriminator between cases and controls. Even more important, multivariate analyses showed that no other measure from the extensive battery of scored components added significantly to the explanation of variance in CHD event rates beyond that accounted for by potential for hostility.

To summarize, the results from both questionnaire-based and SI-based studies make a compelling case for the hostility complex as the major and probably the only aspect of the global TABP that is coronary prone. Manuck, Kaplan, and Matthews (1986) reached a similar conclusion following their extensive review of the literature in this area.

The extensive evidence based on the Cook-Medley Ho scale suggests that a cynical mistrust of others is one aspect of the hostility complex that is coronary prone. The growing body of evidence from studies using components scoring of the SI adds the important aspect of anger expression: In addition to a cynical mistrust (and probably dislike) of people in general, coronary proneness is characterized by a relatively low threshold for the expression of this low regard in which others are held. The SI-based studies have also contributed the important notion that, except for the hostility complex, other aspects of the global TABP have been found not to predict increased CHD risk. In fact, there are strong hints that some TABP components, for example, explosive speech and time pressure, may actually be protective when they are determined not by hostility and anger, but, rather, by a positive, optimistic, and enthusiastic view of the world and the people in it.

To the extent that these aspects of the TABP related to the hostility complex are coronary prone, these effects must be mediated by biological correlates of the hostility complex that are participating in processes of atherogenesis and the precipitation of acute coronary events. This chapter will conclude, therefore, with a consideration of possible biologic pathways whereby various aspects of the hostility complex may be translated into manifestations of CHD.

## BIOLOGIC MECHANISMS OF CORONARY-PRONE BEHAVIOR

It is necessary first to acknowledge that an ultimate understanding of the etiology and pathogenesis of CAD and the various clinical manifestations of CHD that result is not yet available. At the present time, the most widely accepted hypothesis is that the initiation and progression of the pathological lesion of CHD, the atherosclerotic plaque, are determined by various factors that contribute to "injury" of the arterial endothelium (Ross & Glomset,

1976). Thus to the extent that TABP or its hostility complex aspects are coronary prone, it should be possible to demonstrate a relationship between these psychobehavioral characteristics and biological attributes, particularly biological *responses to behavioral challenges*, that appear to be plausible candidates to contribute to processes associated with endothelial injury.

In view of the recentness of the realization that only some aspects of the TABP are coronary prone, it is not surprising that far more research has focused on biological response correlates of the TABP than on biological response correlates of the hostility complex. For the most part, this research suggests that, when Type A men are subjected to experimental conditions that annoy or harass them, or motivate them to accomplish something in a short time, they exhibit cardiovascular and plasma catecholamine responses that are significantly greater than those of Type B men (see Houston, 1986, for a review of this research). With respect to the hostility complex, Dembroski and coworkers have reported positive associations between the PoHo measure from the SI and cardiovascular responses to both psychological and physical (cold pressor) stressors (Dembroski, 1978; Dembroski, MacDougall, Herd, & Shields, 1979).

This research has focused mainly on blood pressure, heart rate, and plasma catecholamine responses. In a recent study, Williams and colleagues (1982) extended this research to include measures of muscle blood flow and other neuroendocrine parameters. During performance of a mental arithmetic task young Type A men showed a greater muscle vasodilatation and greater increases in plasma norepinephrine (NE), epinephrine (EPI), and cortisol than their Type B counterparts. In contrast, during performance of a sensory intake task, there were no A–B differences in plasma NE, EPI, and cortisol responses, but Type A's showed a significantly larger increase in plasma testosterone levels.

A subsequent unpublished study conducted in my laboratory has replicated the larger testosterone response among Type A men during a different sensory intake task. In both studies, the addition of Ho scores to the TABP characterization of subjects resulted in improved discrimination of subjects with respect to testosterone responses; that is, Type B subjects with low Ho scores showed the smallest testosterone increases (or even decreases) and the Type A subjects with high Ho scores showed the largest increases.

How might neuroendocrine response excesses of the sorts found thus far mainly in association with TABP, but in some instances in association with high levels of hostility, play a role in processes involved in endothelial injury or the precipitation of acute CHD events? The effects of catecholamines to mediate both increased cardiovascular function and lipid mobilization from fat depots are quite plausible pathways from TABP and the hostility complex to CHD and must figure prominently in any attempt to understand biobehavioral mechanisms of coronary-prone behavior.

Somewhat less well known, but perhaps of equal if not greater importance, is the potential role of chronic corticosteroid excess. Henry (1983) cites evidence for the following effects of glucocorticoids: (1) increased serum lipids; (2) increased atherosclerosis in dogs fed an atherogenic diet; and (3) increased numbers of dead or injured cells in arterial endothelium. Moreover, the administration of systemic corticosteroids has been associated with the acceleration of arteriosclerosis in patients with rheumatoid arthritis (Kalbak, 1972), and increased plasma cortisol levels during a stressful medical laboratory procedure were associated with more severe CAD in a sample of Air Force personnel undergoing coronary angiography (Troxler, Sprague, Albanese, Fuchs, & Thompson, 1977).

Corticosteroids have several effects (cited in Williams, 1985) that could account for these associations. Cortisol has been shown to increase the activity of catecholamine-synthesizing enzymes in the adrenal medulla and to inhibit the activity of degradative enzymes that terminate the biologic activity of catecholamines. Corticosteroids have also been shown in humans to potentiate alpha-adrenergically mediated vascular responses to catecholamines and to increase beta-adrenergic receptor density on leukocytes.

If Type A men show increased cortisol responding in everyday situations similar to that observed (Williams et al., 1982) when performing a mental work task in the laboratory, such repeated hypercortisolemia could, via the mechanisms outlined earlier, have a variety of consequences that would help to initiate and promote processes of endothelial injury and atherosclerotic plaque formation. That such a sequence of events can occur has been convincingly demonstrated in a study in which cynomolgus monkeys given exogenous cortisol injections and an atherogenic diet developed more severe atherosclerosis than monkeys fed the diet alone (Sprague, Troxler, Peterson, Schmidt, & Young, 1980). Ultimate demonstration of a causal role for cortisol hyperresponsivity will depend, however, upon prospective studies of humans in which cortisol responses to laboratory and naturalistic stressors are evaluated as predictors of subsequent CHD risk.

Another good candidate for involvement in atherogenic processes is the testosterone hyperresponsivity observed in Type A men, particularly those with high Ho scores, during sensory intake behavior. That testosterone excess may be present among Type A men outside the laboratory is suggested by the recent report of Zumoff and colleagues (1984) that Type A men excrete more testosterone glucuronide in the urine during the daytime working hours than their Type B counterparts. The well-known concordance between pubertal increases in male testosterone levels and decreased blood levels of HDL cholesterol provides circumstantial evidence that testosterone excess could play a role in atherogenesis. More directly documenting the potential role of testosterone excess in atherogenesis is the observation that atheroma formation in the rat associated with catheter denudation of the aorta is accelerated by exogenous testosterone administration (Uzunova, Ramey, & Ramwell, 1978).

In addition to these neuroendocrine response mechanisms that might mediate atherogenesis among hostile Type A persons, a recent study employing a different research approach suggests pathways of a somewhat different sort. Instead of subjecting subjects to various forms of behavioral challenge, Muranaka, Williams, Lane, Anderson, and McCown (1986) evaluated physiologic responses of Type A and B men to equipotent infusions (on a μg/kg/min basis) of the beta-adrenergic agonist isoproterenol (Iso). The major finding was that Type A men showed a more prolonged decrease in EKG T-wave amplitude (TWA) than the Type B men in response to the Iso infusion. Since other beta-adrenergically mediated responses, for example, heart rate, forearm blood flow, and cyclic-AMP levels, did not differ between the Type A and B subjects, the difference in TWA responses to the Iso infusion does not appear to result from any A–B differences in beta-receptor function. Another possible explanation for the more rapid TWA recovery during continuing Iso infusion among the Type B subjects is that Type B's have a more robust parasympathetic antagonism (Levy, 1977) of sympathetic effects. Additional analyses of the data of this study supported this interpretation. For example, better TWA recovery during continuing Iso infusion was correlated with a smaller heart rate response to the same continuing infusion. Further research has adduced additional evidence of more robust parasympathetic responses, in this case to stimulation of the dive reflex, among Type B subjects (Muranaka et al., 1987).

It will be important to test more directly this hypothesized increase in parasympathetic antagonism of sympathetic nervous system stimulation among Type B's. Such testing could involve blockade of parasympathetic protection by pretreatment with atropine and stimulation of such protection by pretreatment with the acetylcholinesterase inhibitor edrophonium. If atropine pretreatment abolishes the better TWA recovery among the Type B subjects and edrophonium pretreatment enhances the TWA recovery among the Type A's, it will be strong evidence that, in addition to their enhanced neuroendocrine responsivity, Type A's are placed at greater risk of developing CHD by virtue of a less robust parasympathetic antagonism of sympathetic nervous system effects.

Just as addition of Ho scores provided for a better discrimination of subjects' testosterone responses to sensory intake tasks, addition of Ho scores to the TABP classification of subjects in the Iso infusion study (Muranaka et al., 1986) resulted in better discrimination of subjects with good versus poor TWA recovery during continuing Iso infusion. Although as a group the Type B's showed better TWA recovery than the Type A's, there were four Type B subjects whose TWA recovery overlapped that of the Type A group. Of these four, three had scores above the entire group's mean on the Ho scale, and the fourth had a positive family history of CHD.

In the light of these biological differences between subjects categorized as Type A or Type B, and, in some cases, as high or low on the Ho scale, it is clear that there are several quite plausible pathways whereby these psychobehavioral characteristics have the potential to contribute to processes involved in atherogenesis. Definitive proof of such a causal role must await, as already noted, the conduct of prospective epidemiological studies in which the biological response parameters are evaluated as predictors of subsequent CHD events.

In the meanwhile, one can hypothesize that a person with high levels of cynical mistrust regarding others would spend much of the day in a state of increased vigilance, to be sure that others are not about to mistreat him. With this expectation, it would also be likely that he would see many examples of bad behaviors on the part of others and become angry or even behave aggressively as a result. The vigilance could lead to increased testosterone secretion, and the anger to increased catecholamines and cortisol. Both patterns of neuroendocrine excess could lead, via the effects just reviewed, to increased likelihood of endothelial injury, atherosclerotic progression, and, in the person predisposed by existing coronary atherosclerosis, to acute CHD events. Studies of urinary excretion of these neuroendocrine substances and their metabolites during everyday circumstances in persons characterized with respect to the hostility complex should provide support for this hypothesis.

In addition to their increased neuroendocrine responding, persons with pronounced hostility complex characteristics might also be placed at increased risk by virtue of a reduced parasympathetic antagonism of sympathetic nervous system effects. Support for this mechanism is provided by observations that reduced heart rate responding (which could be due to enhanced parasympathetic antagonism, as well as diminished sympathetic responding) is associated with less severe coronary atherosclerosis in nonhuman primates (see review by Manuck et al., 1986).

Beyond a possible role as biological mediators of the pathophysiological consequences of coronary-prone behavior, it is tempting to speculate that the biological response characteristics just described might themselves also be determinants of the psychobehavioral characteristics that appear to be coronary prone. As Krantz and Durel (1983) and Schmieder, Friedrich, Neus, and Rüddel (1982) have reported, administration of beta-blockers is associated with a diminution of some Type A speech stylistics, as well as potential for hostility. Thus the catecholamine hyperresponsivity that has been so often observed among Type A's might itself be responsible for their typical accelerated and explosive speech and, possibly, some aspects of their hostility.

It is also possible that testosterone hyperresponsivity during sensory intake behaviors might be "hard-wired" (i.e., genetically determined) and thus responsible for some of the other behaviors displayed by Type A persons. For example, the improvement in prediction of testosterone responses to sensory intake tasks when Ho scores are combined with TABP classification may be due to effects of testosterone to increase persistence and narrowing of attentional focus (Thompson & Wright, 1978), to increase dominance behavior (Rose, 1980), and to increase aggressive behavior in man (Ehrenkranz, Bliss, & Sheard, 1974). Thus testosterone excess could be a determinant of increased vigilance and hostility as well as a mediator of increased CHD risk among persons displaying high levels of hostility complex characteristics.

Cortisol could also have effects that potentiate behavioral characteristics of the hostility complex. It is known that CNS adrenergic systems are involved in many aspects of the body's response to stress (Kopin, 1980). Since corticosteroids have been shown to affect the function of brain adrenergic systems (Maas & Mednieks, 1971; Mobley & Sulser, 1980), it is likely that a hard-wired adrenocortical hyperresponsivity to environmental stimuli could have effects upon brain function that could enhance behavioral tendencies associated with the hostility complex.

Finally, the increase in parasympathetic antagonism of sympathetic effects that the Iso infusion study results suggest to be present among low Ho-scoring Type B men calls to mind Gellhorn's (1967) characterization of the behavioral effects observed when the "trophotropic" system is activated as being those of decreased arousal and reactivity to environmental stimuli. Thus low levels of hostility and Type A behavior could just as well be a result as a cause of a more active parasympathetic nervous system.


## CONCLUSIONS AND SUMMARY

A long history of anecdotal observations and clinical experience led to the intuitively attractive hypothesis that certain states of mind, particularly those engendered in "stressful" environmental situations and in persons predisposed to anger easily, are coronary prone. Friedman and Rosenman gave form and substance to this hypothesis when they formulated the TABP construct and documented in a prospective epidemiologic study its prediction of CHD events in previously healthy middle-aged men.

The failure of the global TABP to predict CHD events or correlate with CAD severity in subsequent prospective epidemiologic studies and studies of angiographic populations led to the realization that the TABP hypothesis in its original form—namely, that it is the entire, collective constellation of Type A characteristics taken all together that are coronary prone—was not as robust as was once thought and was in need of refinement.

Subsequent research has resulted in progress toward this refinement, and it now appears to be firmly established that not all aspects of the global TABP are coronary prone. A number of studies carried out by several independent research groups have provided abundant and mutually supportive evidence that, of all the aspects of the TABP originally described by Friedman and Rosenman, only those aspects concerned with the hostility complex are coronary prone. More specifically, the available evidence suggests that a cynical, mistrusting attitude toward others and a willingness to express openly the anger and contempt engendered by such an attitude lie at the heart of coronary-prone behavior.

Just as the original Type A hypothesis has undergone refinement, as reviewed herein, it will be essential in future research to continue to refine our understanding of the hostility complex, with the goal of developing measures that are even more sensitive and specific predictors and correlates of CHD events and CAD severity. At that point we shall be able to drop the general term *hostility complex* and use a more appropriate name to describe those aspects that are coronary prone.

Understanding of the biological mechanisms responsible for transducing the behavioral characteristics of the hostility complex into pathophysiological processes is much less developed. The presently available evidence suggests that increased neuroendocrine and cardiovascular responsivity to environmental stimuli—particularly responses involving the sympathetic nervous system, the hypothalamic–pituitary–adrenal axis, and the pituitary–gonadal axis—and, possibly, decreased responsivity of the parasympathetic nervous system may all represent biological pathways from the hostility complex to CHD. Indeed, it is fascinating to contemplate the possibility that these biological characteristics may themselves be important, perhaps genetically influenced determinants of the extent to which aspects of the hostility complex are expressed in each individual.

It will be essential in future research to increase our understanding of biological mechanisms that underlie the hostility complex and its pathophysiological consequences. Such knowledge will likely offer the best guidelines toward the ultimate goal of all the research in this area: the development of efficient and effective means of preventing CHD.

## REFERENCES

Albright, C. L., King, A. C., Taylor, C. B., Haskell, W. L., & DeBusk, R. F. (1986, March). *Type A, gender, hostility, and increased cardiovascular risk: Relationships with reactivity, cholesterol, fitness, and heart rate variability.* Paper presented at annual meeting, Society of Behavioral Medicine, San Francisco.

Aravanis, C. (1983). The classic risk factors for coronary heart disease: Experience in Europe. *Preventive Medicine, 12,* 16–19.

Barefoot, J. C., Dahlstrom, W. G., & Williams, R. B. (1983). Hostility, CHD incidence and total mortality: A 25-year follow-up study of 255 physicians. *Psychosomatic Medicine, 45,* 59–63.

Barefoot, J. C., Williams, R. B., Dahlstrom, W. G., & Dodge, K. A. (1987, March). *Predicting mortality from scores on the Cook-Medley scale: A follow-up study of 118 lawyers.* Paper presented at the annual meeting of the American Psychosomatic Society, Philadelphia.

Blackburn, H. (1983). Diet and atherosclerosis: Epidemiologic evidence and public health implications. *Preventive Medicine, 22,* 2–10.

Blumenthal, J. A., Williams, R. B., Kong, Y., Schanberg, S. M., & Thompson, L. W. (1978). Type A behavior pattern and coronary atherosclerosis. *Circulation, 258,* 634–639.

Case, R. B., Heller, S. S., Case, N. B., & Moss, A. J. (1985). Type A behavior and survival after acute myocardial infarction. *New England Journal of Medicine, 312,* 737–741.

Cook, W., & Medley, D. (1954). Proposed hostility and pharisaic-virtue scales for the MMPI. *Journal of Applied Psychology, 238,* 414–418.

Costa, P. T., Zonderman, A. B., McCrae, R. R., & Williams, R. B. (1985). Content and comprehensiveness in the MMPI: An item factor analysis in a normal adult sample. *Journal of Personality & Social Psychology, 48,* 925–933.

Costa, P. T., Zonderman, A. B., McCrae, R. R., & Williams, R. B. (1986). Cynicism and paranoid alienation in the Cook and Medley Ho scale. *Psychosomatic Medicine, 248,* 283–285.

Dawber, T. R. (1980). *The Framingham Study: The epidemiology of atherosclerotic disease.* Cambridge, MA: Harvard University Press.

Dembroski, T. M. (1978). Reliability and validity of procedures used to assess coronary-prone behavior. In T. Dembroski, S. Weiss, J. Shields, S. Haynes, & M. Feinleib (Eds.), *Coronary-prone behavior.* New York: Springer-Verlag.

Dembroski, T. M., & MacDougall, J. M. (1983). Behavioral and psychophysiological perspectives on coronary-prone behavior. In T. M. Dembroski, T. H. Schmidt, & G. Blumchen (Eds.), *Biobehavioral bases of coronary heart disease.* New York: Karger.

Dembroski, T. M., & MacDougall, J. M. (1985). Beyond global Type A: Relationships of paralinguistic attributes, hostility, and anger-in to coronary heart disease. In T. Field, P. McAbe, & N. Schneiderman (Eds.), *Stress and coping.* Hillsdale, NJ: Erlbaum.

Dembroski, T. M., MacDougall, J. M., Herd, J. A., & Shields, J. L. (1979). Effect of level of challenge on pressor and heart rate responses in Type A and Type B subjects. *Journal of Applied Social Psychology, 9,* 209–225.

Dembroski, T. M., MacDougall, J. M., Williams, R. B., Haney, T. L., & Blumenthal, J. A. (1985). Components of Type A, hostility, and anger-in: Relationship to angiographic findings. *Psychosomatic Medicine, 247,* 219–233.

Dembroski, T. M., Weiss, S., Shields, J. L., Haynes, S., & Feinleib, M. (Eds.). (1978). *Coronary-prone behavior.* New York: Springer-Verlag.

Diamond, E. L. (1982). The role of anger and hostility in essential hypertension and coronary heart disease. *Psychological Bulletin, 292,* 410–433.

Dimsdale, J. E., Hackett, T. P., Hutter, A. M., Block, P. C., & Catanzano, D. (1979). Type A behavior and angiographic findings. *Journal of Psychosomatic Research, 23,* 273–276.

Ehrenkranz, J., Bliss, E., & Sheard, M. H. (1974). Plasma testosterone: Correlation with aggressive behavior and social dominance in man. *Psychosomatic Medicine, 36*(6), 469–475.

Frank, K. A., Heller, S. S., Kornfeld, D. S., Sporn, A. A., & Weiss, M. B. (1978). Type A behavior pattern and coronary angiographic findings. *Journal of the American Medical Association, 240,* 761–763.

Friedman, M., Brown, M. A., & Rosenman, R. H. (1969). Voice analysis test for detection of behavior pattern. *Journal of the American Medical Association, 208,* 828–836.

Friedman, M., & Rosenman, R. H. (1974). *Type A behavior and your heart.* New York: Knopf.

Friedman, M., Rosenman, R. H., Straus, R., Wurm, M., & Kositchek, R. (1968). The relationship of behavior pattern to the state of the coronary vasculature. A study of 51 autopsy subjects. *American Journal of Medicine, 244,* 525–538.

Gellhorn, E. (1967). *Principles of autonomic-somatic integrations.* Minneapolis: University of Minnesota Press.

Harvey, W. (1928). *Exercitatio anatomica de motu cordis et sanguinis.* London: Baillieve, Tindall & Cox. (Facsimile of original 1628 edition.)

Hecker, M., Frautschi, N., Chesney, M., Black, G., & Rosenman, R. (1985, March). *Components of Type A behavior and coronary heart disease.* Paper presented at the annual meeting of the Society of Behavioral Medicine, New Orleans.

Henry, J. P. (1983). Coronary heart disease and arousal of the adrenal cortical axis. In T. M. Dembroski & T. Schmidt (Eds.), *Biobehavioral bases of coronary heart disease*. Basel: Karger.

Houston, B. K. (1986). Psychological variables and cardiovascular and neuroendocrine reactivity. In K. A. Matthews, S. M. Weiss, T. Detre, T. M. Dembroski, B. Falkner, S. B. Manuck, & R. B. Williams (Eds.), *Handbook of stress, reactivity, and cardiovascular disease*. New York: Wiley.

Hunter, John, in *Dictionary of National Biography* (compact edition) (1975), vol. 10, Sir Leslie Stephen & Sir Sidney Lee (Eds.). London: Oxford University Press.

Jenkins, C. D. (1978). A comparative review of the interview and questionnaire methods in the assessment of the coronary-prone behavior pattern. In T. M. Dembroski, S. M. Weiss, J. L. Shields, S. G. Haynes, & M. Feinleib (Eds.), *Coronary-prone behavior*. New York: Springer-Verlag.

Johnson, J. H., Butcher, J. N., Null, C., & Johnson, K. N. (1984). Replicated item level factor analysis of the full MMPI. *Journal of Personality & Social Psychology, 49*, 105–114.

Kalbak, K. (1972). Incidence of arteriosclerosis in patients with rheumatoid arthritis receiving long-term corticosteroid therapy. *Annals of Rheumatic Disease, 31*, 196–200.

Keys, A. (1970). Coronary heart disease in seven countries: XIII. Multiple variables. *Circulation, 251*, 138–144.

Kopin, I. J. (1980). Catecholamines, adrenal hormones, and stress. In D. J. Krieger & J. C. Hughes (Eds.), *Neuroendocrinology*. New York: Hospital Practice Publishing Co.

Krantz, D., & Durel, L. A. (1983). Psychobiological substrates of the Type A behavior pattern. *Health Psychology, 2*, 393–411.

Levy, M. N. (1977). Parasympathetic control of the heart. In W. C. Randall (Ed.), *Neural regulation of the heart*. New York: Oxford University Press.

Maas, J. W., & Mednieks, M. (1971). Hydrocortisone-mediated increase of norepinephrine uptake by brain slices. *Science, 171*, 178–179.

MacDougall, J. M., Dembroski, T. M., Dimsdale, J. E., & Hackett, T. (1985). Components of Type A hostility, and anger-in: Further relationships to angiographic findings. *Health Psychology, 24*, 137–152.

Manuck, S. B., Kaplan, J. R., & Matthews, K. A. (1986). Behavioral antecedents of coronary heart disease and atherosclerosis. *Atherosclerosis, 6*, 2–14.

Matthews, K. A., Glass, D. C., Rosenman, R. H., & Bortner, R. W. (1977). Competitive drive pattern A, and coronary heart disease: A further analysis of some data from the Western Collaborative Group Study. *Journal of Chronic Diseases, 30*, 489–498.

Matthews, K. A., & Haynes, S. G. (1986). Type A behavior pattern and coronary risk: Update and critical evaluation. *American Journal of Epidemiology, 123*, 923–960.

McCranie, E. W., Watkins, L., Brandsma, J., & Sisson, B. (1986). Hostility, coronary heart disease (CHD) incidence, and total mortality: Lack of association in a 25-year follow-up study of 478 physicians. *Journal of Behavioral Medicine, 29*, 119–125.

Mobley, P. L., & Sulser, F. (1980). Adrenal steroids affect the norepinephrine-sensitive adenylate cyclase system in the rat limbic forebrain. *European Journal of Pharmacology, 65*, 321–323.

Muranaka, M., Lane, J. D., Suarez, E. C., Anderson, N. B., Suzuki, J., & Williams, R. B. (1987, March). *Autonomic balance in Type A and Type B persons: Larger forearm vasoconstriction and vagal reflex in Type B's during cold face stimulus*. Paper presented at the annual meeting of the American Psychosomatic Society, Philadelphia.

Muranaka, M., Williams, R. B., Lane, J. D., Anderson, N. B., & McCown, N. (1986, March). *T-wave amplitude during catecholamine infusion study: A new approach to biological mechanisms of coronary-prone behavior*. Paper presented at the annual meeting of the Society of Behavioral Medicine, San Francisco.

Osler, W. (1910). The Lumliean lectures on angina pectoris. *Lancet*, March 26, pp. 839–844.

Pooling Project Research Group (1978). Relationship of blood pressure, serum cholesterol, smoking habits, relative weight, and ECG abnormalities to incidence of major coronary events: Final report of the pooling project. *Journal of Chronic Diseases, 231,* 201–306.

Ragland, D. R., Brand, R. J., & Rosenman, R. H. (1986). Coronary heart disease in the Western Collaborative Group Study. *American Journal of Epidemiology, 124,* 522.

Review Panel on Coronary-Prone Behavior and Coronary Heart Disease (1981). Coronary-prone behavior and coronary heart disease: A critical review. *Circulation, 63,* 1199–1215.

Rose, R. M. (1980). Endocrine responses to stressful psychological events. In E. J. Sachar (Ed.), *Advances in psychoneuroendocrinology.* Philadelphia: Saunders.

Rosenman, R. H. (in press). Current and past history of Type A behavior pattern. In T. Schmidt, T. M. Dembroski, & G. Blumchen (Eds.), *Biological and psychological factors in cardiovascular disease.* New York: Springer-Verlag.

Rosenman, R. H., Brand, R. J., Jenkins, C. D., Friedman, M., Straus, R., & Wurm, M. (1975). Coronary heart disease in the Western Collaborative Group Study: Final follow-up experience of 8½ years. *Journal of the American Medical Association, 233,* 872–877.

Ross, R., & Glomset, J. (1973). Atherosclerosis and the arterial smooth muscle cell. *Science, 180,* 1332–1339.

Schmieder, R., Friedrich, G., Neus, H., & Rüddel, H. (1982, March). *Effects of beta-blockers on Type A coronary-prone behavior.* Paper presented at the annual meeting of the American Psychosomatic Society, Denver.

Schucker, B., & Jacobs, D. R. (1977). Assessment of behavioral risk of coronary disease by voice characteristics. *Psychosomatic Medicine, 239,* 219–228.

Shekelle, R. B., Gale, M., & Norusis, M. (1985). Type A behavior (Jenkins Activity Survey) and risk of recurrent coronary heart disease in the Aspirin Myocardial Infarction Study. *American Journal of Cardiology, 56,* 221–225.

Shekelle, R. B., Gale, M., Ostfeld, A. M., & Paul, O. (1983). Hostility, risk of coronary disease, and mortality. *Psychosomatic Medicine, 45,* 219–228.

Shekelle, R. B., Hulley, S., Neaton, J., Billings, J., Borhani, N., Gerace, T., Jacobs, D., Lasser, N., Mittlemark, M., Stamler, J., and the MRFIT Research Group (1985). The MRFIT behavioral pattern study: II. Type A behavior pattern and incidence of coronary heart disease. *American Journal of Epidemiology, 122,* 559–570.

Smith, T. W., & Frohm, K. D. (1985). What's so unhealthy about hostility? Construct validity and psychosocial correlates of the Cook and Medley Ho scale. *Health Psychology, 4,* 503–520.

Sprague, E. A., Troxler, R. G., Peterson, D. F., Schmidt, R. E., & Young, J. T. (1980). Effect of cortisol on the development of atherosclerosis in cynomolgus monkeys. In S. S. Kalter (Ed.), *The use of non-human primates in cardiovascular diseases.* Austin: University of Texas Press.

Thompson, W. R., & Wright, J. S. "Persistence" in rats: Effects of testosterone. *Physiological Psychology, 7,* 291–294.

Troxler, R. G., Sprague, E. A., Albanese, R. A., Fuchs, R., & Thompson, A. J. (1977). The association of elevated plasma cortisol and early atherosclerosis as demonstrated by coronary angiography. *Atherosclerosis, 26,* 151–162.

Uzunova, A. D., Ramey, E. R., & Ramwell, P. W. (1978). Gonadal hormones and pathogenesis of occlusive arterial thrombosis. *American Journal of Physiology, 234,* 454–459.

Weidner, G., Sexton, G., McLellarn, R., Matarazzo, J., & Conner, W. (1986, March). *Type A behavior, hostility, and elevated coronary risk in adults of the Family Heart Study.* Paper presented at the annual meeting of the Society of Behavioral Medicine, San Francisco.

Williams, R. B. (1985). Neuroendocrine response patterns and stress: Biobehavioral mechanisms of disease. In R. B. Williams (Ed.), *Perspectives on behavioral medicine: Neuroendocrine control and behavior.* Orlando: Academic Press .

Williams, R. B., Barefoot, J. C., Haney, T. L., Harrell, F. E., Blumenthal, J. A., Pryor, D. B., & Peterson, B. (1986). *Type A behavior and angiographically documented coronary atherosclerosis in a sample of 2,289 patients*. Paper presented at the annual meeting of the American Psychosomatic Society, Baltimore.

Williams, R. B., Barefoot, J. C., & Shekelle, R. B. (1985). The health consequences of hostility. In M. A. Chesney & R. H. Rosenman (Eds.), *Anger, hostility, and behavioral medicine*. New York: Hemisphere.

Williams, R. B., Haney, T. L., Lee, K. L., Kong, Y., Blumenthal, J., & Whalen, R. (1980). Type A behavior, hostility, and coronary atherosclerosis. *Psychosomatic Medicine, 242*, 539–549.

Williams, R. B., Lane, J. D., Kuhn, C. M., Melosh, W., White, A. D., & Schanberg, S. M. (1982). Type A behavior and elevated physiological and neuroendocrine responses to cognitive tasks. *Science, 218*, 483–485.

Zumoff, B., Rosenfeld, R. S., Friedman, M., Byers, S. O., Rosenman, R. H., & Hellman, L. (1984). Elevated daytime excretion of urinary testosterone glucuronide in men with the Type A behavior pattern. *Psychosomatic Medicine, 46*, 223–225.

Zyzanski, S. J., Jenkins, C. D., Ryan, T. J., Flessas, A., Everist, M. (1976). Psychological correlates of coronary angiographic findings. *Archives of Internal Medicine, 136*, 1234–1237.

# 10

## Cardiovascular and Neuroendocrine Reactivity, Global Type A, and Components of Type A Behavior

B. KENT HOUSTON

The pathophysiological mechanisms by which the Type A behavior pattern increases risk for coronary heart disease (CHD) are uncertain. It has been hypothesized that Type A individuals chronically respond to certain situations with greater activity of the sympathetic–adrenomedullary system and perhaps also the pituitary–adrenocortical system (Henry & Meehan, 1981; Williams, 1978; see also Williams & Barefoot, Chapter 9, this volume). Over time such activity may result in increased coronary atherosclerosis and the possibility of a clinical event. Following from this hypothesis, considerable research attention has been given to evaluating possible differences between Type A's and Type B's in their psychophysiological reactivity to various laboratory situations. Studies of this nature are the focus of this chapter.

Specifically, there are three purposes of the present chapter. One is to review the findings from laboratory reactivity studies conducted in the United States in which one of the three major measures of Type A was employed, namely, the Structured Interview (SI; Rosenman, 1978), the Jenkins Activity Survey (JAS; Jenkins, Rosenman, & Zyzanski, 1974), or the Framingham Type A Scale (FTAS; Haynes, Levine, Scotch, Feinleib, & Kannel, 1978). The second purpose is to present some new data regarding how prediction of cardiovascular reactivity by the SI may be influenced by the style in which the SI is administered and by identifying different profiles of SI-derived components via cluster analysis. A third purpose is to review the findings from reactivity studies concerning the relation between SI-derived Type A components and cardiovascular reactivity.

Reactivity has been defined "as the magnitude of an array of physiological responses to discrete, environmental stressors" (Matthews, 1986, p. xi). Foremost in the array of physiological responses investigated in research on reactivity in Type A and Type B individuals are measures of cardiovascular activity, namely, systolic blood pressure (SBP); diastolic blood pressure (DBP); pulse transit time (PTT); heart rate (HR); peripheral vasoconstriction as indexed by finger pulse volume (FPV), finger pulse amplitude (FPA), or skin temperature (ST); and vasodilation–constriction in the muscles as indexed by forearm blood flow (FBF) or forearm vascular resistance (FVR). The second most frequently employed measures in studies of this nature are measures of neuroendocrine activity, for example, epinephrine (E) and norepinephrine (NE). Occasionally, other physiological parameters have been measured as well, for example, cholesterol, triglycerides, and so forth. The aforementioned variables are probably the most relevant to the study of the pathophysiological mechanisms that may increase risk of premature CHD for Type A's. However, some measures have been employed in a few studies (e.g., electrodermal and somatic muscle activity) that do not appear to have much if any significance for the study of pathophysiological mechanisms (see Wright, Contrada, & Glass, 1985). Therefore, these measures will not be included in the review.

The chapter is divided into three major sections: Reactivity studies employing the SI, those employing the JAS, and those employing the FTAS. Within each section the organization of the review of the reactivity studies that involve global or overall Type A reflects the following considerations. One is whether subjects are studied while they are presented alone, that is, by themselves, with a situation that is expected to be arousing (a solitary situation) or as they behave in the presence of others in a situation that is expected to be arousing. Most of the situations with which subjects are presented that are expected to be arousing involve performance of one or more tasks. Thus the majority of laboratory investigations on reactivity have involved studying subjects during task performance, either alone, that is, in a solitary situation, or in the presence of another ostensible subject, frequently a confederate of the experimenter's. When subjects perform a task alone, all the information about the task (e.g., its difficulty) is communicated either by the experimenter or via the subject's own experiences with the task. When subjects perform a task in the presence of another subject, additional information about a task can be obtained via feedback about how well the other person is performing. Moreover, another person may actively or passively provide an additional stimulus to which the subject may react. Occasionally, investigations are focused solely on the responses of subjects to their interacting with another person in the experimental setting.

Another consideration in these investigations is whether potential differences between Type A's and Type B's in reactivity are studied in a single condition or in multiple conditions in which some potentially relevant variable is manipulated independently of the general requirements of the situation or task, for example, conditions in which task difficulty, performance incentive, and so forth are manipulated. Studies that involve multiple conditions have the potential advantage of being able to delineate the circumstances that do and do not elicit differences in reactivity between Type A's and Type B's.

Gender is another consideration in these investigations. Although the majority of studies have been conducted with males, some have been conducted with both males and females, and some with females only. The review of the reactivity studies within each major section below is organized in terms of separate subsections, when there are enough studies to warrant it, that reflect a combination of the aforementioned factors, namely, solitary situation versus behavior in the presence of others, single versus multiple experimental conditions, and gender.

## STUDIES EMPLOYING THE SI

### Global Type A and Reactivity: Review

**Solitary Situations, Single Condition, Males.**   One of the earliest investigations in which subjects were studied while they performed a solitary task was conducted by Dembroski, MacDougall, Shields, Petitto, and Lushene (1978). College males performed three tasks: (1) a reaction-time task that was described as a test of the subject's speed of reaction; (2) an electronic pong game that was described as a test of subject's hand–eye coordination; and (3) a series of difficult anagrams under a time limit. Type A subjects manifested significantly greater SBP and HR responses but not DBP responses across the three tasks than Type B subjects.

In a study by Glass, Krakoff, Contrada, and colleagues (1980, Study II), working adult males performed an electronic pong game under instructions that it was a test of hand–eye coordination. Type A's relative to Type B's were found to respond to the task with significantly greater SBP and DBP and marginally significantly greater HR ($p = .08$) and plasma E ($p = .06$) but not plasma NE.

Type A and Type B males (a combination of college students and working adults) in another study by Glass and associates (Glass, Krakoff, Finkelman et al., 1980) performed a vigilance task and a subsidiary memory task under instructions that emphasized the need for good performance. Type A relative to Type B subjects were found to respond to the tasks with greater increases in SBP ($p < .01$), DBP ($p < .06$), plasma E ($p < .05$), and plasma NE ($p < .07$), but not HR.

Corse, Manuck, Cantwell, Giordani, and Matthews (1982) report a study of adult males who either did or did not have CHD. Subjects performed a difficult concept task, a mental arithmetic task (serial subtraction of 17's), and the Picture Completion subtest of the Wechsler Adult Intelligence Scale. Across CHD categories, Type A's responded to the tasks with significantly greater SBP and DBP than did Type B's.

Male college students' responses to the TAT were assessed in a study by Blumenthal, Lane, and Williams (1985). Relative to Type B's, Type A's exhibited a significantly greater increase in FBF and marginally significantly less increase in FVR ($p < .10$) than type B's during preparation for telling their TAT stories and marginally significantly greater ($p < .10$) increase in FBF during the period that involved recounting their TAT stories. There were no significant differences between Type A's and Type B's in SBP, DBP, or HR during either of these periods.

In a study by Fontana, Rosenberg, Kerns, and Marcus (1986), non-CHD, male medical and surgical patients were investigated while they responded to an unspecified performance test, the JAS, a questionnaire on achievement, and the TAT. Relative to Type B's, Type A's responded with (1) significantly greater SBP but not DBP to the performance test, (2) significantly greater DBP but not SBP to the TAT stories, and (3) significantly greater SBP and DBP to the JAS. Type A's and Type B's did not differ in response to the questionnaire on achievement.

Employed white-collar males' responses during six different tasks were studied by Ward and colleagues (1986). Relative to Type B's, Type A's exhibited significantly greater SBP and DBP but not HR to a concept formation task, significantly greater SBP and HR but not DBP to a reaction-time task, significantly greater HR but not SBP or DBP to a video game, and significantly greater SBP but not DBP or HR to a mental arithmetic (serial subtraction) task. No differences between Type A's and Type B's in SBP, DBP, or HR were found in response to two physical stressors, namely, a handgrip task and the cold pressor test.

In a study of male college students by Allen and colleagues (1987), subjects' cardiovascular responses were measured while they performed a reading comprehension test, a virtually impossible digit span recall task, the cold pressor test, and a handgrip task. Type A's exhibited significantly greater HR responses across all the tasks and significantly greater DBP to the cold pressor test than Type B's. There were no other differences in DBP responses to the tasks between Type A's and Type B's and no significant main effects of A–B Type for SBP or PTT.

In contrast to the foregoing studies, the following investigations did not obtain differences in psychophysiological reactivity between Type A and Type B males. Scherwitz, Berton, and Leventhal (1978) report a study in which male college subjects were exposed to a physical stressor, namely, the cold pressor test, a mental arithmetic task (serial subtraction of 17's), a maze-learning task, and a task involving the generation of emotions. Following these tasks, the Structured Interview was also administered. Type A's relative to Type B's did not differ in SBP, DBP, or HR responses but manifested significantly more FPV (indicating less arousal) across all the rest periods and the task periods. It should be noted, however, that no mention was made of any instructions that would have provided subjects with incentive for performing well on the tasks.

In a study by Glass, Lake, Contrada, Kehoe, and Erlanger (1983), adult, employed males were given a mental arithmetic task (serial subtraction of 13's) and a modified Stroop task with instructions to perform quickly and accurately. Type A's did not differ from Type B's in SBP, DBP, or HR responses to either task or in NE or E responses to the modified Stroop task.

Male college students' responses to three tasks, namely, the cold pressor test, the presentation of a snake, and mental arithmetic (serial addition and subtraction), each accompanied by instructions designed to increase stress, were investigated by Lake, Suarez, Schneiderman, and Tocci (1985). Type A's and Type B's did not differ significantly in SBP, DBP, or HR responses to any of the three tasks.

In a study of medical students by Lovallo, Pincomb, and Wilson (1986b), subjects' psychophysiological responses were assessed during two tasks. One was the cold pressor test, given purposefully without special instructions. The second was a reaction-time task with monetary incentive for good performance. Type A's and Type B's were not found to differ in HR responses to the cold pressor test or in SBP, DBP, HR, plasma cortisol, or NE response to the reaction-time task. This lack of differences between A's and B's in response to the reaction-time task may have been due to the incentive increasing the level of motivation and arousal of Type B's to that of Type A's. This interpretation is buttressed by the findings of a study reviewed in a subsequent section in which differences between Type A's and Type B's were found in a low-incentive but not a high-incentive condition (Blumenthal, et al., 1983).

*Summary.*    In a substantial majority of the investigations in which subjects' responses to potentially arousing, solitary situations were studied, SI-defined Type A's exhibited greater cardiovascular and/or neuroendocrine reactivity than Type B's. Generally, the kinds of tasks that elicit A–B differences are those that involve time pressure and are moderately high in difficulty, that is, having a reasonably high likelihood of failure, for example, reaction-time tasks, video pong games, concept formation tasks, and so on. However, A–B differences tend not to be found for tasks that are highly difficult, for example, mental arithmetic tasks that involve serial subtraction, and perhaps addition. For these tasks, the majority of studies reviewed did not find A–B differences in reactivity. Such tasks are highly difficult in the sense that mistakes (failures) occur readily.

A–B differences in reactivity also tend to be found during reasonably structured tasks that are emotionally evocative, such as the TAT. In contrast, A–B differences in reactivity tend not to be found for physical stressors, for example, the cold pressor test, isometric exercise, and so forth, or physical threats, for example, presentation of a snake.

**Solitary Situations, Multiple Conditions, Males.**   The earliest investigation in which multiple conditions were used in the study of subjects while they performed a solitary task was conducted by Dembroski, MacDougall, Herd, and Shields (1979). Subjects were exposed to the cold pressor test and a reaction-time task under high- and low-challenge conditions. The difficulty of the respective tasks was emphasized in the high-challenge but not low-challenge conditions. The results indicated that the challenge manipulation differentially affected the responses of Type A's and Type B's to the cold pressor test but not the reaction-time task. Type A's relative to Type B's exhibited significantly greater SBP and HR responses to the cold pressor test in the high- but not low-challenge condition. However, across challenge conditions Type A's relative to Type B's exhibited significantly greater SBP and HR responses to the reaction-time task. There were no significant differences between A's and B's for DBP for either task.

College males performed a concept formation task in either a high-incentive condition ($5.00 for good performance) or a low-incentive condition (no monetary inducement) in a study by Blumenthal and colleagues (1983). Type A's relative to Type B's exhibited significantly greater SBP and HR responses to the task in the low-incentive condition but not in the high-incentive condition. This pattern of results was due to the incentive manipulation influencing Type B's but not Type A's. Type B's exhibited greater SBP and HR in the high- than low-incentive condition, but Type A's exhibited the same high SBP and HR responses across incentive conditions. Finally, across conditions Type A's exhibited less FVR ($p < .07$) and greater FBF ($p < .05$) than Type B's. No significant differences between A's and B's were found for DBP. Although the no-monetary-inducement condition was labeled for expository purposes as low incentive, it was clear to the subjects that the task was one of inductive reasoning; hence preservation or enhancement of self-esteem was an incentive for good performance. Thus it seems that this condition in actuality involved a moderate degree of incentive.

In a study by Contrada and colleagues (1982) of adult employed males, subjects performed a reaction-time task while they were exposed to high-intensity noise that increased over trials plus occasional shocks that decreased over trials or to low-intensity noise plus occasional shocks, both of which decreased over trials. Half of the subjects within each aversive stimulation condition were led to believe that avoidance of the aversive stimulation was contingent upon their performance on the reaction-time task, while the other half of the subjects were led to believe that avoidance of the aversive stimulation was not contingent upon their performance. Across conditions, Type A's exhibited significantly greater HR responses than Type B's. The analyses also revealed complicated higher-order interactions for SBP, DBP, and both plasma E and NE levels. These interactions were probably due to the complexity of the procedures involved in the study and, unfortunately, are difficult to interpret.

A study by Lovallo and Pishkin (1980) obtained anomalous results of a different nature. Male medical and dental students performed two tasks, a pattern recognition task and an anagram task, that were either easily or nearly unsolvable. Then all subjects performed a fairly difficult concept formation task. Independent of the level of difficulty of the first two tasks, across all three tasks, Type A's relative to Type B's responded with significantly greater FPV (indicating less arousal) but not HR. No significant differences between Type A and Type B subjects in SBP, DBP, cholesterol, or triglycerides were found for any of these tasks, though it should be noted that these measures were obtained following rather than during task performance.

In another study of medical students (Lovallo, Pincomb, & Wilson, 1986a), subjects' responses were assessed during two tasks. One was the cold pressor test, given purposefully without special instructions. The second was a task in which subjects were given noise and shock, and during one period they were led to believe that they could avoid aversive stimulation, and during another period they were led to believe that aversive stimulation was unavoidable. Type A's and Type B's did not differ in HR responses to the cold pressor test or in SBP, DBP, HR, plasma cortisol, NE, E, or free fatty acids to either of the avoidable or unavoidable aversive stimulation tasks. Differences in responses between Type A's and Type B's would not have been expected for either the cold pressor test, because it was not accompanied by challenging instructions, or the unavoidable aversive stimulation task, because there was no incentive for Type A's to try harder to control the situation than Type B's. However, the reason is unclear for the absence of A–B differences in response to the avoidable aversive stimulation task.

A rather complex study was conducted by Jennings and Choi (1981) with male executives. Initially, all subjects performed the same reaction-time task; then they performed the reaction-time task twice at four different speeds, once during a training period and again during an experimental period. There were no reactivity differences between Type A's and Type B's in SBP, DBP, FPV, or interbeat interval (HR). It should be noted that blood pressure was measured at the end rather than during performance periods, and the design and full results of the analyses were not described.

In a similar study by Jennings (1984), male college subjects performed a reaction-time task with instructions for fast and accurate performance; then they performed the reaction-time task at five different speed criteria during practice and under both high- and low-monetary-incentive conditions. Over the various experimental periods, Type A's and Type B's did not differ significantly in SBP, DBP, or interbeat interval (HR). However, blood pressure was measured at the end of performance blocks rather than during task performance, the experiment involved from three to five 2-hour sessions across as many as 3 days, and the overall design and results of the statistical analysis were not described. The complexity and length of the study could easily have obscured differences in reactivity between Type A's and Type B's.

*Summary.*   The results of the investigations in which multiple conditions were used in the study of subjects' responses to solitary situations were somewhat disappointing. The complexity of the designs precludes drawing conclusions from several of the studies. However, at least one conclusion is warranted from the other studies.

Differences between Type A's and Type B's in reactivity are obtained when there is moderate incentive for task performance, but not when there is high incentive. Under high-incentive conditions, Type B's appear to become as aroused as Type A's, thereby eliminating differences in reactivity between them.

**Behavior in the Presence of Others, Males.**   The earliest investigation in which subjects were studied while they performed a task in the presence of another person was conducted on employed males by Friedman, Byers, Diamant, and Rosenman (1975). A pair of subjects (one Type A and one Type B) were presented with a complex puzzle and told that the first member of the pair to solve the puzzle would receive a bottle of French wine. Type A relative to Type B subjects were found to respond to the task with a significantly greater increase in plasma NE but not greater plasma E.

In a study of adult, employed males by Glass, Krakoff, Contrada, and colleagues (1980, Study I), a confederate made a series of harassing remarks to the subject (harass condition) or was silent (no-harass condition) while they competed on an electronic pong game. Further, in both conditions, the subject failed to win on two-thirds of the games and consequently lost a prize. Type A subjects in the harass condition responded with significantly greater increases in SBP, HR, and plasma E, but not DBP or NE, than Type B subjects in the harass condition or either Type A or B subjects in the no-harass condition. Thus it appears that Type A subjects were differentially aroused specifically by the harassing comments made by the confederate. There were no significant differences in SBP, DBP, HR, E, or NE between Type A and Type B subjects in response to the task in the no-harass condition. This may have been due to Type A subjects perceiving that it was too difficult to be successful in the situation because the task itself was too hard and/or the confederate was too good.

Male college students competed with a confederate on a video pong game in one of three conditions in a study by Diamond and colleagues (1984). In one condition, the subject and confederate merely competed for 15 minutes. In a frustration condition, the experimenter asked distracting questions and frustrated the subject in his desire to win the game. In a harassment condition, the confederate made derogatory remarks to the subject while he performed the task. There were no significant differences between Type A's and Type B's in the harassment condition for DBP or HR, but there appears to have been a significant difference for SBP, although the statistical analysis is unclear. There were no significant differences between Type A's and Type B's in SBP, DBP, or HR in the other two conditions.

Male college students' responses to two competitive card games were investigated by Lake and colleagues (1985). During one card game, the subject was harassed by a confederate, and during the second card game, the subject was harassed by the confederate and the experimenter. Relative to Type B's, Type A's exhibited greater HR reactivity during the second card game. Type A's and Type B's did not differ in SBP and DBP responses during the second card game or in SBP, DBP, or HR responses during the first card game.

Several studies have investigated the psychophysiological responses of Type A and Type B subjects during the SI. Dembroski, MacDougall, and Lushene (1979) found significantly greater SBP and DBP but not HR responses for Type A relative to Type B male subjects during the latter two-thirds of the SI. Similarly, Krantz and colleagues (1981) reported finding greater SBP and HR responses but not DBP responses on the part of Type A than Type B coronary patients during the latter two-thirds of the SI. In the study by Lake and colleagues (1985) of college males just mentioned, Type A's were found to exhibit greater SBP and DBP but not HR responses during the SI than Type B's.

Male college students' responses during the SI were assessed in a study by Blumenthal and colleagues (1985). Type A's responded with significantly less FVR than Type B's, but A's and B's did not differ significantly in SBP, DBP, HR, or FBF.

Non-CHD, male medical and surgical patients were investigated while they responded to the SI in the study by Fontana and colleagues (1986) mentioned earlier. Relative to Type B's, Type A's responded with significantly greater DBP but not SBP to the SI.

In contrast to the foregoing studies, Scherwitz and colleagues (1978) found no significant differences in SBP, DBP, HR, or FPV between Type A and Type B male college subjects during the SI. However, the SI is typically given as an isolated procedure, yet in Scherwitz and colleagues' study the SI followed several apparently unchallenging tasks. It is possible that having preceded the SI with several tasks reduced the SI's impact, or the unchallenging nature of the preceding tasks may have generalized to the SI itself.

*Summary.*    Three summary statements can be made concerning the investigations in which subjects were studied as they behaved in some situation in the presence of others. One is that harassment tends to evoke greater reactivity in Type A's than in Type B's. This is not unexpected considering that easily evoked hostility is regarded as one of the primary characteristics of Type A (Rosenman, 1978).

A second summary statement is that differences in reactivity between A's and B's are found during the SI. This is also not surprising because the SI is meant to be somewhat provocative and to elicit Type A behaviors (Chesney, Eagleston, & Rosenman, 1980). It is curious, however, that there is such inconsistency across studies in the physiological parameters on which Type A's and Type B's were found to differ during the SI. Assuming that the SI is a reasonably standardized procedure, one would expect considerable consistency in the psychophysiological measures on which Type A's and Type B's differed. The lack of consistency may be due to differences in the kinds of Type A behaviors that were elicited by the interviews (e.g., amount of hostility evoked), differences in stimulus value of the interviewers, effects of preceding tasks or anticipation of subsequent tasks, unreliability and/or inaccuracy of the physiological measuring techniques, and so forth. Together, these findings call into question how well the SI is, or can be, standardized as an assessment procedure.

The third summary statement about the studies in this section is that differences in reactivity between Type A's and Type B's were not found in two (Diamond et al., 1984; Glass, Krakoff, Contrada, et al., 1980, Study I) out of the three studies (the third being by Friedman et al., 1975) in which subjects competed on a task with another person. In Friedman and colleagues' study subjects did not receive feedback on their performance, while in the two studies in which reactivity differences were not found, subjects received a fair amount of negative feedback about their performance. Perhaps Type A subjects in these two studies perceived the task as too difficult or the competitor as too good for them to be successful, and hence Type A's did not try harder and thus did not respond to the tasks differently than Type B's.

**Studies Employing Females.**    Very few studies have been conducted in which the relation between SI-defined Type A and reactivity for females has been investigated. Thus these studies will not be reviewed under different subsections.

Type A and reactivity were investigated in two studies of college females reported by MacDougall, Dembroski, and Krantz (1981). Subjects in the first study were exposed to the cold pressor test and a reaction-time task.

Instructions for both tasks emphasized the tasks' difficulty. No differences between Type A's and Type B's in SBP, DBP, or HR responses to either task were found. Subjects in the second study had cardiovascular responses measured during their performance of a reaction-time task with monetary incentive for good performance. No differences between Type A's and Type B's were found in SBP, DBP, or HR responses to this task, either.

In another study of college females by Lawler, Schmied, Mitchell, and Rixse (1984), subjects were presented with three tasks, a mental arithmetic task (addition and multiplication) and two sets of Raven's Progressive Matrices problems. No significant differences were found between Type A's and Type B's in their SBP, DBP, or HR responses to the experimental tasks.

A sample of both blue-collar and white-collar employed women were instructed to perform a mental addition task as quickly as possible in a study by Mayes, Sime, and Ganster (1984). No significant differences between Type A's and Type B's, using either a two-category or a four-category classification procedure, were found for SBP, DBP, HR, or ST responses to the task. Similarly, no significant differences between Type A's and Type B's were found in SBP, DBP, or HR responses to a mental arithmetic task (serial subtraction) in a study of employed Black females by Anderson and colleagues (1986).

In a study of college females during administration of the SI, MacDougall and colleagues (1981, Study II) found greater SBP but not greater DBP or HR on the part of Type A's compared to Type B's in response to the SI. Similarly, Type A's compared to Type B's were found to manifest significantly greater SBP and DBP but not HR responses to the SI in the study of employed Black women by Anderson and colleagues (1986). However, in a study of Black inner-city women by Smyth, Call, Hansell, Sparacino, and Strodtbeck (1978), no significant differences in SBP or DBP were found between Type A's and Type B's to a modified SI. Why this occurred is unclear, though possibly the small sample size and the modifications to the SI could have obscured A–B differences in reactivity.

*Summary.* Collectively, the studies on Type A and reactivity that have been conducted with females have been few and their results disappointing. The only differences in reactivity that have been found between SI-defined Type A and Type B females have been in response to verbal exchanges such as the SI. SI-defined Type A for females has not been found to be related to reactivity to the kinds of tasks for which Type A–Type B reactivity differences have been found for males. Reiterating what has been suggested previously (Houston, 1983; MacDougall et al., 1981), sex-role expectations may help explain these findings. Because of sex-role expectations (Lenney, 1977; Maccoby & Jacklin, 1974) many women may be uncertain whether they can adequately perform difficult cognitive (as in Lawler et al., 1984) or motor tasks (e.g., reaction-time tasks, as in MacDougall et al., 1981).

Thus Type A females may perceive the probability of failure on such tasks as quite high and therefore do not respond to them any more vigorously than Type B females; consequently, no differences in physiological responses are obtained. However, verbal situations may appear more sex role appropriate for females, and therefore Type A women may become more engaged in such situations, which in turn leads to differences in psychophysiological response being observed between Type A and Type B females.

Another possible explanation for the lack of differences in reactivity between Type A and Type B females derives from evidence that cardiovascular reactivity in women varies across the menstrual cycle (Hastrup & Light, 1984; Little & Zahn, 1974). Such variability would tend to obscure potential differences in reactivity between Type A and Type B females.

Yet another possible explanation is that the concept of global Type A, that is, the constellation of behaviors that are regarded as Type A, or the measurement of global Type A, both of which were developed from observations and research on middle-class, middle-aged men, may not be as pertinent or valid for females as it is for males. This is a point to which we will return later.

Conclusion.    A review of the reactivity studies in which global Type A was measured by the SI suggests the following. Generally, the SI is not nearly as predictive of reactivity for females as it is for males. For females, SI-defined Type A is most likely to be related to reactivity in verbal exchanges such as the SI. For males, SI-defined Type A is most likely to be related to reactivity in situations in which the individual is annoyed or harassed or in situations in which there is moderate incentive for individuals, under time pressure, to accomplish something that is viewed as moderately high in difficulty. The reason for using that adjective *moderate* is that, in situations in which there is high incentive for individuals in general to accomplish something, Type B's appear to become as aroused as Type A's (cf. Blumenthal et al., 1983). Further, the reason for using the phrase *moderately high* with difficulty is that, in situations in which accomplishing something is viewed as highly difficult, Type A's typically do not become more aroused than Type B's, perhaps because the perceived probability of success or avoidance of failure is so low. Time pressure appears to be an important element in the situations that are likely to evoke differences in reactivity between Type A's and Type B's, perhaps because it contributes to the perceived difficulty of accomplishing something and/or the incentive to accomplish it. Finally, in regard to cardiovascular responses, differences between male Type A's and Type B's are most frequently found for SBP, second most frequently found for HR, and third most frequently found for DBP. In regard to neuroendocrine measures, differences between male Type A's and Type B's are slightly more frequently found for E than for NE.

Several studies of males have employed tasks that would be expected to elicit significant A–B differences in reactivity, but such differences were not found, for example, on the Stroop task in Glass and colleagues' study (1983), the maze-learning task in Scherwitz and colleagues' study (1978), and so on. There are probably many other studies of this nature, but they do not get into print. One likely reason for studies not finding significant SI-defined A–B differences has to do with sampling error in conjunction with a relation that is not very strong. Although correlations between SI-defined Type A and measures of reactivity are rarely reported, the correlations that have been reported have been in the .30s (Dembroski et al., 1978; Dembroski, MacDougall, & Lushene, 1979). These correlations are probably higher than those in the population at large because studies that do not obtain statistically significant relations between A–B type and measures of reactivity are less likely to be published. Whether the correlation between A–B type and indices of reactivity in the general population is .30, or more realistically closer to .20 (see Houston, 1983), the point is the same. In a certain proportion of the samples of subjects that are studied, the differences in reactivity between Type A's and Type B's will not be found to be significant. This is particularly true considering the relatively small sample sizes that are typically employed.

## Cluster Analysis of Type A Components and Reactivity

Another reason why global Type A–Type B is not more consistently found to be predictive of reactivity for males or females may be due to the heterogeneity of people who are classified as Type A. Traditionally, individuals are categorized as Type A, in contrast to Type B, on the basis of their exhibiting several of a number of Type A characteristics in the SI, specifically, more rapid and/or emphatic speech, quicker responses, louder voice, evidence of hostility, more verbal competitiveness, and so on. However, individuals who exhibit different combinations of these characteristics all wind up being categorized as Type A. This procedure assumes a certain amount of equivalence between Type A characteristics. Perhaps prediction of reactivity, as well perhaps as prediction of CHD, can be enhanced by assigning people who exhibit different combinations of Type A characteristics to different categories rather than combining them in the same category.

This was done in two studies that were conducted in our laboratory, one with males (Kelly & Houston, 1985) and one with females (Pace & Houston, 1986). Individuals with different patterns of Type A characteristics were identified and then were compared in regard to cardiovascular reactivity.

The same method was employed in both studies. Eighty-four males were given the SI by a female interviewer in the first study and 101 females were given the SI by a female interviewer in the second study. SBP, DBP, and HR were monitored during the SI and during a subsequent task involving remembering and reciting digits backward. The interviews were rated for global A–B type and the following Type A components: latency of response, rate and loudness of speaking, emphases, potential for hostility, and verbal competition. Cluster analyses of individuals were then performed employing the data for the Type A component characteristics for each gender separately. Simply put, cluster analysis of people is a technique for identifying individuals who have similar patterns of characteristics. Thus cluster analysis will identify a group of people who have a similar profile of characteristics and who are different from other groups of people who have different profiles of characteristics.

**Cluster Analysis Study of Males: Results and Discussion.**    The cluster analysis revealed three clusters. The profiles of the characteristics for the clusters are displayed in Figure 10.1. Basically, one cluster of subjects is relatively high on all the Type A characteristics, so this group was labeled High A's. The second cluster of subjects are relatively intermediate on all the characteristics, so this group was labeled Moderate A's. And the third cluster of subjects is relatively low on all the characteristics, and so this group was labeled Non A's.

To evaluate relations between cluster membership and reactivity to the SI and digits-backward task, 3 (Clusters: High A, Moderate A, Non A) × 2 (Tasks) analyses of covariance testing for linear trends for cluster mem-

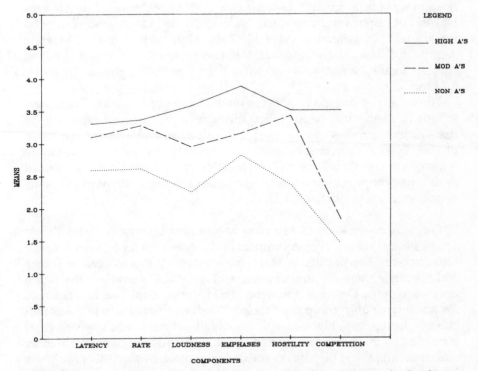

FIGURE 10.1.    Profiles of Type A components for empirically derived clusters of male subjects.

bership (High A > Moderate A > Non A) were performed on SBP, DBP, and HR change scores with base level values as covariates (Benjamin, 1967; Wilder, 1968). In addition, because global Type A ratings are the benchmark against which to compare some other procedure for classifying individuals, analyses were also performed to evaluate relations between Type A–Type B classifications and reactivity to the SI and digits-backward task. Specifically, 3 (Type A1, A2, B) × 2 (Tasks) analyses of covariance testing for linear trends for A–B type were performed on SBP, DBP, and HR change scores with base level values as covariates.

Considering first the analyses employing A–B type classifications, no significant relations emerged for the SBP or HR data. However, there was a significant linear, negative relation between A–B classification and DBP reactivity scores, $F(1,76) = 4.82$, $p < .04$. Means, adjusted for baseline values, for the DBP data across tasks for A–B type classification are as follows: A1 = 2.56 mm Hg; A2 = 6.20 mm Hg; and B = 5.72 mm Hg. No significant interactions between A–B type and tasks were found for the SBP, DBP, or HR data. The findings, then, indicate that Type A males did not respond with greater reactivity than Type B's to situations that would be expected to elicit such differences, namely, the SI and a difficult but not exceedingly difficult memory task.

Considering next the analyses employing cluster groupings, a significant relation was found for SBP responses, $F(1,79) = 8.49$, $p < .005$, but not for DBP or HR responses. Across tasks, subjects in the High A group exhibited the greatest SBP responses ($M = 12.77$ mm Hg), subjects in the Moderate A group exhibited the next highest SBP responses ($M = 9.86$ mm Hg), and subjects in the Non A group exhibited the least SBP responsivity ($M = 6.82$ mm Hg).

The results of this study point to the following conclusions. For males, groups of people can be identified through cluster analysis who, on the basis of their profiles of characteristics, can be ordered roughly in terms of how Type A they are. Assigning individuals to groups that are more homogeneous in their Type A characteristics than is found in the traditional A–B type groupings improves prediction of reactivity. Perhaps the same might occur for predicting CHD.

**Cluster Analysis Study of Females: Results and Discussion.** The cluster analysis based on the Type A component characteristics for females revealed four clusters. The profiles of their characteristics are displayed in Figure 10.2. Because there are four clusters and the profiles overlap, the figure appears complex. One cluster is highest on loudness, emphases, and potential for hostility, so this group was labeled "loud, emphatic, hostile." Another cluster of subjects is highest, or at least high, on the various speech characteristics, so this group was labeled "quick, vigorous" speakers. Yet another cluster of subjects is highest on verbal competitiveness, so this group was labeled "verbally competitive." And the final cluster of subjects are relatively

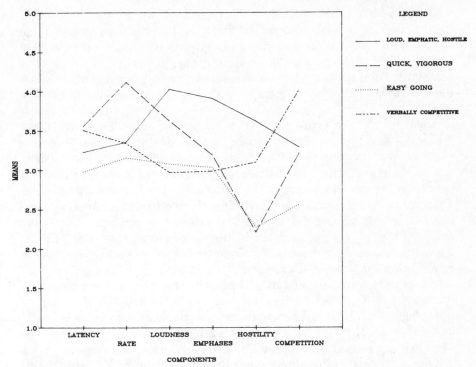

**FIGURE 10.2.** Profiles of Type A components for empirically derived clusters of female subjects.

low on all the characteristics, so this group was labeled "easy going," which is the same as Non A.

To evaluate relations between cluster membership and reactivity to the SI and digits backward task, 4 (Clusters) × 2 (Tasks) analyses of covariance were performed on SBP, DBP, and HR change scores with base level values as covariates (Benjamin, 1967; Wilder, 1968). Again, because global Type A ratings are the benchmark against which to compare some other procedure for classifying individuals, analyses were also performed to evaluate relations between Type A–Type B classifications and reactivity to the SI and digits-backward task. Specifically, 3 (Type A1, A2, B) × 2 (Tasks) analyses of covariance were performed on SBP, DBP, and HR change scores with base level values as covariates.

Considering first the analyses employing A–B type classifications, none of the main effects for A–B type classification even approached significance, all $F$'s < 1. None of the interactions involving task were significant either, all $F$'s < 1.60. Thus Type A females did not respond with greater reactivity than Type B's to the SI and/or digits-backward task.

Considering next the analyses employing cluster groupings, main effects emerged in the analyses for each cardiovascular measure, $F(3,97) = 4.04$,

$p < .01$ for SBP, $F(3,97) = 2.44$, $p < .07$ for DBP, and $F(3,96) = 2.25$, $p < .09$ for HR, respectively. The means for these data are presented in Table 10.1. Across tasks, subjects in the "quick, vigorous" cluster were the most reactive while subjects in the other three groups basically did not differ in reactivity. Thus the use of cluster analysis to assign females to Type A–derived categories resulted in the identification of a group that was more reactive than other groups.

The results of this study point to the following conclusions. One is that the profiles of Type A characteristics for females differed from those for males. It was mentioned in the review of reactivity studies that the SI is not nearly as predictive of reactivity for females as for males. Perhaps this is because females do not fit as well into categories that range from more Type A-like to less Type A-like, which is done when individuals are categorized as A1, A2, and B. It may be that a different categorization scheme employing Type A characteristics is more predictive for women. This is what occurred in the present study. Compared to the prediction of reactivity by assigning females to A–B categories, prediction of reactivity was improved when females were assigned to groups that (1) were more homogeneous in their Type A characteristics than is found in the traditional A–B type groupings, and (2) have different profiles of characteristics than are found in the traditional A–B type groupings. Perhaps prediction of CHD by the SI for women would be improved by using a similar procedure.

One additional thing about these data should be noted. The "loud, emphatic, hostile" group that might be expected to be particularly reactive was not more reactive than the other groups. Why this occurred is unclear. As will be seen later in the review of the data for Type A components and reactivity, prediction of reactivity by ratings of potential for hostility has been inconsistent. Moreover, it is uncertain how "toxic" potential for hostility as assessed via the SI is for women. It should be noted that only male subjects were employed in the studies emanating from the WCGS in which potential for hostility was related to incidence of CHD (Matthews, Glass,

**TABLE 10.1.   REACTIVITY SCORES FOR SYSTOLIC BLOOD PRESSURE, DIASTOLIC BLOOD PRESSURE, HEART RATE, AND CLUSTER CLASSIFICATION OF SUBJECTS**

|  | Cluster Classification | | | |
|---|---|---|---|---|
| Measure | Quick, Vigorous | Easy Going | Loud, Emphatic, Hostile | Verbally Competitive |
| SBP | $14.58^a$ | $8.94^b$ | $9.14^b$ | $9.26^b$ |
| DBP | $11.07^a$ | $8.27^{ab}$ | $6.45^b$ | $8.17^{ab}$ |
| HR | $6.48^a$ | $4.17^{ab}$ | $1.08^b$ | $3.06^{ab}$ |

*Note:* Means are adjusted for baseline values. Means across rows that do not share the same superscript differ significantly ($p < .05$).

Rosenman, & Bortner, 1977; see also Chesney, Hecker, & Black, Chapter 8, this volume) and of the two studies in which potential for hostility has been related to severity of coronary atherosclerosis, one study contained all males (MacDougall, Dembroski, Dimsdale, & Hackett, 1985) and 75 percent of the subjects in the second study were males (Dembroski, MacDougall, Williams, Haney, & Blumenthal, 1985).

## Style of Administering the SI and Reactivity

The question has been raised recently by Scherwitz (1984; see also Scherwitz, Chapter 3, this volume) whether the style of administering the SI influences the prediction of CHD by Type A. Specifically, from a reassessment of the Multiple Risk Factor Intervention Trial (MRFIT) data, Scherwitz proposes that Type A ratings that are derived from interviewers whose style (termed *facilitative*) involves speaking more slowly and being less emphatic are predictive of CHD, while Type A ratings that are derived from interviewers whose style (termed *disruptive*) involves speaking more rapidly and rushing and interrupting the interviewee tend to be negatively predictive of CHD. Congruent with this notion, one can question whether a facilitative style of administering the SI may result in A–B classifications that predict reactivity better than A–B classifications based on a disruptive style of administering the SI. We undertook the following study to address this question.

Male subjects were randomly assigned to receive the SI in either a facilitative or a disruptive fashion. The disruptive style basically involved administering the SI in the challenging manner that has been recommended in recent years (Chesney et al., 1980). The interviewer, a female, spoke relatively rapidly, interrupted the speaker frequently, tried to hurry the speaker, and resumed talking quickly after the interviewee had finished speaking. In the facilitative style condition, the interviewer spoke more slowly, did not interrupt the speaker, did not hurry the speaker, and waited longer after the interviewee had finished speaking before she resumed talking. In a separate session, the subjects were given the Stroop task and a mirror-tracing task while SBP, DBP, and HR were monitored. In yet another session, subjects were given the JAS and FTAS. The reason for giving these measures was to determine whether style of administering the SI influenced the relations between SI-defined A–B and A–B type as defined by other measures, namely, either the JAS or FTAS.

Subjects were categorized as to Type A or Type B without regard to condition. Next, Type A subjects were separated into those who had been administered the SI with the facilitative style and those who had been administered the SI with the disruptive style. The same was done for Type B subjects. This resulted in a 2 (A–B Type) × 2 (Style of Administering the SI) factorial design. Analyses of the dependent measures revealed interactions between A–B type and style of administering the SI for DBP, $F(1,69) = 5.11$, $p < .03$, and for FTAS, $F(1,63) = 4.79$, $p < .04$. (Missing data were responsible for the variation in degrees of freedom.) The three-way interactions involving tasks were not significant in any of the analyses.

Inspection of the significant interactions revealed the following. Subjects identified as Type A via the facilitative style exhibited greater DBP responses ($M$ = 12.69 mm Hg) to the experimental tasks than subjects identified as Type B ($M$ = 8.88 mm Hg), but subjects identified as Type A via the disruptive style evidenced less DBP responsivity ($M$ = 11.63 mm Hg) than Type B's ($M$ = 16.37 mm Hg). These findings are congruent with the results of Scherwitz's (1984) reassessment of the MRFIT study in which the Type A ratings from facilitative interviewers were found to be predictive of CHD while the Type A ratings from some of the disruptive interviewers were found to be negatively predictive of CHD.

Additionally, subjects identified as Type A via the facilitative style had higher scores on the FTAS ($M$ = .70) than subjects identified as B ($M$ = .57). However, subjects identified as Type A via the disruptive style tended to exhibit lower FTAS scores ($M$ = .60) than Type B's ($M$ = .67). The pattern of results for the JAS scores was similar to that for the FTAS, but the interaction was not significant. Thus the results for the questionnaire measures of Type A, the FTAS in particular, provide additional support for categorizing subjects as Type A and Type B on the basis of the SI administered in a facilitative style.

The results of this study revealed the following. A positive relation between reactivity and Type A was found only when the SI was administered in a facilitative style. Moreover, a positive relation between FTAS scores and SI-defined Type A was found only when the facilitative style of administering the SI was employed. Collectively, then, these results are congruent with the notion that a facilitative style of giving the interview is necessary for obtaining Type A ratings that predict CHD.

## SI Components and Reactivity

A fair amount of interest has been focused recently on the relation between individual SI-derived Type A components and cardiovascular reactivity. Interest in this area sprang from research in which SI-derived Type A components have been examined separately for their relation to cardiovascular disease (Matthews et al., 1977; see also Chesney, Hecker, & Black, Chapter 8, this volume). This area of research on reactivity also embraces the hypothesis that chronic, exaggerated sympathetic–adrenomedullary activity mediates the association with CHD.

The purpose of this section is to summarize briefly the findings concerning the relation between SI-derived Type A components and cardiovascular reactivity. The findings are summarized in Tables 10.2, 10.3, and 10.4. In each table, the author(s) of the study, subject gender, and task or tasks are presented in the first three columns. Diamond and colleagues' (1984) study presented in Tables 10.2 and 10.3 contained three conditions, so the

**TABLE 10.2. TYPE A COMPONENTS AND REACTIVITY: I**

| Study | Gender | Task[a] | Latency | Rate | Loudness | Emphasis | Loud–Explosive (loudness and emphasis) |
|---|---|---|---|---|---|---|---|
| Dembroski et al., 1978 | Male | (RT, pong, and anagrams) | 0 | +SBP** | | | 0 |
| Glass et al., 1983 | Male | Modified Stroop | 0 | +DBP** | | | 0 |
| Allen et al., 1984 | Male | RCR | −SBP**, +PTT** | 0 | | 0 | |
| | | RCQ | −SBP**, −DBP* | 0 | 0 | 0 | |
| | | DB | 0 | 0 | 0 | 0 | |
| | | CP | 0 | 0 | 0 | 0 | |
| | | IH | 0 | 0 | 0 | 0 | |
| Diamond et al., 1984 | Male | Pong | | | | | |
| | | Competition | 0' | 0' | | | 0' |
| | | Frustration | 0' | 0' | | | 0' |
| | | Harassment | 0' | 0' | | | 0' |
| MacDougall et al., 1981 | | | | | | | |
| Study I | Female | CP | 0' | 0' | | | 0' |
| | | RT | 0' | 0' | | | 0' |
| Study II | Female | SI | 0' | 0' | | | 0' |
| | | RT | 0' | 0' | | | 0' |
| Anderson et al., 1986 | Female | SI | 0 | +SBP** +DBP** | +SBP** +DBP** | +SBP** +DBP** | 0 |
| | | MA | 0 | | | | |

[a] RT = reaction time; SI = Structured Interview; DB = digits backward; CP = cold pressor; MA = mental arithmetic; RCR = reading comprehension reading phase; RCQ = reading comprehension questioning phase; IH = isometric handgrip.
*$p < .10$
**$p < .05$.

231

## TABLE 10.3. TYPE A COMPONENTS AND REACTIVITY: II

| Study | Subject Gender | Task[a] | Potential for Hostility | Verbal Competitiveness |
|---|---|---|---|---|
| Dembroski et al., 1978 | Male | (RT, pong, and anagrams) | +SBP**, +HR** | +SBP** |
| Glass et al., 1983 | Male | Modified Stroop | −SBP*, −DBP** | −DBP* |
| Allen et al., 1984 | Male | RCR | 0 | 0 |
| | | RCQ | 0 | +HR** |
| | | DB | +HR**, −PTT* | +HR** |
| | | CP | +SBP**, +DBP* | +SBP** |
| | | IH | +SBP*, +DBP** | 0 |
| Diamond et al., 1984 | Male | Pong | | |
| | | Competition | 0 | 0' |
| | | Frustration | 0 | 0' |
| | | Harassment | 0 | 0' |
| MacDougall et al., 1981 | | | | |
| Study I | Female | CP | 0 | 0' |
| | | RT | +SBP**, +HR** | 0' |
| Study II | Female | SI | +SBP** | 0' |
| | | RT | −HR** | 0' |
| Anderson et al., 1986 | Female | SI | 0 | 0 |
| | | MA | 0 | +DBP** |

[a]RT = reaction time; SI = Structured Interview; DB = digits backward; CP = cold pressor; MA = mental arithmetic; RCR = reading comprehension reading phase; RCQ = reading comprehension questioning phase; IH = isometric handgrip.
*$p < .10$.
**$p < .05$.

data for each condition are presented. Because all of these studies also assessed global Type A, more information about any one of them can be obtained by referring back to the review of studies on global Type A and reactivity.

A plus (+) preceding the abbreviation for a cardiovascular measure indicates that there is a positive relation between the component in question and that measure of reactivity. For example, in the first study presented in Table 10.2—the one by Dembroski and colleagues (1978)—the faster the speaking rate, the greater the SBP and DBP responses across the three tasks. A minus sign (−) preceding the abbreviation for a cardiovascular

TABLE 10.4.   TYPE A COMPONENTS AND REACTIVITY: III

| Study | Subject Gender | Task[a] | Stylistic Vigor (loud–explosive and rapid and latency) | Hostility–Competition (hostility and verbal competitiveness) |
|---|---|---|---|---|
| Dembroski, MacDougall, Herd, & Shields, 1979 | Male | CP—high-low challenge | +SBP**—high +HR** challenge | +HR**—high challenge +SBP**, +DBP**—low challenge |
| | | RT—high-low challenge | +SBP**—high and low challenge | +SBP**—high and low challenge |
| Dembroski, MacDougall, & Lushene, 1979 | Male | SI | +SBP** +DBP** | +SBP** |

[a]RT = reaction time; SI = Structured Interview; CP = cold pressor.
*$p < .10$
**$p < .05$.

measure indicates that there is a negative relation between the component in question and that measure of reactivity. For example, in the Latency column, the more quickly the interviewees responded to the interviewers' questions, the less SBP reactivity they showed in Allen and colleagues' (1984) study. A zero (0) means that the component in question was not found to be associated with any measure of cardiovascular reactivity. A zero-prime (0') means that the component is assumed not to be related to any measure of cardiovascular reactivity because, although the component was scored and measures of cardiovascular reactivity were obtained, no results were reported. A blank means that the component in question was not investigated in a particular study.

In Table 10.2, looking down the columns indicates few relations between reactivity and latency of response, rate of speech, loudness of speech, emphatic speech, or loud–explosive speech. Table 10.3 summarizes additional information for these same studies. Potential for hostility is of particular interest because it has been found to be related to CHD (Matthews et al., 1977; see also Chesney et al., Chapter 8, this volume) as well as coronary atherosclerosis (Dembroski et al., 1985; MacDougall et al., 1985). However, as can be seen, the findings for the relation between ratings of potential for hostility and reactivity are somewhat inconsistent. Most of the investigations in which potential for hostility has been found to be significantly, positively related to reactivity are those studies conducted by Dembroski, MacDougall, and colleagues. Perhaps Dembroski and colleagues are picking up on subtle cues with regard to potential for hostility that need to be more clearly articulated and taught to raters. The results for verbal competition are too inconsistent to draw any conclusions.

In a pair of studies by Dembroski and MacDougall and their colleagues (Dembroski, MacDougall, Herd, & Shields, 1979; Dembroski, MacDougall, & Lushene, 1979), the SI components were combined into two categories, namely, stylistic vigor and hostility–competition. As can be seen from Table 10.4, each combination was predictive of reactivity. The implications of these results are unclear, however. Did the combination of components derive their predictiveness because of a single, highly predictive component, an additive effect of weak predictors, an interaction effect, or what? Also, because components were combined, information concerning the capacity of individual components to predict reactivity is lost. Thus knowledge concerning the individual SI-derived components is not advanced by this ad hoc procedure for agglutinizing components.

In summary, the findings for relations between SI-derived components and reactivity are disappointing. The results for potential for hostility are the most promising, although positive relations between potential for hostility and reactivity were found for less than half of the experimental situations that were investigated.

Measurement problems may be partly responsible for this state of affairs. More clear criteria and supervised training for raters may be necessary for scoring the components, in particular, the more subjective components, for example, potential for hostility, verbal competition, and so on (see Chapter 8 by Chesney et al. for careful work in this regard). Additionally, perhaps the use of automated devices, such as employed by Howland and Siegman (1982), may be desirable for quantifying latency of response, rate of speaking, and so on.

Another possibility is that the experimental arrangement may inadvertently obscure relations. Take individuals who are high in potential for hostility as an example. Hostile individuals may feel threatened by, disgusted with, or in some other way disenchanted by the experimenter or some unforeseen aspects of the experimental situation. In turn, such individuals may withdraw from involvement in the experiment and therefore be less responsive to the experimental task or situation then they otherwise would be. Careful postexperimental inquiry may be needed to identify circumstances such as this.

## STUDIES EMPLOYING THE JAS

### Global Type A and Reactivity: Review

**Solitary Situations, Single Conditions, Males.**    Perhaps the first methodologically sound investigation of reactivity in which subjects were studied as they performed tasks by themselves was conducted by Dembroski and colleagues (1978). In this study, described earlier because it also employed the SI, college male subjects performed a reaction-time task that was described as a test of the subject's speed of reaction, an electronic pong game that was described as a test of subject's hand–eye coordination, and a series of difficult anagrams under a time limit. Type A subjects manifested significantly greater SBP and DBP but not HR responses across the three tasks than Type B subjects.

In a study by Newlin and Levinson (1982), male college students performed a shock avoidance reaction-time task, a Stroop task with interpolated encouragement to respond quickly, and an isometric handgrip task. Type A's responded with greater DBP than B's to all three tasks. Type B's responded with greater SBP than A's to the isometric handgrip task. There were no differences between Type A's and Type B's in interbeat interval (HR) or FPA responses to any of these tasks.

Male college students performed a task involving remembering and reciting digits backward in a study by Smith, Houston, and Stucky (1984). The analyses revealed that by the end of the task Type A's manifested significantly greater PR responses than Type B's, although no differences were found at the beginning of the task. No significant A–B main effects or interactions with task periods were found for SBP or DBP.

Investigators who included both males and females, as in the next two studies, typically either did not find interactions with gender or apparently did not include gender as a factor in their analyses of the data. Studies employing both males and females will be discussed in both this section and the section on females.

College males and females performed the Stroop Color-Word Interference Test, a mental arithmetic task (serial subtraction of 7's), and a difficult shock-avoidance task in a study by Jorgensen and Houston (1981). Relative to Type B's, Type A's exhibited significantly greater DBP responses to the Stroop task and marginally significantly ($p < .06$) greater DBP responses to the shock avoidance task. There were no differences between Type A's and Type B's in SBP or HR responses to these two tasks or in SBP, DBP, or HR responses to the mental arithmetic task.

A sample of men and women who ranged in age from 21 to 64 were studied by Hull, Young, and Ziegler (1984) while they performed the Stroop task, watched an industrial accident film, were exposed to the cold pressor test, and exercised on a treadmill until exhausted. Relative to Type B's, Type A's exhibited significantly greater HR responses to the Stroop but not greater SBP, DBP, or plasma NE or E. Type A's and Type B's did not differ on any of the physiological measures during the accident film, the cold pressor test, or the treadmill test.

Male college students were selected on the basis of extreme scores on the JAS by Essau and Jamieson (1987) and performed a digit-recall task while their HR responses were monitored. Type A's were found to exhibit a greater increase in HR to the task than Type B's.

In contrast to the aforementioned studies, several investigations have failed to find differences in reactivity between JAS-defined Type A's and Type B's. Type A and Type B male attorneys were administered a difficult concept formation task with purposefully low-incentive instructions in a study by Manuck, Corse, and Winkelman (1979). Type A was not related to SBP, DBP, or HR responses to the task. However, the attorneys as a group scored well into the Type A range on the JAS; hence it may have been difficult to find cardiovascular differences bettween subject groups because of the restricted range of scores. Moreover, there may have been insufficient incentive in this situation for attorneys to perform well on the task, and therefore cardiovascular differences between more and less Type A subjects did not emerge.

Male college students were selected on the basis of extreme scores on the JAS in a study by Diamond and Carver (1980). Subjects were given a mental subtraction task (serial subtraction of 12's) and a task that involved recognizing words that were projected blurry, backward, and upside-down on a screen. On both tasks, subjects were encouraged to perform as quickly and accurately as possible. No differences between Type A's and Type B's were found in SBP, DBP, HR, or FPV.

Goldband (1980, II) conducted a study in which male college subjects blew up balloons until they burst and also were exposed to the cold pressor test. To demonstrate that tasks such as these by themselves do not differentially evoke A–B differences, subjects were not given any incentive to perform well on either task, nor were they led to believe that either task was difficult. Congruent wth expectation, no differences in HR or PTT were found between Type A's and Type B's for either task.

In a study of male college students by Cornelius and Averill (1980), subjects could influence the time at which a shock would occur but not whether or for how long it would occur. No differences in HR responses were found between Type A and Type B subjects. Perhaps this occurred because there was no incentive, for example, negative reinforcement, for task performance since subjects were not able to avoid or escape the shock.

Lott and Gatchel (1978) found no differences between Type A and Type B college male and female subjects in SBP, DBP, or HR reactions to a cold pressor test. However, there is no indication that the subjects were given incentive to perform well or that subjects were led to believe that the task was difficult.

Male and female patients and staff from a large medical practice served as subjects in an investigation by Goldstein, Edelberg, Meier, Orzano, and Blaufuss (1985). Subjects were studied while they performed a reaction-time task and a paced arithmetic task that involved mental addition and subtraction. Type A's and Type B's did not differ significantly in SBP, DBP, or HR responses to the tasks. However, interpretation of the results is complicated by the fact that half of the subjects were diagnosed as mild hypertensives and no mention is made of how these individuals were distributed across Type A and Type B categories.

College males selected on the basis of extreme JAS scores performed a shock avoidance, reaction-time task in a study by Stoney, Langer, Sutterer, and Gelling (1987). No significant differences between Type A's and Type B's were found for subjects in SBP, DBP, or HR responses to the task in either a control condition or two biofeedback conditions.

There are a few studies that were described previously because they employed the SI as well as the JAS that failed to find differences in reactivity between JAS-defined Type A's and Type B's. In a study by Scherwitz and colleagues (1978) of male college students, subjects were exposed to the cold pressor test, a mental arithmetic task, a maze-learning task, and a task involving the generation of emotions. As mentioned earlier, it does not appear, however, that any instructions were given that would have provided subjects with incentive for performing well on the tasks. Type A's relative to Type B's evidenced significantly higher SBP across all the rest periods and across all the task periods, although there were no differences in reactivity.

Adult males who either did or did not have CHD performed a difficult concept task, a mental arithmetic task (serial subtraction of 17's), and the Picture Completion subtest of the Wechsler Adult Intelligence Scale in a study by Corse and colleagues (1982). There were no significant differences in SBP, DBP, or HR responses to the tasks between Type A and Type B subjects.

Male subjects from the fire and police departments were given a mental arithmetic task (serial subtraction of 13's) and a modified Stroop task to perform with instructions to perform quickly and accurately in a study by Glass and colleagues (1983). Type A's did not differ from Type B's in SBP, DBP, or HR responses to either task or in NE or E responses to the modified Stroop task.

In an investigation by Fontana and colleagues (1986), male, non-CHD medical and surgical patients were studied while they responded to an unspecified performance test, the JAS, a questionnaire on achievement, and the TAT. There were no significant differences between Type A's and Type B's in SBP or DBP responses to any of the tasks.

In a study of male college students by Allen and colleagues (1987), no significant main effects for A–B type were found for SBP, DBP, HR, or PTT responses to a reading comprehension test, a virtually impossible digit span task, the cold pressor test, or a handgrip task.

*Summary.*    There were certain expected consistencies and some troublesome inconsistencies in the results of investigations in which male subjects' responses to solitary situations were studied. Type A–Type B differences in reactivity were found for reaction-time tasks and the Stroop task in the majority of studies in which these tasks were included. Both kinds of tasks require speed and involve a moderate probability of failure. Consistently, no differences between Type A's and Type B's were found in response to performing serial subtraction tasks. As suggested earlier, because this task is very difficult, both JAS-defined and SI-defined Type A's may perceive that the probability of failure is too great and thus they are not motivated to try harder than B's. Consistently also, no differences between A's and B's were found in response to physical stressors, for example, the cold pressor, exercise, and so on. These results are not surprising because there is no reason to expect such tasks to engage the characteristics of Type A's or arouse them more than Type B's.

It is noteworthy, however, that in three studies in which both the SI and JAS were included, SI-defined A–B differences in reactivity were found in response to a variety of tasks, namely, the concept formation and picture completion tasks in the study by Corse and colleagues (1982), a performance test in the study by Fontana and colleagues (1986), various tasks including a reading comprehension test in the study by Allen and colleagues (1987), while JAS-defined A–B differences in reactivity were not found. On the other hand, in two other studies in which both the SI and JAS were employed (Dembroski et al., 1978; Glass et al., 1983), the presence or lack of reactivity differences between JAS-defined Type A's and Type B's were basically the same as for SI-defined Type A's and Type B's. A reasonable explanation for these findings is that SI-defined Type A is more strongly related to reactivity than JAS-defined Type A; hence in some but not all studies in which both the SI and the JAS are employed, statistically significant differences in reactivity will be found for SI-defined Type A's and Type B's but not JAS-defined Type A's and Type B's.

**Solitary Situations, Multiple Conditions, Males.** Male and female college students selected on the basis of extreme JAS scores were given either solvable or unsolvable anagrams on which to work in a study by Gastorf (1981). Half of the subjects in both the solvable and unsolvable conditions were told that the anagrams were easy to solve, while the other half were told that the anagrams were difficult to solve. Type A relative to Type B subjects (1) did not differ significantly in SBP or DBP responses to the solvable anagrams that had been described as easy, but (2) did manifest significantly greater SBP responses but not DBP responses to the anagrams in the other three conditions. Thus Type A's and Type B's differed in reactivity to the tasks when they were told or found through their own experience that it was difficult. Because of the brevity of the tasks and the ambiguity of the anagrams, it is unlikely that subjects accurately perceived the true difficulty of the unsolvable anagrams.

Male college students selected on the basis of extreme JAS scores served as subjects in a study by Holmes, McGilley, and Houston (1984). Subjects were assigned to one of three conditions in which they were given six sets of digits to remember and repeat backward. The number of digits in each of the six sets varied across the low-, medium-, and high-difficulty conditions. Type A's exhibited greater SBP responses than Type B's only in the high-difficulty condition. There were no differences between Type A's and B's in DBP, HR, or FPV.

In a study of college males by Dembroski, MacDougall, Herd, and Shields (1979) described earlier, subjects performed a cold pressor test and a reaction-time task under high- and low-challenge conditions. The difficulty of the respective tasks was emphasized in the high-challenge but not low-challenge condition. Type A's relative to Type B's responded with significantly greater SBP and less FPV but no differences in DBP or HR to the reaction-time task in the low-challenge but not high-challenge condition. Type A's and Type B's did not differ in SBP, DBP, HR, or FPV to the cold pressor test in either condition.

Subjects performed a reaction-time task under either high- or low-challenge conditions in a study by Goldband (1980, Study I). In the high-challenge condition, subjects were exhorted to do their very best on the tasks and subsequently were given two kinds of failure feedback. One kind of failure feedback was that they missed the time deadline for the task on half of the trials, and the second was performance feedback that ultimately indicated that they had failed the task relative to the "average subject." There were no differences in HR or PTT between Type A's and Type B's in this condition, possibly because the task was perceived as being highly difficult. In the low-challenge condition, subjects received no instructions to perform well, and they received feedback that they were performing successfully. There were apparently no HR or PTT differences between Type A and Type B males in this condition, possibly because of the lack of incentive or low difficulty of the task.

In a study by Manuck and Garland (1979), college males peformed a difficult concept formation task either in a high-incentive condition with monetary inducement for correct responses or a low-incentive condition without monetary inducements. SBP and HR responses, but not DBP responses, were significantly, positively correlated with JAS scores in the low- but not high-incentive condition.

College males were selected on the basis of extreme scores on the JAS in a study by Blumenthal and colleagues (1983). Subjects performed a concept formation task in either a high-incentive condition (monetary inducement for good performance) or low-incentive condition (no monetary inducement). Type A's and Type B's did not differ significantly on SBP, DBP, HR, FVR, or FBF in response to the task.

In a study by Perkins (1984), male college students were selected for extreme scores on the JAS and performed a reaction-time task in conditions that varied from 90 percent to 0 percent failure feedback and in response cost for poor performance (losing money, points, or nothing). Although tests of simple main effects were not made following a significant A–B Type × Response Cost interaction, it appears that Type A's responded with greater HR to the task than B's when subjects lost money but not points for poor performance. Curiously, Type A's relative to Type B's also manifested greater HR responses to the task when they neither received failure feedback nor expected to lose anything if they performed poorly.

In a study employing college males by Jennings (1984), subjects performed a reaction-time task with instructions for fast and accurate performance and then performed the reaction-time task at five different speed criteria during practice and under both high- and low-monetary-incentive conditions. Overall, Type A's and Type B's were not reported to differ significantly in SBP, DBP, or interbeat interval (HR). However, no report was made of the overall design of the statistical analyses or the results therefrom, blood pressure was measured at the end of performance blocks rather than during task performance, and the experiment involved from three to five 2-hour sessions across as many as 3 days. The complexity and length of the study could easily have obscured A–B type differences in reactivity.

*Summary.* The following summary statements can be made about the results of the studies in which multiple conditions were used in the study of subjects while they performed a solitary task. Differences between JAS-defined Type A's and Type B's are more likely to be observed when the task is viewed as high but not extremely high in difficulty. Moreover, the results of the studies involving levels of challenge on incentive suggest that JAS-defined Type A's are more likely to respond with greater reactivity than Type B's in situations involving moderate incentive. Comparing studies in which the SI and JAS have been used to measure Type A, it appears that a lower level of incentive may trigger differences in reactivity between JAS-defined Type A's and Type B's than SI-defined Type A's and B's. This may occur because evidence of individuals' achievement striving contributes more to high JAS scores than a designation of Type A via the SI. However, neither incentive nor additional challenge seems to elicit differences in reactivity between JAS-defined Type A's and B's to physical stressors, like the cold pressor test.

**Behavior in the Presence of Others, Males.** In three investigations, Van Egeren (1979a, 1979b) and colleagues (Van Egeren, Sniderman, & Roggelin, 1982) studied male and female subjects in mixed-motive games. Basically, the goal of such games is for the subject to gain as many points as possible by behaving in a competitive or cooperative manner with another person (via pushbuttons) with the realization that the point payoff also depends on how competitively or cooperatively the other person behaves. In one study (Van Egeren, 1979a) male and female Type A relative to Type B subjects exhibited significantly greater HR, though also more FPV (indicating less arousal), in a condition in which the other person (actually a computer) acted very competitively. In a condition in which the subject's opponent ostensibly acted very cooperatively, there were no significant differences in HR or FPV responses between Type A and Type B subjects. Perhaps in this condition Type A's perceived it as being very easy to gain as many points as they wanted because the other ostensible subject was very un-competitive; therefore, they did not work harder and thus did not exhibit greater psychophysiological arousal than Type B's.

In a second study (Van Egeren, 1979b), each subject's opponent was a real subject. However, male and female subjects were paired such that half of the Type A subjects interacted with another Type A while the other half interacted with a Type B; similarly, half of the Type B subjects interacted with a Type A and the other half interacted with another Type B. During the interaction, Type A subjects exhibited more arousal as indexed by less FPV, but not by HR, when they interacted with another Type A or a Type B than when two Type B's interacted. In addition, when interacting with Type A's, Type B's exhibited nearly as much arousal, as indexed by FPV, as when Type A's interacted with either Type A's or Type B's. However, these results should be regarded cautiously because they failed to replicate in the study by Van Egeren and colleagues (1982).

Male college students were selected on the basis of extreme scores on the JAS in a study by Diamond and colleagues (1984) that was described earlier. Subjects were assigned to one of three conditions in which they competed on a video game with a confederate. The confederate made harassing comments to the subject in one condition but was silent in another condition, and in a third condition, the experimenter frustrated the subject's winning the game. There were no significant differences between Type A's and Type B's in SBP, DBP, or HR in any of the conditions.

In a study by Zurawski and Houston (1983), male college students performed a perceptual motor task twice with a confederate in either an anger provocation condition or nonanger condition. The first time the task was performed, the confederate was cooperative, which resulted in his winning a prize. The second time, the confederate either was again cooperative (which helped the subject win a prize) or was uncooperative and critical (which prevented the subject from winning a prize). Although there was a main effect for DBP and self-reported anger indicating that the manipulation of anger was effective, Type A's and Type B's did not differ significantly in SBP, DBP, or HR in either condition.

In a study by Holmes and Will (1985), male college students performed a perceptual motor task with a confederate in either an anger provocation condition in which the confederate was uncooperative and derogatory or a nonanger condition in which the confederate was cooperative and sup-portive. Although there were significant main effects for SBP, DBP, and HR indicating that the manipulation of anger was effective, Type A's and Type B's did not differ significantly in SBP, DBP, or HR in either condition.

In two studies, the responses of JAS-defined Type A's and Type B's to the SI were investigated. No differences between Type A's and Type B's in SBP, DBP, HR, or FPV were found in a study of male college students by Scherwitz and colleagues (1978). Similarly, no significant differences between Type A's and Type B's in SBP or DBP responses to the SI were found in a study of male, non-CHD medical and surgical patients by Fontana and colleagues (1986).

*Summary.*   The investigations in which subjects' behaviors were studied in the presence of others revealed little evidence of differences between JAS-defined Type A's and Type B's in response to interpersonal competition, harassment, or other provocation. This may be due to the paucity of anger-related items on the JAS (Matthews, 1982; Zurawski & Houston, 1983), which may reduce not only the sensitivity of the JAS for measuring the hostility component of Type A but also the kind of competitiveness that may be motivated by hostility.

### Solitary Task Performance, Single Condition, Females.

Somewhat more studies have been conducted of potential differences in reactivity between Type A and Type B females in which the JAS was employed than for the SI. There are enough such studies that they will be reviewed in separate sections, as was done for males. However, each subsection will not have its own summary; rather there is one overall summary at the end of the review of the reactivity studies in which females were employed as subjects.

No cardiovascular differences between A's and B's were obtained in the following five investigations in which college females were studied in regard to their responses to performing solitary tasks. Two studies of college females, which were described earlier because the SI was also employed, were reported by MacDougall and colleagues (1981). Subjects in the first study were exposed to two tasks: the cold pressor test and a reaction-time task. Instructions for both tasks emphasized the tasks' difficulty. No differences between Type A's and Type B's were found for SBP, DBP, or HR responses to either task. Subjects in the second study performed a reaction-time task with monetary incentive for good performance. Type A's and Type B's were not found to differ significantly in SBP, DBP, or HR responses to this task.

Subjects were presented with three tasks, a mental arithmetic task (addition and multiplication) and two sets of Raven's Progressive Matrices problems in a study by Lawler and colleagues (1984). No significant differences were found between Type A's and Type B's in their SBP, DBP, or HR responses to the experimental tasks.

College females who were selected on the basis of extreme scores on the JAS performed a mental arithmetic task (serial subtraction of 13's) in a study by Lane, White, and Williams (1984). No significant differences were found between Type A's and Type B's in FBF or FVR or in their SBP, DBP, or HR responses to the mental arithmetic task.

In another investigation of college women by Lawler and Schmied (1986), subjects were studied while they performed the Stroop test. No differences between Type A's and Type B's in SBP, DBP, or HR were found.

The following two studies, described earlier, employed both college males and females as subjects. Lott and Gatchel (1978) found no differences in Type A and B male and female subjects' SBP, DBP, or HR reactions to a cold pressor test. However, as mentioned earlier, there is no indication that the subjects were given incentive to perform well or that subjects were led to believe that the task was difficult. Moreover, as has been described before, differences in reactivity between A's and B's are rarely found for physical stressors.

In a study by Jorgensen and Houston (1981), college males and females performed the Stroop Color-Word Interference Test, a mental arithmetic task (serial subtraction of 7's), and a difficult shock avoidance task. Relative to Type B's, Type A's exhibited significantly greater DBP responses to the Stroop task and marginally significantly ($p < .06$) greater DBP responses to the shock avoidance task. There were no differences in SBP or HR response between A's and B's to these two tasks. Additionally, Type A's and B's did not differ significantly in SBP, DBP, or HR responses to the mental arithmetic task. Although none of the A–B by gender interactions were significant in this study, a reexamination of the analyses for the DBP data for the Stroop and shock avoidance tasks indicated that the differences between Type A's and Type B's for females were half as great as those found for males. Thus the A–B differences for females were weak but were counterbalanced in the overall analyses by stronger differences for males.

In contrast to the general lack of reactivity differences for Type A and Type B college females, studies of noncollege women have been somewhat more promising. Lawler, Rixse, and Allen (1983) studied cardiovascular reactivity for both women employed outside the home in professional or executive positions and homemakers. Subjects performed three tasks, a mental arithmetic task (addition and multiplication) and two sets of Raven's Progressive Matrices problems. Type A relative to Type B homemakers exhibited significantly greater SBP and DBP but no differences in HR responses across the tasks. However, all the women employed outside the home scored in the Type A range on the JAS, which precluded the comparison of Type A with Type B employed women in their responses to the experimental tasks.

Adult employed women were instructed to perform a mental addition task as quickly as possible in a study by Mayes and colleagues (1984). Relative to Type B's, Type A's exhibited a significantly greater decrease in ST but did not differ in SBP, DBP, or HR responses to the task. In contrast, in a study of employed Black women by Anderson and colleagues (1986) described earlier, no significant relations were found between A–B type and SBP, DBP, or HR responses to a mental arithmetic (serial subtraction) task.

The following two studies, described earlier, employed both noncollege males and females as subjects. A sample of men and women who ranged in age from 21 to 64 were studied by Hull and colleagues (1984) while they performed the Stroop task, watched an industrial accident film, were exposed to the cold pressor test, and exercised on a treadmill until exhausted. Relative to Type B's, Type A's responded to the Stroop with significantly greater HR but not greater SBP, DBP, or plasma NE or E. Type A's and Type B's did not differ on any of these physiological measures during the accident film, the cold pressor test, or the treadmill test.

Male and female patients and staff from a large medical practice served as subjects in an investigation by Goldstein and colleagues (1985). Subjects were studied while they performed a reaction-time task and a paced arithmetic task that involved mental addition and subtraction. Type A's and Type B's did not differ significantly in SBP, DBP, or HR responses to the tasks. However, as mentioned earlier, interpretation of the results is complicated by the fact that half of the subjects were diagnosed as mild hypertensives and no mention is made of how these individuals were distributed across Type A and Type B categories.

**Solitary Task Performance, Multiple Conditions, Females.**    In a study of college females by Weidner and Matthews (1978), subjects performed an arithmetic task while being exposed to either predictable or unpredictable loud noise. Type A relative to Type B subjects evidenced significantly higher SBP in the predictable noise condition but not in the unpredictable noise condition. There were no differences in DBP or ST between A's and B's. The presence of unpredictable noise is usually regarded by subjects as much more disruptive than predictable noise (Weidner & Matthews, 1978). Type A's may have worked harder and hence been more aroused than Type B's in the predictable noise condition. However, the disruptive, unpredictable noise may have made the situation appear too complex or difficult for Type A's, and hence they may not have tried harder and thus no differences in arousal between Type A's and Type B's emerged in the unpredictable noise condition.

In a study of college females by Morell (1985, Study II), subjects performed a reaction-time task under either high- or low-challenge conditions. In both conditions, subjects were encouraged to respond as quickly and accurately as possible. Additionally, in the high-challenge condition, subjects were told that task performance was related to ability and they were given failure feedback on half of the trials. No significant differences in interbeat interval (HR) or PTT were found between Type A's and Type B's in either condition.

In a study of women from the community by Morell (1985, Study I), subjects performed a reaction-time task under the same high- or low-challenge conditions as in the study of college females (Morell, 1985, Study II). No significant differences in interbeat interval (HR) or PTT were found between Type A's and Type B's in either condition. It should be noted that over 40 percent of this sample was composed of professional women, and more of the Type A's held master's and doctoral degrees than the Type B's. As may have occurred on the part of the Type A male attorneys in Manuck and colleagues' (1979) study, perhaps the laboratory task in the present study did not seem sufficiently important to the highly educated, Type A professional women to engage them differentially; hence differences in reactivity were not observed.

Male and female college students were given either solvable or unsolvable anagrams on which to work in a study by Gastorf (1982) described earlier. Half of the subjects in both the solvable and unsolvable conditions were told that the anagrams were easy to solve, while the other half were told that the anagrams were difficult to solve. Type A relative to Type B subjects (1) did not differ significantly in SBP or DBP responses to the solvable anagrams that had been described as easy, but (2) did manifest significantly greater SBP responses but not DBP responses to the anagrams in the other three conditions. As mentioned before, because of the brevity of the tasks and the ambiguity of the anagrams, it is unlikely that subjects accurately perceived the true difficulty of the unsolvable anagrams.

**Behavior in the Presence of Others, Females.**    In three studies described previously, Van Egeren (1979a, 1979b) and colleagues (Van Egeren et al., 1982) studied male and female college subjects in mixed-motive games. In one study (Van Egeren, 1979a), male and female Type A relative to Type B subjects exhibited significantly greater HR, though also more FPV (indicating less arousal), in a condition in which the other person (actually a computer) acted very competitively. In a condition in which the subject's opponent ostensibly acted very cooperatively, there were no significant differences in HR or FPV responses between Type A and Type B subjects. The results for the physiological measures in the second study (Van Egeren, 1979b) were not replicated by Van Egeren and colleagues (1982); hence they will not be recapped here.

In a study by MacDougall and colleagues (1981, Study II) of college females mentioned earlier, subjects had cardiovascular responses measured during the SI and a brief though difficult oral American history quiz. Type A's and Type B's did not differ significantly in their SBP, DBP, or HR responses to these tasks. Similarly, no significant differences between Type A's and Type B's were found in SBP, DBP, or HR response to the SI in a study of employed Black women by Anderson and colleagues (1986).

In an investigation of college women by Lawler and Schmied (1986), subjects were studied while they were orally given an American history quiz, a procedure that was interpreted as an interpersonal stressor. No differences between Type A's and Type B's in SBP, DBP, or HR responses were found.

**Summary for Studies Employing Females.**    The results of the investigations in which potential differences in reactivity between Type A and Type B females were studied are perplexing. On the one hand, it is not surprising that no differences in reactivity were found between Type A's and Type

B's to physical stressors, for example, the cold pressor, or to serial subtraction tasks in studies containing only college women because neither kind of task is often found to elicit differences in reactivity between Type A and Type B males.

On the other hand, in studies containing only college females, no differences between Type A's and Type B's were found in reactivity even for those tasks or situations that can be regarded as congruent with sex-role expectations, for example, verbal tasks such as the Stroop (Lawler & Schmied, 1986), challenging verbal interaction (Lawler & Schmied, 1986; MacDougall et al., 1981, Study II), and so forth. Moreover, in the studies that included both college males and females uncertainty exists concerning the strength of the relation between Type A and the responses by females to various tasks including those that can be regarded as congruent with sex-role expectations, for example, the Stroop (Jorgensen & Houston, 1981), and other verbal tasks such as anagrams (Gastorf, 1981), and so on.

In contrast to the fairly consistent negative results for college females, the results for the small number of investigations in which noncollege females have been studied are somewhat more promising and suggest that differences in cardiovascular reactivity tend to be found for JAS-defined Type A and Type B females even for tasks that would not be regarded as congruent with sex-role expectations, namely, mental arithmetic and Raven's Progressive Matrices. Perhaps the JAS is less appropriate for college females than noncollege females because of differences in age and attendant life experiences. The noncollege female subjects in the studies reviewed tended to be older than the college female subjects. Perhaps because of more and broader life experiences, the Type A's among noncollege women may not have been as concerned as college women about sex-role expectations for the tasks with which they were confronted.

**Conclusion.** A review of the reactivity studies in which global Type A was measured by the JAS suggests the following. For males, JAS-defined Type A's are most likely to exhibit greater reactivity than Type B's to tasks that require speed of response, are difficult but not highly difficult, and involve a moderate degree of incentive for performance. Unlike what was said about SI-defined Type A for males, however, JAS-defined Type A does not appear to be related to reactivity in situations in which the individual is annoyed or harassed. Moreover, differences between JAS-defined male Type A's and Type B's are slightly more frequently found for SBP than HR, and least frequently found for DBP. No differences between JAS-defined Type A's and Type B's have been found for plasma E or NE, although neuroendocrine measures have infrequently been included in studies of reactivity that involve the JAS.

For college females, there is not much evidence that JAS-defined Type A is related to reactivity. For noncollege females, there is some preliminary evidence that JAS-defined Type A is related to reactivity for the same kinds of tasks as those for males.

## STUDIES EMPLOYING THE FTAS

### Global Type A and Reactivity: Review

The FTAS has been related to reactivity in very few studies, and so they do not need to be reviewed under different subsections. In a study of college males by Dembroski, MacDougall, Herd, and Shields (1979), described earlier, subjects underwent the cold pressor test and performed a reaction-time task under high- or low-challenge conditions. The difficulty of the respective tasks was emphasized in the high-challenge but not low-challenge conditions. Type A's relative to Type B's responded to the reaction-time task in the low-challenge condition with significantly less FPV but not greater SBP, DBP, or HR. There were no significant differences between Type A's and Type B's in SBP, DBP, HR, or FPV in the high-challenge condition or either high- or low-challenge conditions for the cold pressor test.

The relation between FTAS scores and reactivity was investigated in two studies of college females by MacDougall and colleagues (1981) described earlier. In both studies, subjects performed a reaction-time task and in the first study, subjects also underwent the cold pressor test. Instructions for both tasks emphasized the tasks' difficulty. Subjects' responses to the SI were also investigated in the second study. No differences between Type A's and Type B's were found for SBP, DBP, or HR responses to any of the tasks.

In a study by Smith, Houston, and Zurawski (1985), male and female college subjects responded to videotaped questions from the SI and a brief though difficult American history quiz adapted from Dembroski, MacDougall and Lushene (1979). Comparing subjects selected on the basis of extreme FTAS scores, Type A's relative to Type B's were found to respond with significantly greater SBP but not DBP, HR, or FPV.

It is difficult to draw many inferences with confidence from so few studies, particularly since the findings were neither strong nor consistent. At present, it seems reasonable to conclude tentatively that the relation between FTAS-defined A–B type and reactivity is weak at best.

## CONCLUSIONS

In this chapter studies have been reviewed that were conducted in the United States on the relation between reactivity and global Type A as measured by the SI, JAS, and FTAS. For males, the kinds of solitary tasks that elicit differences in reactivity between SI-defined Type A's and Type B's and JAS-defined Type A's and Type B's appear to be similar. However, the prediction of reactivity is substantially stronger when the SI is used to measure A–B type than when the JAS is used. Moreover, only SI-defined Type A predicts reactivity in situations in which subjects are annoyed or harassed by others. Because the SI measures subjects' behavior in a situation in which they are annoyed by another person, it makes sense that the SI should predict reactivity better than the JAS in situations in which subjects are annoyed or harassed by others. Moreover, it was mentioned earlier that the JAS may be deficient in measuring hostility and the kind of competitiveness that may be motivated by hostility.

The results of the reactivity studies for males may help to explain why the SI predicts CHD and coronary atherosclerosis better than the JAS. The SI not only predicts reactivity more strongly than the JAS, it predicts reactivity to a wider array of situations, for instance, those that elicit hostility. The latter may be particularly significant considering the importance that hostility has been found to play in predicting CHD and coronary atherosclerosis (see Chesney et al., Chapter 8, Williams & Barefoot, Chapter 9, this volume). In sum, one would expect SI-defined Type A's compared to JAS-defined Type A's to experience more frequent and more intense physiological arousal in their daily lives, which is the mechanism that has been proposed for linking Type A with CHD (Henry & Meehan, 1981; Williams, 1978; see also Williams & Barefoot, Chapter 9, this volume).

Compared to that for males, prediction of reactivity for females appears to be much more limited, namely, to certain kinds of situations for SI-defined Type A's and Type B's and perhaps to certain kinds of populations for JAS-defined Type A's and Type B's. The relation between scores on the FTAS and reactivity for males and/or females is meager.

The implication of these findings for females is that the prediction of CHD or coronary atherosclerosis by global Type A as measured by the SI, JAS, or the FTAS would be weak. This implication is supported by the research on Type A and CHD or coronary atherosclerosis that has been conducted with women (see Eaker & Castelli, Chapter 5, Haynes & Matthews, Chapter 4, this volume).

The other data presented in the chapter suggest the following summary statements. One is that to improve prediction of reactivity and perhaps cardiovascular disease via the SI: (1) a facilitative style of administering the SI is preferable to a disruptive, challenging style (see also Scherwitz, Chapter 3, this volume); (2) males and females should be assigned to categories that are more homogeneous in their SI-defined Type A characteristics than is found in the traditional SI-defined Type A and Type B groupings; and (3) females, at least, should be assigned to groups that have different profiles of SI-defined Type A characteristics than are found in the traditional SI-defined Type A and Type B groupings. Second, research on SI-defined

Type A components and reactivity needs strengthening in terms of measurement and more careful attention being given to how subjects view the experimental arrangements.

The future directions for research on Type A and reactivity will probably mirror several of the current and emerging issues in this general research area. One issue is how Type A is best measured. Because the SI seems to be the best measure of global Type A in terms of predicting reactivity, additional research is needed to determine how the style with which the SI is administered influences prediction of reactivity by Type A ratings, components, and other characteristics, for example, self-referencing. In addition, attention needs to be given to the gender of the interviewer and how it may interact with the gender of the interviewee in influencing prediction of reactivity by Type A ratings.

There is also an emerging emphasis on how the milieu may influence risk of CHD for Type A's (see Haynes & Matthews, Chapter 4, this volume). Further research thus is needed wherein the context is varied in which subjects perform different kinds of tasks to simulate variations in job milieu, and interpersonal interactions are varied to simulate variations in interpersonal milieu. Along the latter line, studies in which reactivity is measured during interaction between different combinations of Type A and Type B husbands and wives would be interesting.

There is a flourishing interest in the components of Type A, hostility in particular (see Chesney et al., Chapter 8, Williams & Barefoot, Chapter 9, this volume). Thus more research is needed on carefully and consistently measuring Type A components and related characteristics (e.g., self-referencing) and relating them to reactivity. Such research also should include investigation of the influence on reactivity of the context in which the participant is studied, as was mentioned in the preceding paragraph.

Further research needs to be focused on reactivity and Type A in women. Perhaps, as was suggested earlier, a configuration of Type A components and related characteristics that is different from that for men needs to be considered in such research.

Two topics that were not covered in the review in this chapter also deserve further research. One is Type A, associated components, and reactivity in children (see Thoresen & Pattillo, Chapter 6, this volume). The second is the use of reactivity as a dependent measure in intervention studies of Type A and associated components (see Price, Chapter 12, this volume).

## REFERENCES

Allen, T. A., Lawler, K. A., Matthews, K. A., & Rakaczky, C. J. (1984). Speech stylistic components of the structured interview and cardiovascular reactivity in college males. *Psychophysiology, 21*, 567–568. (Abstract)

Allen, M. T., Lawler, K. A., Mitchell, V. P., Matthews, K. A., Rakaczky, C. J., & Jamison, W. (1987). Type A behavior pattern, parental history of hypertension, and cardiovascular reactivity in college males. *Health Psychology, 6*, 113–130.

Anderson, N. B., Williams, R. B., Jr., Lane, J. D., Haney, T., Simpson, S., & Houseworth, S. J. (1986). Type A behavior, family history of hypertension, and cardiovascular responsivity among Black women. *Health Psychology, 5*, 393–406.

Benjamin, L. S. (1967). Facts and artifacts in using analysis of covariance to "undo" the law of intial values. *Psychophysiology, 4*, 187–206.

Blumenthal, J. A., Lane, J. D., & Williams, R. B., Jr. (1985). The inhibited power motive, Type A behavior, and patterns of cardiovascular response during the structured interview and Thematic Apperception Test. *Journal of Human Stress, 11*(2), 89–92.

Blumenthal, J. A., Lane, J. D., Williams, R. B., McKee, D. C., Haney, T., & White, A. (1983). Effects of task incentive on cardiovascular response in Type A and Type B individuals. *Psychophysiology, 20*, 63–70.

Chesney, M. A., Eagleston, J. R., & Rosenman, R. H. (1980). The Type A Structured Interview: A behavioral assessment in the rough. *Journal of Behavioral Assessment, 2*, 255–272.

Contrada, R. J., Glass, D. C., Krakoff, L. R., Krantz, D. S., Kehoe, K., Isecke, W., Collins, C., & Elting, E. (1982). Effects of control over aversive stimulation and Type A behavior on cardiovascular and plasma catecholamine responses. *Psychophysiology, 19*, 408–419.

Cornelius, R. R., & Averill, J. R. (1980). The influence of various types of control on psychophysiological stress reactions. *Journal of Research in Personality, 14*, 503–517.

Corse, C. D., Manuck, S. B., Cantwell, J. D., Giordani, B., & Matthews, K. A. (1982). Coronary-prone behavior pattern and cardiovascular response in persons with and without coronary heart disease. *Psychosomatic Medicine, 44*, 449–459.

Dembroski, T. M., MacDougall, J. M., Herd, J. A., & Shields, J. L. (1979). Effect of level of challenge on pressor and heart rate responses in Type A and B subjects. *Journal of Applied Social Psychology, 9*, 209–228.

Dembroski, T. M., MacDougall, J. M., & Lushene, R. (1979). Interpersonal interaction and cardiovascular response in Type A subjects and coronary patients. *Journal of Human Stress, 5*(4), 28–36.

Dembroski, T. M., MacDougall, J. M., Shields, J. L., Petitto, J., & Lushene, R. (1978). Components of the Type A coronary-prone behavior pattern and cardiovascular responses to psychomotor performance challenge. *Journal of Behavioral Medicine, 1*, 159–175.

Dembroski, T. M., MacDougall, J. M., Williams, R. B., Jr., Haney, T. L., & Blumenthal, J. A. (1985). Components of Type A, hostility and anger-in: Relationship to angiographic findings. *Psychosomatic Medicine, 47*, 219–233.

Diamond, E. L., & Carver, C. S. (1980). Sensory processing, cardiovascular reactivity, and the Type A coronary-prone behavior pattern. *Biological Psychology, 10*, 265–275.

Diamond, E. L., Schneiderman, N., Schwartz, D., Smith, J. C., Vorp, R., & Pasin, R. D. (1984). Harassment, hostility, and Type A as determinants of cardiovascular reactivity during competition. *Journal of Behavioral Medicine, 7*, 171–189.

Essau, C. A., & Jamieson, J. L. (1987). Heart rate perception in the Type A personality. *Health Psychology, 6*, 43–54.

Fontana, A. F., Rosenberg, R. L., Kerns, R. D., & Marcus, J. L. (1986). Social insecurity, the Type A behavior pattern, and sympathetic arousal. *Journal of Behavioral Medicine, 9*, 79–88.

Friedman, M., Byers, S. O., Diamant, J., & Rosenman, R. H. (1975). Plasma catecholamine response of coronary-prone subjects (Type A) to a specific challenge. *Metabolism, 4*, 205–210.

Gastorf, J. W. (1981). Physiologic reaction of Type As to objective and subjective challenge. *Journal of Human Stress, 7*(1), 16–20.

Glass, D. C., Krakoff, L. R., Contrada, R., Hilton, W. F., Kehoe, K., Mannucci, E. G., Collins, C., Snow, B., & Elting, E. (1980). Effect of harassment and competition upon cardiovascular and plasma catecholamine responses in Type A and Type B individuals. *Psychophysiology, 17*, 453–463.

Glass, D. C., Krakoff, L. R., Finkelman, J., Snow, B., Contrada, R., Kehoe, K., Mannucci, E. G., Isecke, W., Collins, C., Hilton, W. F., & Elting, E. (1980). Effect of task overload upon cardiovascular and plasma catecholamine responses in Type A and B individuals. *Basic & Applied Social Psychology, 1*, 199–218.

Glass, D. C., Lake, C. R., Contrada, R. J., Kehoe, K., & Erlanger, L. R. (1983). Stability of individual differences in physiological responses to stress. *Health Psychology, 2*, 317–341.

Goldband, S. (1980). Stimulus specificity of physiological response to stress and the Type A coronary-prone behavior pattern. *Journal of Personality & Social Psychology, 39*, 670–679.

Goldstein, H. S., Edelberg, R., Meier, C. F., Orzano, J. A., & Blaufuss, L. (1985). The paradoxical relation between diastolic blood pressure change under stress and the H factor of the Jenkins Activity Survey. *Journal of Psychosomatic Research, 29*, 419–425.

Hastrup, J. L., & Light, K. C. (1984). Sex differences in cardiovascular stress responses: Modulation as a function of menstrual cycle phases. *Journal of Psychosomatic Research, 28*, 475–483.

Haynes, S. G., Levine, S., Scotch, N., Feinleib, M., & Kannel, W. B. (1978). The relationship of psychosocial factors to coronary heart disease in the Framingham study: I. Methods and risk factors. *American Journal of Epidemiology, 107*, 362–383.

Henry, J. P., & Meehan, J. P. (1981). Psychosocial stimuli, physiological specificity, and cardiovascular disease. In H. Weiner, M. A. Hofer, & A. J. Stunkard (Eds.), *Brain, behavior, and bodily disease*. New York: Raven.

Holmes, D. S., McGilley, B. M., & Houston, B. K. (1984). Task-related arousal of Type A and Type B persons: Level of challenge and response specificity. *Journal of Personality & Social Psychology, 46*, 1322–1327.

Holmes, D. S., & Will, M. J. (1985). Expression of interpersonal aggression by angered and nonangered persons with the Type A and Type B behavior patterns. *Journal of Personality & Social Psychology, 48*, 723–727.

Houston, B. K. (1983). Psychophysiological responsivity and the Type A behavior pattern. *Journal of Research in Personality, 17*, 22–39.

Howland, E. W., & Siegman, A. W. (1982). Toward the automated measurement of the Type A behavior pattern. *Journal of Behavioral Medicine, 5*, 37–54.

Hull, E. M., Young, S. H., & Ziegler, M. G. (1984). Aerobic fitness affects cardiovascular and catecholamine responses to stressors. *Psychophysiology, 21*, 353–360.

Jenkins, C. D., Rosenman, R. H., & Zyzanski, S. J. (1974). Prediction of clinical coronary heart disease by a test for the coronary-prone behavior pattern. *New England Journal of Medicine, 290*, 1271–1275.

Jennings, J. R. (1984). Cardiovascular reactions and impatience in Type A and B college students. *Psychosomatic Medicine, 46*, 424–440.

Jennings, J. R., & Choi, S. (1981). Type A components and psychophysiological responses to an attention-demanding performance task. *Psychosomatic Medicine, 43*, 475–487.

Jorgensen, R. S., & Houston, B. K. (1981). The Type A behavior pattern, sex differences, and cardiovascular response to and recovery from stress. *Motivation & Emotion, 5*, 201–214.

Kelly, K. E., & Houston, B. K. (1985). *Type A components and cardiovascular reactivity*. Paper presented at the meeting of the American Psychological Association, Los Angeles.

Krantz, D. S., Schaeffer, M. A., Davia, J. E., Dembroski, T. M., MacDougall, J. M., & Shaffer, R. T. (1981). Extent of coronary atherosclerosis, Type A behavior, and cardiovascular response to social interaction. *Psychophysiology, 18,* 654–664.

Lake, B., Suarez, E. C., Schneiderman, N., & Tocci, N. (1985). The Type A behavior pattern, physical fitness, and psychophysiological reactivity. *Health Psychology, 4,* 169–187.

Lane, J. D., White, A. D., & Williams, R. B., Jr. (1984). Cardiovascular effects of mental arithmetic in Type A and Type B females. *Psychophysiology, 21,* 39–46.

Lawler, K. A., Rixse, A., & Allen, M. T. (1983). Type A behavior and psychophysiological responses in adult women. *Psychophysiology, 20,* 343–350.

Lawler, K. A., & Schmied, L. A. (1986). Cardiovascular responsivity, Type A behavior, and parental history of heart disease in young women. *Psychophysiology, 23,* 28–32.

Lawler, K. A., Schmied, L., Mitchell, V. P., & Rixse, A. (1984). Type A behavior and physiological responsivity in young women. *Journal of Psychosomatic Research, 28,* 197–204.

Lenney, E. (1977). Women's self-confidence in achievement settings. *Psychological Bulletin, 84,* 1–13.

Little, B. C., & Zahn, T. P. (1974). Changes in mood and autonomic function during the menstrual cycle. *Psychophysiology, 11,* 579–590.

Lott, G. G., & Gatchel, R. J. (1978). A multi-response analysis of learned heart rate control. *Psychophysiology, 15,* 576–581.

Lovallo, W. R., Pincomb, G. A., & Wilson, M. F. (1986a). Heart rate reactivity and Type A behavior as modifiers of physiological response to active and passive coping. *Psychophysiology, 23,* 105–112.

Lovallo, W. R., Pincomb, G. A., & Wilson, M. F. (1986b). Predicting response to a reaction time task: Heart rate reactivity compared with Type A behavior. *Psychophysiology, 23,* 648–656.

Lovallo, W. R., & Pishkin, V. (1980). A psychophysiological comparison of Type A and B men exposed to failure and uncontrollable noise. *Psychophysiology, 17,* 29–36.

Maccoby, E. E., & Jacklin, C. N. (1974). *The psychology of sex differences.* Stanford, CA: Stanford University Press.

MacDougall, J. M., Dembroski, T. M., Dimsdale, J. E., & Hackett, T. P. (1985). Components of Type A, hostility, and anger-in: Further relationships to angiographic findings. *Health Psychology, 4,* 137–152.

MacDougall, J. M., Dembroski, T. M., & Krantz, D. S. (1981). Effects of types of challenge on pressor and heart rate response in Type A and B women. *Psychophysiology, 18,* 1–9.

Manuck, S. B., Corse, C. D., & Winkelman, P. A. (1979). Behavioral correlates of individual differences in blood pressure reactivity. *Journal of Psychosomatic Research, 23,* 281–288.

Manuck, S. B., & Garland, F. N. (1979). Coronary-prone behavior pattern, task incentive, and cardiovascular response. *Psychophysiology, 16,* 136–142.

Matthews, K. A. (1982). Psychological perspectives on the Type A behavior pattern. *Psychological Bulletin, 91,* 293–323.

Matthews, K. A. (1986). Preface (pp. xi–xii). In K. A. Matthews, S. M. Weiss, T. Detre, T. M. Dembroski, B. Falkner, S. B. Manuck, & R. B. Williams, Jr. (Eds.), *Handbook of stress, reactivity, and cardiovascular disease.* New York: Wiley.

Matthews, K. A., Glass, D. C., Rosenman, R. H., & Bortner, R. W. (1977). Competitive drive, pattern A, and coronary heart disease: A further analysis of some data from the Western Collaborative Group Study. *Journal of Chronic Diseases, 30,* 489–498.

Mayes, B. T., Sime, W. E., & Ganster, D. C. (1984). Convergent validity of Type A behavior pattern scales and their ability to predict physiological responsiveness in a sample of female public employees. *Journal of Behavioral Medicine, 7,* 83–108.

Morell, M. A. (1985, August). Psychophysiologic stress reactivity in Type A and B community women and female college students. In B. K. Houston (Chair), *Type A in women*. Symposium presented at the meeting of the American Psychological Association, Los Angeles.

Newlin, D. B., & Levenson, R. W. (1982). Cardiovascular responses of individuals with Type A behavior pattern and parental coronary heart disease. *Journal of Psychosomatic Research, 26*, 393–402.

Pace, L., & Houston, B. K. (1986). *Type A components and cardiovascular reactivity*. Unpublished manuscript, University of Kansas, Lawrence, KS.

Perkins, K. A. (1984). Heart rate change in Type A and Type B males as a function of response cost and task difficulty. *Psychophysiology, 21*, 14–21.

Rosenman, R. H. (1978). The interview method of assessment of the coronary-prone behavior pattern. In T. M. Dembroski, S. M. Weiss, J. L. Shields, S. G. Haynes, & M. Feinleib (Eds.), *Coronary-prone behavior*. New York: Springer-Verlag.

Scherwitz, L. (1984). Reply to Dr. Krantz. *Psychosomatic Medicine, 46*, 67–68.

Scherwitz, L., Berton, K., & Leventhal, H. (1978). Type A behavior, self-involvement, and cardiovascular response. *Psychosomatic Medicine, 40*, 593–609.

Smith, T. W., Houston, B. K., & Zurawski, R. M. (1985). The Framingham Type A Scale: Cardiovascular and cognitive–behavioral responses to interpersonal challenge. *Motivation & Emotion, 9*, 123–134.

Smith, T. W., Houston, B. K., & Stucky, R. J. (1984). Type A behavior, irritability, and cardiovascular response. *Motivation & Emotion, 8*, 221–230.

Smyth, K., Call, J., Hansell, S., Sparacino, J., & Strodtbeck, F. L. (1978). Type A behavior pattern and hypertension among inner-city Black women. *Nursing Research, 27*, 30–35.

Stoney, C. M., Langer, A. W., Sutterer, J. R., & Gelling, P. D. (1987). A comparison of biofeedback-assisted cardiodeceleration in Type A and B men: Modification of stress-associated cardiopulmonary and hemodynamic adjustments. *Psychosomatic Medicine, 49*, 79–87.

Van Egeren, L. F. (1979a). Cardiovascular changes during social competition in a mixed-motive game. *Journal of Personality & Social Psychology, 37*, 858–864.

Van Egeren, L. F. (1979b). Social interactions, communications, and the coronary-prone behavior pattern: A psychophysiological study. *Psychosomatic Medicine, 41*, 2–18.

Van Egeren, L. F., Sniderman, L. D., & Roggelin, M. S. (1982). Competitive two-person interactions of Type-A and Type-B individuals. *Journal of Behavioral Medicine, 5*, 55–66.

Ward, M. M., Chesney, M. A., Swan, G. E., Black, G. W., Parker, S. D., & Rosenman, R. H. (1986). Cardiovascular responses of Type A and Type B men to a series of stressors. *Journal of Behavioral Medicine, 9*, 43–49.

Weidner, G., & Matthews, K. A. (1978). Reported physical symptoms elicited by unpredictable events and the Type A coronary-prone behavior pattern. *Journal of Personality & Social Psychology, 36*, 213–220.

Wilder, J. F. (1968). *Stimulus and response: The law of initial values*. Baltimore: Williams & Wilkins.

Williams, R. B., Jr. (1978). Psychophysiological processes, the coronary-prone behavior pattern, and coronary heart disease. In T. M. Dembroski, S. M. Weiss, J. L. Shields, S. G. Haynes, & M. Feinleib (Eds.), *Coronary-prone behavior*. New York: Springer-Verlag.

Wright, R. A., Contrada, R. J., & Glass, D. C. (1985). Psychophysiologic correlates of Type A behavior. In E. S. Katkin & S. M. Manuck (Eds.), *Advances in behavioral medicine*. Greenwich, CT: JAI.

Zurawski, R. M., & Houston, B. K. (1983). The Jenkins Activity Survey measure of Type A and frustration-induced anger. *Motivation & Emotion, 7*, 301–312.

# 11

## Type A Behavior, Emotion, and Psychophysiologic Reactivity: Psychological and Biological Interactions

RICHARD J. CONTRADA, DAVID S. KRANTZ,
AND D. ROBIN HILL

The sensitivity of the sympathetic nervous system to psychological influences has been of long-standing interest to biological and behavioral researchers (Cannon, 1929; Mason, 1972). In recent years, increased attention has been devoted to this area, and it has been hypothesized that behaviorally induced physiologic responses (reactivity) may be a marker for processes involved in the etiology of coronary heart disease and hypertension (Krantz & Manuck, 1984; Matthews et al., 1986). The measurement of reactivity

Preparation of this article was assisted by NIH grant HL31514 and USUHS grant RO7233. The opinions and assertions expressed herein are not to be construed as reflecting those of the DoD or the USUHS.

involves the assessment of physiologic *changes* in response to stress, as opposed to the sole assessment of resting levels of physiologic function. In addition to being a possible marker of risk for cardiovascular disorders, reactivity may operate as a pathway mediating the risk-enhancing effects of other psychosocial variables, such as stress and Type A behavior.

Currently, an active research area has examined differences between Type A and Type B subjects in physiological responses to psychological stressors (see Houston, Chapter 10, this volume). The aim of this research has been to understand the psychophysiological mechanisms linking Type A to coronary disease, and the nature of situations that elicit increased responding in Type A subjects (cf. Matthews, 1982). In a more general sense, investigators have also sought to identify the types of situations and stressors that elicit reactivity, and the patterns of physiologic responses produced by different stressors. This approach is illustrated by the arrows moving from left to right in Figure 11.1. There is considerable evidence that psychological and behavioral factors influence reactivity, and some evidence that reactivity can have subsequent effects on coronary disease (Krantz & Manuck, 1984; Matthews et al., 1986).

However, there is also evidence that reactivity can affect behavior. A question bearing on this issue that has been of long-standing interest to researchers on emotion is the extent to which peripheral or visceral responses contribute to the intensity of affective experience (Cannon, 1929; James, 1884; Schachter & Singer, 1962). Drugs that selectively block or stimulate sympathetic nervous system responses allow researchers to examine in a new way the role of bodily responses in generating emotional reactions. That is, if peripheral reactions of the sympathetic nervous system are im-portant for generating the subjective experience of certain emotions, a blockade of these physiologic responses should reduce psychological and behavioral correlates of emotion. Similarly, stimulation of such responses should tend to increase such emotional reactions.

Recent research indicates that aspects of Type A behavior may be lessened by beta-adrenergic blocking drugs that operate to inhibit selected responses of the sympathetic nervous system (Schmieder, Friedrich, Neus, Rüddel, & Von Eiff, 1983; Zanchetti & Turner, 1985). This evidence was derived, in part, from a research perspective that views the Type A behavior pattern

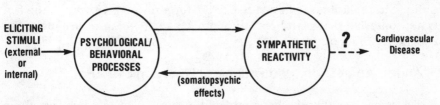

**FIGURE 11.1.** Model illustrating bidirectional relationships between physiologic reactivity and behavior.

as involving both physiological and psychological elements acting together. These data further raise the possibility that, just as physiologic responses heighten emotion, physiologic reactivity may contribute to the expression of Type A behavior and anger. This perspective is illustrated by the arrow pointing from right to left in Figure 11.1, and has generated research that will constitute the focus of our review.

This chapter will describe research suggesting that components of Type A behavior reflect heightened sympathetic nervous system reactivity, and review the results of recent studies that have tested this hypothesis. This idea is closely related to the notion that bodily activity can contribute to emotional experience, and recent research on the effects of beta-blockers on emotional behavior that suggests parallels between the mechanisms of their effects on anxiety and on Type A. To provide necessary background before discussing research on sympathetic nervous system activity as an antecedent of Type A behavior, we will describe evidence for the role of peripheral sympathetic nervous system responses in the experience of emotion.

## THE ROLE OF PERIPHERAL SYMPATHETIC RESPONSES IN ANGER AND ANXIETY

Early theories of emotion proposed by James (1884) and Lange (1885/1922) maintained that emotions reflect the perception of visceral, skeletal, and muscular responses. Later, Schachter and Singer (1962) argued that the production of emotion requires both the perception of peripheral sympathetic responses and the cognitive interpretation or labeling of these responses in terms of emotional cues derived from the social environment. In this view, a state of sympathetic arousal is affectively neutral, gaining its emotional quality from the individual's perceptions of the circumstances in which it occurs. Thus when subjects injected with epinephrine had no ready explanation for why they were aroused, their emotional state could be manipulated by variations in social context. In the presence of an angry confederate, subjects behaved more angrily, whereas the presence of a euphoric confederate caused subjects to behave in a more euphoric manner (Schachter & Singer, 1962). The role of peripheral arousal in emotion has been a matter of controversy, and aspects of the Schachter study have been difficult to replicate (see Leventhal, 1980, for a review). However, the fact is not contested that peripheral autonomic responses can contribute to the experience of emotion.

### Anger, Aggression, and Peripheral Physiologic Arousal

The Schachter theory has stimulated a number of research programs investigating the determinants of anger-related emotional behavior. For example, Zillman demonstrated that undissipated physiologic arousal generated by strenuous exercise or exposure to erotic stimuli led to increased aggressive behavior in subjects who previously had been provoked (Zillman, 1971; Zillman, Johnson, & Day, 1974). Aggressiveness was affected only when arousal had dissipated somewhat and held no cues (e.g., heavy breathing) linking it to its actual source. This finding supports the notion that physiologic arousal per se does not automatically induce emotional behavior. Only when environmental conditions justified the labeling of arousal in terms of anger was aggressiveness potentiated.

In a related line of research, Konečni (1975a, 1975b) demonstrated increases in aggressive behavior following exposure to physiologically arousing auditory stimuli among subjects previously insulted by a confederate. As in the Zillman studies, subjects not provoked showed no such increase in aggressive behavior when aroused. It is important to note that, once again, increases in aggression were seen only among subjects who both were aroused and had available to them anger-relevant cues. Taken together with the Schachter and Singer (1962) experiment, the work of Zillman, Johnson, and Day (1974) and Konečni (1975a, 1975b) strongly suggests that emotionally relevant cognitive cues and autonomic arousal interact in the production of angry emotional responses.

It should be noted that, while the aforementioned research was primarily concerned with emotional *behavior* (e.g., aggression), other work suggests that self-rated *affect* can also be manipulated by varying the explanation that subjects attach to a particular state of physiologic arousal. For example, Erdmann and Janke (1978) investigated the effects on mood of the sympathomimetic agent ephedrine, and a situational manipulation offering cues for the interpretation of arousal in terms of anxiety, anger, or happiness. Neither sympathetic arousal nor manipulation of emotionally relevant cues alone had a significant impact on mood ratings. However, as expected, mood scores indicated greater negative affect in the anger-inducing as compared to happiness-inducing condition among subjects receiving ephedrine, but not among those receiving placebo. Geen and associates (Geen, Rakosky, & Pigg, 1972) also found that self-rated anger can be manipulated by varying the explanation that subjects attach to a particular state of physiological arousal.

Because the research just reviewed was concerned exclusively with the induction of emotion in the laboratory setting, questions may be raised with respect to the ecological validity of the findings. However, several field studies reinforce the notion that peripheral autonomic reactions are very much a part of the naturalistic experience of anger (Averill, 1982; Davitz, 1969; Gates, 1926). For example, data suggest that a significant proportion of individuals experience anger and anxiety in terms of symptoms such as quickened and forceful heartbeat, tense musculature, and rapid breathing (Davitz, 1969; Gates, 1926). While there is considerable individual variability in the actual and experienced autonomic correlates of emotion

(Averill, 1982), these naturalistic data do support the idea that autonomic responses play a role in the experience of anger and other emotion at least for some people. Additional evidence to support this hypothesis is reviewed in a later section on beta-adrenergic blocking drugs.

## A PSYCHOBIOLOGICAL MODEL OF TYPE A BEHAVIOR

The previous review of physiologic antecedents of anger is relevant to Type A behavior—a construct with anger and hostility as major components. Type A has been conceived as the outcome of a person–situation interaction (Friedman & Rosenman, 1959; Glass, 1977). That is, Type A behaviors are thought to emerge in certain individuals when they encounter appropriately stressful or challenging situations. The Structured Interview (SI) technique used to assess Type A behavior (Rosenman, 1978) is based on this principle: Questions are asked in a deliberately provocative fashion in order to elicit Type A behaviors. Thus the interview may itself be considered a challenging situation that elicits Type A behavior in susceptible individuals.

### Type A and Physiologic Reactivity

Because Type A appears to be related to CHD even after controlling for the standard risk factors (Review Panel, 1981), the hypothesis has been advanced that behaviors evidenced by Type A persons are accompanied by pathogenic cardiovascular and neuroendocrine responses that act upon the cardiovascular system to promote atherosclerosis or precipitate clinical coronary heart disease (see Houston, Chapter 10, this volume). The relationship between Type A and reactivity is only moderate, with some components of Type A behavior, such as anger and hostility, apparently showing stronger relationships with physiologic responsiveness than others (e.g., Dembroski, MacDougall, Herd, & Shields, 1979). The evidence indicates that Type A–Type B differences in reactivity are most pronounced while subjects are actively engaged in stressful or challenging situations, and seldom are observed while subjects are at rest (Contrada, Wright, & Glass, 1985; Houston, 1983; Wright, Contrada, & Glass, 1985). For example, research by Glass and colleagues involved a situation where subjects competed with either a hostile or nonhostile competitor (Glass et al., 1980). Under conditions of hostile competition, Type A's showed greater cardiovascular and catecholamine responses than Type B's. However, where competition was not hostile, there were no significant differences between Type A's and Type B's.

### Coronary Bypass Studies

As noted, most studies suggest that Type A behaviors and their physiologic correlates emerge only when individuals encounter situations perceived as threatening or demanding. This view is challenged by a study (Kahn, Kornfeld, Frank, Heller, & Hoar, 1980) that found that while under general anesthesia for coronary artery bypass surgery Type A patients with coronary disease evidenced greater increases over admission blood pressure than their Type B counterparts. Admission blood pressure measurements had been taken by a physician upon entry into the hospital when patients were fully awake.

These results suggest that there may be, in part, an underlying psychobiological or "constitutional" basis for Type A–Type B differences in cardiovascular reactivity because these responses are observed among coronary patients undergoing general anesthesia. However, the calculation of peak operative increases over admission blood pressure used in this study places some qualification on this conclusion. It is not possible to determine from these data whether increases reflected elevations occurring entirely during surgery (while patients were anesthetized), as opposed to elevations over admission blood pressure occurring prior to surgery when patients were fully awake.

Given this difficulty in interpretation, Krantz, Arabian, Davia, and Parker (1982) undertook to replicate and extend these findings, obtaining an additional measure of blood pressure at onset of surgery (first operative blood pressure). Three reactivity measures were calculated: (1) operative increase over admission, as in Kahn and colleagues' (1980) study; (2) peak operative increase over first operative; and (3) peak operative increase from admission to first operative. The results indicated that intensity of Type A behavior was positively related to the second measure (intraoperative increases in systolic blood pressure occurring during surgery while patients were anesthetized). In contrast, Type A behavior was not related to physiologic changes occurring prior to surgery. The previous finding of a positive relationship of Type A intensity to operative increases over admission also was replicated, and it was shown that the SI, but not the Jenkins Activity Survey (JAS), was related to intraoperative changes. Taken together, therefore, it would appear that the findings of both Kahn and colleagues (1980) and Krantz, Arabian, Davia, and Parker (1982) reflect physiologic hyperreactivity among Type A coronary patients under conditions in which conscious mediation was minimized.

Recently, Kornfeld and colleagues (1985) sought to determine whether Type A behavior is associated with intraoperative blood pressure elevations among patients with no history of coronary heart disease undergoing general surgery. For the sample as a whole, there was no evidence of a relationship between SI ratings and intraoperative blood pressure increases. Subgroup analyses were conducted to explore the possibility that the expected association was in evidence for patients with a positive family history of coronary heart disease. Results for this subgroup indicated respectable associations between global SI ratings and intraoperative elevations in systolic blood pressure ($r = .49$), as well as between SI-derived ratings of "pressured drive" and intraoperative diastolic changes ($r = .48$). Several other correlations involving SI Type A variables and intraoperative blood pressure reactivity were on the order of .30. However, because of the small number of subjects with a positive family history ($N = 11$), none of the reported coefficients attained acceptable significance levels. Therefore, the question of whether Type A behavior is associated with intraoperative blood pressure reactivity among noncoronary patients, with or without a family history of coronary heart disease, must be considered an open one, pending further research employing larger samples.

## Twin Studies of Type A

Research has examined the heritability of global Type A and components as measured in the Structured Interview. Clearly, a finding of significant heritability would be consistent with a biological contribution to Type A behavior. An earlier report (Rahe, Hervig, & Rosenman, 1978) found no significant heritability for global Type A. However, some of the self-report inventories significantly correlated with global Type A do show significant heritability (e.g., the Thurstone Temperament Schedule). A reanalysis of these data examined components of Type A related to speech stylistics and potential for hostility, and found these components to be heritable (Matthews, Rosenman, Dembroski, Harris, & MacDougall, 1984). These results add weight to the suggestion that speech stylistics and potential for hostility may reflect a constitutional hyperresponsivity to environmental challenge. Recent evidence also indicates that cardiovascular hyperreactivity to stress also may have a heritable base (Rose, Grim, & Miller, 1984). Perhaps, then, underlying certain Type A components may be a temperamental tendency to respond physiologically and behaviorally to stress.

## EFFECTS OF BETA-ADRENERGIC BLOCKING DRUGS ON TYPE A BEHAVIOR

The results of the studies of intraoperative physiologic responses suggest that, at least among coronary patients, there may be a psychobiologic, or constitutional, basis for the physiologic hyperreactivity of Type A individuals. That is, the impatience, hostility, and speech patterns exhibited by Type A individuals may *reflect* an underlying sympathetic nervous system responsivity. Although this possibility is different from the idea that Type A appraisals or behaviors *produce* elevated sympathetic responses, the two views are not mutually exclusive. Moreover, if Type A is a consequence of sympathetic hyperreactivity, then Type A behavior might be suppressed by treatment techniques that act to decrease sympathetic responsiveness.

Beta-blockers are drugs that antagonize certain sympathetic nervous system responses that would otherwise be activated by epinephrine or norepinephrine. These responses occur primarily in organs such as the heart, and in smooth muscle of the blood vessels and lungs, but there are also metabolic effects of beta-blockers. Accordingly, several studies have examined the effects of beta-adrenergic blocking drugs—medications commonly used for the treatment of cardiovascular disorders—on Type A behavior. Some of these studies, conducted on hypertensive or coronary patient samples, have found that beta-blockers decrease elements of Type A behavior. However, there are methodological shortcomings in these studies, and there have also been failures to obtain this effect. The results of these studies are summarized in Table 11.1, and will be described.

In a correlational study, Krantz, Durel, and colleagues (1982) found that patients receiving the beta-blocker propranolol as part of their usual medical program were lower in several components of interview-rated Type A behavior (speech stylistics and potential for hostility) when compared to patients not receiving propranolol. Patients taking propranolol were also found to be less reactive on heart rate and blood pressure, when compared to patients who were not taking this particular medication.

Additional evidence that chronic beta-blocker therapy might decrease Type A behavior comes from an experiment by the German investigators Schmieder and colleagues (1983). In this study, seven hypertensive patients received the beta-blocker atenolol, and nine patients received a thiazide diuretic to lower blood pressure. After 4 to 10 weeks, only the atenolol-treated group showed a decrease in intensity of interview-rated Type A behavior. Speech stylistics associated with Type A appeared to be lessened by blockade of beta-adrenergic reactivity with atenolol. The diuretic-treated patients, by contrast, showed a nonsignificant tendency toward increased Type A behavior. These data are particularly interesting because the behavioral effects were obtained with the beta-blocker atenolol, which is believed to penetrate poorly into the brain. Schmieder and colleagues (1983) also report that patients taking atenolol were less reactive on cardiovascular measures to the Structured Interview. In a similar long-term follow-up of patients after 1.5 years, beta-blocked patients were still showing significant attenuation of potential for hostility, assessed from the Structured Interview (Schmieder, Neus, Rüddel, & Von Eiff, 1985).

An additional recent study by these investigators compared the effects on Type A behavior of a beta-blocker (oxprenolol) with that of a calcium channel blocker (Rüddel, Schmieder, Langewitz, & Otten, 1986). Calcium channel blockers are also used in the treatment of cardiovascular disorders, but do not directly affect the sympathetic nervous system. Eighty hypertensive patients were treated for 6 months, and the Thurstone Activity Scale (which correlates well with the SI) and the Framingham Type A Scale were given before treatment and at 3-month intervals. The Structured Interview was given at the 6-month testing session. Results indicated that after 3 months the Type A questionnaire scores in the beta-blocker group were significantly lower. Drug group differences after 6 months were weakened, but still

**TABLE 11.1. STUDIES EXAMINING THE EFFECTS OF CHRONIC BETA-BLOCKER MEDICATION UPON TYPE A BEHAVIOR**

| Study | Subjects | Design | Results and Comment |
|---|---|---|---|
| Krantz et al., 1982 | Patients referred for coronary arteriography due to prior MI, chest pain, abnormal EKG; N = 88 | Correlational, no placebo control; patients receiving propranolol compared to those receiving non-beta-blocker therapy; mean daily dose of propranolol = 112 mg | Propranolol: lower global SI ratings, hostility, and speech stylistics; no difference for JAS |
| Schmieder, Friedrich, et al., 1983 | Hypertensives without complications | Experimental, no placebo control; subjects received either 100 mg per day of atenolol (N = 7) or 50 mg per day of hydrochlorothiazide and 50 mg per day of amiloride (N = 9); SI given prior to and after 4 to 10 weeks of therapy | Atenolol: 1 subject changed toward Type A, 1 no change, 5 toward Type B; diuretics: 4 toward Type A, 5 no change, none toward Type B; speech stylistics lower for atenolol compared to diuretics after therapy |
| Schmieder, Neus, et al., 1985 | Hypertensives without complications | Experimental, no placebo control; subjects received either atenolol (N = 9) or diuretics (N = 11) in same dosages used in previous study; SI given prior to and after 1 to 1.5 years of therapy | Atenolol: 2 subjects changed toward Type A, 4 no change, 5 toward Type B; diuretics: 3 toward Type A, 6 no change, none toward Type B; hostility ratings lower for atenolol compared to diuretics after therapy |

| Rüddel et al., 1986 | Hypertensives without complications | Experimental, no placebo control; subjects received 160 mg per day of oxprenolol (N = 11) or 20 mg per day of nitrendipine (N = 7); dose doubled if BP remained ≥140/90; SI given after 6 months of therapy | Hostility ratings lower for oxprenolol compared to nitrendipine after therapy; could reflect selective attrition since subjects with high scores on Type A questionnaires were more likely to drop out of beta-blocker group |
|---|---|---|---|
| Schneider et al., 1985 | Normotensives | Experimental, placebo-controlled; subjects received 50 mg per day of metoprolol (N = 15) or placebo (N = 13) for 6 weeks | Metoprolol: 1 subject showed increased hostility, 11 showed no change, and 3 decreased; placebo: 4 increased, 8 no change, and 1 decreased |
| Krantz et al., unpublished data | Hypertensives without complications | Experimental placebo-controlled; subjects received 50 mg per day of atenolol (N = 12), 80 mg per day of propranolol (N = 12), 50 mg per day of hydrochlorothiazide (N = 10), or placebo (N = 12); dose of beta-blockers doubled after 2 weeks of therapy; SI given prior to and after 6 weeks of therapy | Propranolol: 7 subjects (58%) showed decreased global Type A behavior, little effect on hostility; all other drug conditions: no evidence for decreased Type A behavior, majority of subjects (79%) showed a slight increase or no change; reductions for propranolol but not atenolol suggest central mechanism may mediate effects on Type A behavior |

were maintained for the Framingham Type A Scale. It further appears that Type A subjects were more likely to drop out of the beta-blocker group at 6-month follow-up—suggesting that Type A behavior may be associated with risk of dropout of antihypertensive therapy with beta-blockers. However, the results of the study have to be regarded as equivocal for that reason.

So far, the drug studies reviewed in this section have utilized patients with cardiovascular disease as subjects. A recent study compared the effects of a low-dose beta-blocker (metoprolol) with those of placebo on Type A behavior in normotensive subjects (Schneider, Julius, & Moss, 1985). They found little evidence that the beta-blocker affected Type A behavior over a 6-week period, with the exception of a nonsignificant trend toward a lessening of hostility with the beta-blocker. These negative results may have been due to the low drug dose utilized, or the effects of beta-blockers on Type A behavior may be confined to coronary patients or patients with high blood pressure.

None of the studies that have shown a reduction in Type A components among hypertensive patients produced by beta-blockers have utilized placebo control groups, so that it is not possible to determine to what extent the effects obtained are attributable to decreases in Type A with the beta-blocker or to increases in Type A produced by the other drugs (diuretics or calcium channel blockers) utilized for comparison. In addition, these studies have reported effects of several beta-blockers, regardless of the extent to which these drugs penetrate the brain. For example, Schmieder and colleagues (1983) found that in a small sample, atenolol, which has low central nervous system (CNS) penetration, had the apparent effect of reducing Type A when compared to a diuretic (see also Schmieder, Neus, Friedrich, & Rüddel, 1985). In a later study using a larger sample, oxprenolol, which readily penetrates the brain, was found to have similar effects (Rüddel et al., 1986). Because of this, a prospective placebo-controlled study was conducted by Contrada and colleagues (1987) to compare the effects of two beta-blockers differing in degree of CNS penetration to placebo.

In a double-blind study, 46 mild hypertensives were randomly assigned to receive either propranolol, a beta-blocker that penetrates the central nervous system highly, atenolol, which is very low in CNS penetration, placebo, or a diuretic (hydrochlorothiazide) for 6 weeks. Subjects were administered parallel forms of the Structured Interview and performed mental arithmetic and an abstract reasoning task prior to treatment and at the end of the study. Systolic and diastolic blood pressure and heart rate were monitored during rest and task performance. For analyses of Type A behavior and cardiovascular reactivity, data for placebo and diuretic did not differ and were combined into a single control group. Both beta-blockers produced a significant reduction in heart rate reactivity ($p < .02$), which was strongest for mental arithmetic. No change in reactivity was seen in the control group.

Covariance analysis of change-scores for SI components indicated a reduction only in ratings of explosive speech for the beta-blockers versus controls ($p = .05$). For global Type A ratings we classified subjects according to whether or not they decreased in Type A as a result of treatment, and compared the control, propranolol, and atenolol conditions. In the control group, most subjects (18 of 22, or 72 percent) either remained the same or increased in interview-rated Type A. Of subjects who received propranolol, seven out of 12 subjects (58 percent) showed a reduction in global Type A, the rest showing no change or an increase. By contrast, only three of 12 atenolol subjects (18 percent) changed in the Type B direction ($\chi^2 = 6.14$, $df = 2$, $p < .05$). These results suggest that beta-blockers that readily penetrate the brain, such as propranolol, have a more potent effect in lessening Type A behavior, and central nervous system mechanisms are probably important in producing these effects. However, it is important to note that the effects of the drugs on Type A in this study were relatively weak.

## BEHAVIORAL EFFECTS OF BETA-BLOCKERS: MECHANISMS AND ISSUES

An understanding of the mechanisms responsible for the effects of beta-blockers on Type A must take into account what is known about the psychological effects of these drugs. Because beta-blockers have come to be widely used in the treatment of cardiovascular disorders, a variety of behavioral and psychological effects have been observed. One of the most commonly noted beneficial effects is the reduction of anxiety in certain patient groups (Durel, Krantz, Eisold, & Lazar, 1985; Frishman, Razin, Swencionis, & Sonnenblick, 1981). For example, when given to patients who characterize their anxiety in *somatic* terms, such as palpitations and tremor, beta-blockers are effective antianxiety agents. However, among patients with predominantly cognitive symptoms such as worry or mental tension, beta-blockers seem to be relatively ineffective. In addition, beta-blockers appear to be useful for decreasing the anxiety of healthy subjects in acutely stressful situations such as public speaking, examinations, or stage fright, where bodily symptoms of anxiety might interfere with performance (Frishman et al., 1981).

### An Animal Model of Antianxiety Effects

Recent animal model data in this area may permit a closer examination of the mechanism mediating the antianxiety effects of beta-blockers. A study conducted by Lynn Durel and colleagues (Durel, Krantz, & Barrett, 1986) utilized a conflict paradigm to study the effects of beta-blockers in pigeons. In this paradigm, which is commonly used by behavioral pharmacologists to study the effects of benzodiazepines (e.g., Valium), responses are simultaneously reinforced and punished. Durel and colleagues (1986) showed that suppression of responding with punishment is released by several types of beta-blockers—an effect that occurs with benzodiazepines—and that propranolol produced a considerably larger effect than atenolol.

Decreases in heart rate and contractility are the physiologic effects of beta-blockers believed to be most relevant to cardiac treatment and to anxiety reduction. To determine whether heart rate could be related to the behavioral effects obtained, in a follow-up study Durel (1986) recorded EKGs during similar experimental sessions. Under control (no drug) conditions, heart rate increases during unpunished responding exceeded increases during punished responding. Although heart rate tended to be positively related to response rate, during punished responding high heart rate usually accompanies low response rate. Under the effective doses of propranolol, Durel (1986) found that heart rate increases associated with both types of behavior were substantially limited. Thus it is plausible that a peripheral feedback mechanism may be involved in the behavioral effects of beta-blockers in pigeons.

The precise means by which beta-blockers reduce anxiety are not entirely clear. Although all the commonly used beta-blockers penetrate the blood–brain barrier to some extent, they vary widely in this characteristic. Those agents that are lipid soluble (e.g., propranolol) accumulate in brain tissue to a far greater extent than do those that are water soluble. Nevertheless, it is important to note that the ability to penetrate the brain does not prove that this is the site of drug action. In fact, it is widely believed that the peripheral actions of beta-blockers can explain many of their anxiolytic effects. This mechanism may involve the role of bodily changes in the subjective experience of emotion, a mechanism that has been described in detail in a previous section of this chapter. Beta-blockers are thought to act by inhibiting selected physiological responses, thus interrupting the feedback loop from bodily responses to psychological reactions, and reducing the emotional intensity of anxiety. However, it should be noted that the degree to which peripheral as opposed to CNS (brain) mechanisms are involved in the anxiety-reducing and other psychological effects of beta-blockers is far from a settled issue (Durel et al., 1985; Patel & Turner, 1981).

## Relevance to Type A Behavior

How might the aforementioned discussion of beta-blockers and anxiety be relevant to an understanding of mechanisms underlying Type A behavior? At first glance, it may seem irrelevant because research indicates that Type A behavior as defined by Rosenman's interview is largely unrelated to psychometric measures of anxiety and distress. However, the descriptive and observable features of Type A behavior (such as anger, hostility, irritability, vigorous mannerisms, etc.) do represent forms of emotional behavior apart from anxiety. Thus the chronic beta-blocker studies reviewed earlier lead us to speculate that certain speech stylistics (such as loud–explosive and rapid–accelerated speech)—which were sensitive to beta-blocking medication in the aforementioned study—might reflect underlying physiological processes. The attitudes that the patients expressed, that is, their interview answers (unrelated to beta-blockade), might be more heavily linked to psychological factors. By lessening sympathetic responses, beta-blockers may reduce the intensity of Type A.

Taken together, these findings suggest that dampening of beta-adrenergically mediated responses produces a similar reduction in Type A behavior. However, this conclusion must be tempered by the correlational nature of one of the studies, and by the fact that only one of the experimental studies included a placebo control group. In addition, it has not been shown that components of Type A behavior can be potentiated by any pharmacological agent. The present line of reasoning would gain added support were it to be shown that aspects of Type A behavior are potentiated by acute administration of a drug such as isoproterenol, which acts peripherally and increases beta-adrenergic activity, and diminished by acute administration of propranolol, which decreases beta-adrenergic responses.

## EFFECTS OF ACUTE BETA-ADRENERGIC STIMULATION AND BLOCKADE

To examine some of the effects of sympathetic nervous system activity on behavior, a recent study (Krantz et al., in press) administered a beta-adrenergic agonist (stimulant), isoproterenol, and antagonist, propranolol, at different times in the same subjects. Of possible sympathetic agonists that could have been utilized (e.g., epinephrine, norepinephrine), isoproterenol was chosen because it stimulates only beta-receptors and, like the aforementioned catecholamines, does not cross the blood–brain barrier. The two drugs, as well as placebo, were given intravenously to study the effect of sympathetically mediated cardiovascular activity on Type A behavior and emotional responses to the Structured Interview.

### Substance–Stress Interactions and Reactivity

In the context of studying the effects of sympathetic nervous system drugs on behavior, it was also of interest to examine their influence upon cardiovascular reactivity. There has been growing interest in modulators and stimulators of psychophysiological responses to mental stressors (Dembroski, 1984). These studies have often reported that caffeine and nicotine, when given prior to having the subject engage in mental stress tasks, act to increase the psychophysiologic response to the stressors. In some studies, the effect of stress and substance is additive, and in other studies, stress and substances have an interactive effect. Among the variables that have been studied are substances (e.g., caffeine and nicotine) that have actions at various sites, including the central and autonomic nervous systems, receptors, and end-organs. The study of drugs such as beta-adrenergic agonists and antagonists, whose pharmacological effects are relatively specific, may shed light on physiological mechanisms underlying certain substance–stress interactions. Moreover, as suggested earlier in the discussion of beta-blockers and behavior, drugs that affect reactions to mental stressors also may operate through psychological processes, such as when the subject perceives and interprets bodily changes in a way that influences emotionality.

## Predictions and Obtained Results

The expectation in conducting this study was that the increase in cardiovascular activity caused by isoproterenol, and the dampening of this activity caused by propranolol, would be accompanied by parallel changes in Type A behavior and in self-reported anger and anxiety. We also expected that propranolol would decrease the magnitude of heart rate and blood pressure responses to mental stress, and that, perhaps, isoproterenol would increase heart rate and systolic blood pressure reactivity to stress.

The physiologic results obtained were generally as expected. However, the results for the effects of the drugs on Type A were surprising. Instead of isoproterenol infusion increasing the intensity of various Type A components, scores on these variables, presented in Table 11.2, were lower for this drug than for placebo. For anger and anxiety as measured by affect rating scales, isoproterenol ratings were significantly higher than ratings taken during placebo infusion.

The effects of isoproterenol on affect ratings can be explained in terms of the effects of the drug on peripheral autonomic responses. Subjects no doubt became aware of the marked increases in heart rate and tremor, and consequently may have perceived themselves as more anxious or angry.

For the measures of cardiovascular reactivity to the stressors, despite the fact that resting levels were predictably altered by the drugs, changes in both heart rate and blood pressure were significantly decreased by propranolol and significantly increased by isoproterenol. (The results for heart rate are presented in Fig. 11.2; comparable results were obtained for systolic blood pressure.) This enhancement of physiologic reactivity to the tasks with the beta-adrenergic agonist isoproterenol might be explained with reference to the effects of the drug at certain sympathetic nervous system receptors. More specifically, recent pharmacologic research indicates that there are beta-2 receptors at sympathetic nerve endings that, when stimulated, act to facilitate the release of norepinephrine at these nerve terminals (Adler-Graschinsky & Langer, 1975; Brown & Macquin, 1982). By activating this

**TABLE 11.2.   MEAN TYPE A RATINGS DURING ACUTE INFUSION OF EACH DRUG**

|                        | Placebo | Propranolol | Isoproterenol |
|------------------------|---------|-------------|---------------|
| Loud                   | 2.98    | 3.02        | 2.67          |
|                        | (.69)   | (.79)       | (.91)         |
| Explosive              | 2.85    | 2.81        | 2.56          |
|                        | (.78)   | (.78)       | (.75)         |
| Rapid–accelerated      | 3.19    | 3.15        | 2.77          |
|                        | (.76)   | (.98)       | (.75)         |
| Short response latency | 3.06    | 2.88        | 2.88          |
|                        | (.68)   | (.61)       | (.80)         |
| Hostility-potential    | 2.48    | 2.75        | 2.35          |
|                        | (.62)   | (.75)       | (.74)         |
| Verbal competition     | 2.54    | 2.46        | 1.96          |
|                        | (.82)   | (.62)       | (.66)         |
| Global Type A          | 2.06    | 2.04        | 1.67          |
|                        | (.75)   | (.86)       | (.78)         |

*Note:* Standard deviations are given in parentheses. Placebo values are computed as the average of both placebo conditions.

*Source:* Krantz et al., 1987.

mechanism, isoproterenol—a potent agonist at both beta-1 and beta-2 receptors—might increase synaptic norepinephrine output and result in greater cardiovascular responses to the tasks than were produced by the mental stress alone. On the other hand, psychologic mechanisms as well could have contributed to these effects. The increased anger and anxiety produced by the peripheral manifestations of the drugs may have heightened the perceived stressfulness of the tasks, thereby leading to increased reactivity.

In contrast to the cardiovascular measures, as noted earlier, SI-derived measures of Type A behavior responded to drug administration in a manner counter (decreases in some components with isoproterenol; see Table 11.2) to what would be predicted by a psychobiologic model, which called for increases in Type A with isoproterenol and reductions in Type A with propranolol. Regarding this model, these data suggest two possible conclusions. One is that the somatopsychic sequence for some elements of Type A behavior is not correct. However, this chapter has reviewed the body of data—including two prospective studies—supporting this theory. Alternatively, the intravenous drug infusion paradigm of this study may not have been a satisfactory one for testing the psychobiologic model. For example, with intravenous lines and EKG leads attached, subjects were placed in a passive situation. If this were so, they may have been constrained from responding to the situation in an aggressive Type A manner.

Also of relevance are the particular physiological effects of intravenous isoproterenol, compared to the effects of other sympathetic drugs that could

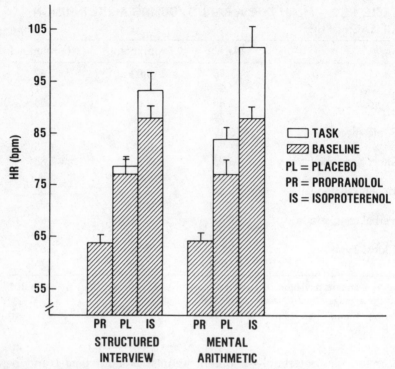

**FIGURE 11.2.** Effects of infusion of isoproterenol, propranolol, and placebo on resting heart rate and heart rate reactivity to mental stress. (From Krantz et al., in press.)

have been utilized (e.g., norepinephrine, epinephrine). When infused in humans, isoproterenol and epinephrine result in markedly increased heart rate and systolic blood pressure, and decreased diastolic blood pressure (Weiner, 1980). By contrast exogenous norepinephrine produces increased blood pressure, with little increase or even a decrease in heart rate. It is conceivable, therefore, that the tachycardia and tremor produced by isoproterenol resulted in perceptions of anxiety that are incompatible with Type A speech stylistics, and that different effects would have been produced by norepinephrine. Indeed, in a review of the effects of anxiety on speech tempo, Siegman (1978) found evidence of an inverted-U relationship, with speech rate increasing with moderate anxiety and decreasing with intense anxiety. Since anxiety ratings appear to have been increased markedly in the present study, it is possible that this emotion acted to decrease the SI-assessed speech characteristics as well.

In sum, this study clearly demonstrates that increasing reactivity with drugs has the effect of increasing the intensity of emotions such as anger and anxiety. However, paradoxical effects on Type A were obtained with isoproterenol—a drug that increases rate and forcefulness of heartbeat, tremor, and skin flushing. Whether similar results would have been obtained with norepinephrine—another beta-adrenergic agonist that produces different peripheral symptoms—is yet to be determined. Such a study would seem important to give a fair test to the hypothesis that reactivity is a contributor to Type A behavior.

## SUMMARY AND CONCLUSIONS

This chapter has presented current evidence concerning the role of sympathetic nervous system reactivity in contributing to Type A behavior and, more generally, the relationships between physiologic reactivity and emotional behavior. In light of this evidence, the initial hypotheses about Type A that were advanced based on studies of coronary bypass patients and earlier studies of the effects of beta-blockers on Type A (Krantz, Durel, et al., 1982; Krantz & Durel, 1983; Schmieder et al., 1983) may need to be revised or at least qualified.

Existing studies of the effects of chronic use of beta-blocking medications on Type A have obtained inconsistent results, with some studies of hypertensive and coronary patient samples finding that beta-blockers decrease the intensity of global Type A and certain Type A components. It should also be noted that at least one study utilizing a nonpatient population has failed to confirm this effect. Beta-blocking agents could well be expected to have different effects on normotensives and hypertensives, since the autonomic nervous system is involved in mild hypertension (Julius & Esler, 1975; Schmieder, Neus, Rüddel, & von Eiff, 1985).

Furthermore, the results of a study of the acute effects of beta-adrenergic stimulation on Type A manifestations in the Structured Interview are not supportive of the psychobiologic hypothesis that Type A behaviors are a consequence of *peripheral* physiologic responding. Results did indicate, however, that beta-adrenergic stimulation did increase anxiety, anger, and cardiovascular reactivity to mental stress. Because, like the catecholamines, isoproterenol does not cross the blood–brain barrier, these results argue against a role of peripheral physiologic responses in producing Type A behavior. However, the results of the acute study do not address the issue of the role of CNS mechanisms in contributing to Type A. Moreover, these findings are not incompatible with the results of the placebo-controlled study comparing the effects of propranolol (a beta-blocker that freely penetrates the brain) with those of atenolol (which shows considerably less CNS penetration). This study indicated that a lessening of Type A was found only with propranolol, and suggests that central nervous system mechanisms may play an important role in producing these effects.

The data presented in this chapter illustrate how pharmacologic techniques have been used to examine research issues concerning the relationship of psychophysiologic reactivity to behavior. Despite some very suggestive findings, cardiovascular reactivity per se cannot yet be regarded as a proven risk factor for coronary disease. Nevertheless, the complex two-way relationship between reactivity and behavior is not in doubt, and provides an important area for future research on both Type A behavior and emotion.

## REFERENCES

Adler-Graschinsky, E., & Langer, S. Z. (1975). Possible role of beta-adrenoceptors in the regulation of noradrenaline release by nerve stimulation through a positive feedback mechanism. *British Journal of Pharmacology, 53,* 43–50.

Averill, J. R. (1982). *Anger and aggression: An essay on emotion.* New York: Springer-Verlag.

Brown, M. J., & Macquin, I. (1982). Catecholamine neurotransmitters and the heart. *Acta Medica Scandinavica* (Suppl. 660), 34–39.

Cannon, W. (1929). *Bodily changes on pain, hunger, fear, and rage.* New York: Appleton-Century-Crofts.

Contrada, R. J., Krantz, D. S., Friedler, E., Durel, L. A., Hill, D. R., & Lazar, J. D. (1987). Effects of different beta-blockers on Type A behavior and cardiovascular reactivity in hypertensives. *Psychosomatic Medicine, 49,* 207–208. (Abstract).

Contrada, R. J., Wright, R. A., & Glass, D. C. (1985). Psychophysiologic correlates of Type A behavior: Comments on Houston (1983) and Holmes (1983). *Journal of Research in Personality, 19,* 12–30.

Davitz, J. R. (1969). *The language of emotion.* New York: Academic.

Dembroski, T. M. (1984). Stress and substance interaction effects on risk factors and reactivity. *Behavioral Medicine Update, 6,* 16–20.

Dembroski, T. M., MacDougall, J. M., Herd, J. A., & Shields, J. L. (1979). Effects of level of challenge on pressor and heart rate responses in Type A and B subjects. *Journal of Applied Social Psychology, 9,* 209–228.

Durel, L. A. (1986). *The effects of beta-blockers on punished responding and on heart rate in pigeons.* Unpublished doctoral dissertation, Uniformed Services University of the Health Sciences.

Durel, L. A., Krantz, D. S., & Barrett, J. A. (1986), The anti-anxiety effects of beta-blockers on punished responding. *Pharmacology Biochemistry & Behavior, 25,* 371–374.

Durel, L. A., Krantz, D. S., Eisold, J. F., & Lazar, J. D. (1985). Behavioral effects of beta-blockers: Reduction of anxiety, acute stress, and Type A behavior. *Journal of Cardiopulmonary Rehabilitation, 5,* 257–273.

Erdmann, G., & Janke, W. (1978). Interaction between physiological and cognitive determinants of emotions: Experimental studies on Schachter's theory of emotions. *Biological Psychology, 6,* 61–74.

Friedman, M., & Rosenman, R. H. (1959). Association of specific overt behavior pattern with blood and cardiovascular findings: Blood cholesterol level, blood clotting time, incidence of arcus senilis and clinical coronary artery disease. *Journal of the American Medical Association, 169,* 1286–1296.

Frishman, W. H., Razin, A., Swencionis, C., & Sonnenblick, E. (1981). Beta-adrenoceptor blockade in anxiety states: New approach to therapy? *Cardiovascular Reviews & Reports, 2,* 447–459.

Gates, G. S. (1926). An observational study of anger. *Journal of Experimental Psychology, 9,* 235–331.

Geen, R. G., Rakosky, J. J., & Pigg, R. (1972). Awareness of arousal and its relation to aggression. *British Journal of Social & Clinical Psychology, 11,* 115–121.

Glass, D. C. (1977). *Behavior patterns, stress, and coronary disease.* Hillsdale, NJ: Erlbaum.

Glass, D. C., Krakoff, L. R., Contrada, R. J., Hilton, W. F., Kehoe, K., Mannucci, E. G., Collins, C., Snow, B., & Elting, E. (1980). Effects of harassment and competition on cardiovascular and plasma catecholamine responses in Type A and B individuals. *Psychophysiology, 17,* 453–463.

Houston, B. K. (1983). Psychophysiological reactivity and the Type A behavior pattern. *Journal of Research in Personality, 17,* 22–39.

James, W. (1884). What is an emotion? *Mind, 9,* 188–205.

Julius, S., & Esler, M. (1975). Autonomic nervous cardiovascular regulation in borderline hypertension. *American Journal of Cardiology, 36,* 685–696.

Kahn, J. P., Kornfeld, D. S., Frank, K. A., Heller, S. S., & Hoar, P. F. (1980). Type A behavior and blood pressure during coronary bypass surgery. *Psychosomatic Medicine, 42,* 407–414.

Konečni, V. J. (1975a). Annoyance, type and duration of postannoyance activity, and aggression. *Journal of Experimental Psychology: General, 104,* 75–102.

Konečni, V. J. (1975b). The mediation of aggressive behavior: Arousal level versus anger and cognitive labeling. *Journal of Personality & Social Psychology, 32,* 706–712.

Kornfeld, D. S., Kahn, J. P., Frank, K. A., Heller, S., Freeman, P., & Keller-Epstein, W. (1985). Type A behavior and blood pressure during general surgery. *Psychosomatic Medicine, 47,* 214–241.

Krantz, D. S., Arabian, J. M., Davia, J. E., & Parker, J. S. (1982). Type A behavior and coronary artery bypass surgery: Intraoperative blood pressure and perioperative complications. *Psychosomatic Medicine, 44,* 273–284.

Krantz, D. S., Contrada, R. J., LaRiccia, P., Anderson, J., Durel, L. A., & Dembroski, T. M. (1987). Effects of acute beta-adrenergic stimulation and blockade on cardiovascular reactivity, affect, and Type A behavior. *Psychosomatic Medicine, 49,* 146–158.

Krantz, D. S., Durel, L. A., Davia, J. E., Shaffer, R., Arabian, J. M. Dembroski, T. M., & MacDougall, J. M. (1982). Propranolol medication among coronary patients: Relationship to Type A behavior and cardiovascular response. *Journal of Human Stress, 8(3),* 4–12.

Krantz, D. S., & Durel, L. A. (1983). Psychobiological substrates of the Type A behavior pattern. *Health Psychology, 2,* 393–411.

Krantz, D. S., & Manuck, S. B. (1984). Acute psychophysiologic reactivity and risk of cardiovascular disease: A review and methodologic critique. *Psychological Bulletin, 96,* 435–464.

Lange, C. G. (1885/1922). *The emotions.* Baltimore: Williams and Wilkins.

Leventhal, H. (1980). Toward a comprehensive theory of emotion. In L. Berkowitz (Ed.), *Advances in experimental social psychology.* New York: Academic.

Mason, J. W. (1972). Organization of psychoendocrine systems: A review and reconsideration of research. In N. S. Greenfield & R. A. Sternbach (Eds.), *Handbook of psychophysiology.* New York: Holt, Rinehart, & Winston.

Matthews, K. A. (1982). Psychological perspectives on the Type A behavior pattern. *Psychological Bulletin, 91,* 293–323.

Matthews, K. A., Rosenman, R. H., Dembroski, T. M., Harris, E. L., & MacDougall, J. M. (1984). Familial resemblance in components of the Type A behavior pattern: A reanalysis of the California Type A twin study. *Psychosomatic Medicine, 46,* 512–522.

Matthews, K. A., Weiss, S. M., Detre, T., Dembroski, T. M., Falkner, B., Manuck, S. B., & Williams, R. B. (1986). *Handbook of stress, reactivity, and cardiovascular disease.* New York: Wiley.

Patel, L., & Turner, P. (1981). Central actions of beta-adrenoceptor blocking drugs in man. *Medicinal Research Reviews, 1,* 387–410.

Rahe, R. H., Hervig, L., & Rosenman, R. H. (1978). The heritability of Type A behavior. *Psychosomatic Medicine, 40,* 478–486.

Review Panel. (1981). Coronary-prone behavior and coronary heart disease: A critical review. *Circulation, 63,* 1199–1215.

Rose, R. J., Grim, C. J., & Miller, J. Z. (1984). Familial influences on cardiovascular stress reactivity: Studies of normotensive twins. *Behavioral Medicine Update, 6,* 21–24.

Rosenman, R. H. (1978). The interview method of assessment of the coronary-prone behavior pattern. In T. M. Dembroski, S. M. Weiss, J. L. Shields, S. G. Haynes, & M. Feinleib (Eds.), *Coronary-prone behavior.* New York: Springer-Verlag.

Rüddel, H., Schmieder, R., Langewitz, W., & Otten, H. (1986). Effect of antihypertensive therapy with beta-blockers on Type A behavior and hostility. *Psychosomatic Medicine, 48,* 295 (Abstract).

Schachter, S., & Singer, J. E. (1962). Cognitive, social, and physiological determinants of emotional state. *Psychological Review, 69,* 379–399.

Schmieder, R., Friedrich, G., Neus, H., Rüddel, H., & Von Eiff, A. W. (1983). The influence of beta-blockers on cardiovascular reactivity and Type A behavior pattern in hypertensives. *Psychosomatic Medicine, 45,* 417–424.

Schmieder, R., Neus, H., Friedrich, G., & Rüddel, H. (1985). Beta-blockers and Type A behavior: Long-term effect and methodological problems. *Psychophysiology, 20,* 470 (Abstract).

Schmieder, R., Neus, H., Rüddel, H., & von Eiff, A. W. (1985). Attenuation of Type A behavior in hypertensives: A comparison between beta-blockers, diuretics, and calcium antagonists. In A. Zanchetti & P. Turner (Eds.), *Towards preventive treatment of coronary-prone behavior.* Toronto: Hans Huber.

Schneider, R., Julius, S., & Moss, G. (1985). Physiological correlates of the Type A coronary-prone behavior pattern and the influence of metoprolol (Lopressor): A preliminary report. In A. Zanchetti & P. Turner (Eds.), *Towards a preventive approach to coronary-prone behavior.* Berne: Hans Huber.

Siegman, A. W. (1978). The telltale voice: Nonverbal messages of verbal communication. In A. W. Siegman & S. Feldstein (Eds.), *Nonverbal behavior and communication.* Hillsdale, NJ: Erlbaum.

Weiner, N. (1980). Drugs that inhibit adrenergic nerves and block adrenergic receptors. In A. G. Goodman-Gilman, L. S. Goodman, & A. Gilman (Eds.), *The pharmacologic basis of therapeutics* (6th ed.). New York: Macmillan.

Wright, R. A., Contrada, R. J., & Glass, D. C. (1985). Psychophysiologic correlates of Type A behavior. In E. S. Katkin & S. B. Manuck (Eds.), *Advances in behavioral medicine.* Greenwich, CT: JAI.

Zanchetti, A., & Turner, P. (Eds.). (1985). *Towards preventive treatment of coronary-prone behavior.* Berne: Hans Huber.

Zillman, D. (1971). Excitation transfer in communication-mediated aggressive behavior. *Journal of Experimental Social Psychology, 7,* 419–434.

Zillman, D., Johnson, R. C., & Day, K. D. (1974). Attribution of apparent arousal and proficiency of recovery from sympathetic activation affecting excitation transfer to aggressive behavior. *Journal of Experimental Social Psychology, 10,* 503–515.

# 12

## Research and Clinical Issues in Treating Type A Behavior

VIRGINIA A. PRICE

### INTRODUCTION TO TYPE A TREATMENT RESEARCH

The basic issue for investigators interested in conducting research on modifying Type A behavior is: Why do it? What can be learned about the Type A behavior pattern from conducting treatment intervention studies? Is it premature to try to modify the Type A pattern when there is not yet full agreement among researchers on just what the behavior pattern is or how to measure it, including how to measure possible changes that occur as a result of treatment?

Treatment research to date suggests that, despite the limitations in our present knowledge of Type A and the problems inherent in clinical research, carefully designed and controlled treatment studies may provide researchers with more intimate views of the Type A behavior pattern than can be gained through epidemiological or laboratory research alone. Clinical efforts to modify Type A behavior can reveal information about both the remote and the immediate antecedents and consequences of the Type A behavior pattern that would otherwise be difficult to obtain. For example, our knowledge about the environmental factors that promote and maintain Type A behavior, including significant early relationships and current family and job circumstances, can be improved through clinical research on Type A behavior. Clinical research also offers us a unique opportunity to learn more about the cognitive factors associated with observable Type A behavior. Ultimately, we may also be able to add to our knowledge about the biophysiological effects of Type A by examining differences in these variables before and after treatment. Thus, through treatment research, it may be possible to gain more thorough knowledge about the nature of the Type A behavior pattern, clearer insights into its possible causes, better ideas about how to "cure" it, and an improved understanding of its effects on cardiovascular health.

"Hard facts" and clinical impressions obtained from treatment research can be studied further—and confirmed or disconfirmed—through other methods of scientific inquiry, including laboratory and epidemiological research. It seems reasonable to expect that a better understanding of the behavior pattern will grow out of a synthesis of data, collected through a variety of different scientific methodologies including treatment intervention research.

## Review of Type A Treatment Studies

A number of studies testing the feasibility of modifying Type A behavior have already been completed. Among them are six preliminary, small-scale studies done in the seventies and early eighties (Blumenthal, Williams, Williams, & Wallace, 1980; Jenni & Wollersheim, 1979; Levenkron, Cohen, Mueller, & Fisher, 1983; Roskies, Spevack, Surkis, Cohen, & Gilman, 1978; Suinn, 1975; Suinn & Bloom, 1978) and three more recent, large-scale investigations, including the Recurrent Coronary Prevention Project (RCPP) (M. Friedman et al., 1986), the United States Army War College study (USAWC) (Gill et al., 1985), and the Montreal Type A Intervention Project (MTAIP) (Roskies et al., 1986). Although the six early studies helped launch research on treating Type A behavior, most of them had rather serious conceptual and methodological limitations, which the three more recent treatment studies have tried to overcome. This research has been extensively and thoughtfully reviewed elsewhere (Levenkron et al., 1983; Price, 1982; Roskies, 1979; Suinn, 1980; Thoresen, Telch, & Eagleston, 1981). Four of the limitations common to most of these studies will be discussed here.

**Duration of Treatment.**    One limitation of all the early studies was their short duration. The maximum length of treatment was 14 hours over a 20-week period (Roskies et al., 1978). Considering how many years this pattern of behavior takes to develop, how pervasive it is in a person's life, and how intractable it is reputed to be (M. Friedman, 1979), we may be overly optimistic to expect these short treatments to achieve lasting changes. By contrast, the RCPP offered 50 hours of treatment over a 4.5-year period and the USAWC program offered 32 hours of treatment over 9 months.

**Treatment Components.**   A second issue has to do with the nature of the treatment itself. In several of the early studies (Blumenthal et al., 1980; Suinn, 1975; Suinn & Bloom, 1978) the treatment was limited to reducing stress and tension. Relaxation, physical exercise, and other coping techniques were used, but little or no attention was paid to modifying any of the specific components of the Type A behavior pattern, such as time urgency and hostility. Yet M. Friedman and Rosenman (1974) have contended that reducing Type A requires the use of specific behavioral methods aimed at modifying specific, habitual Type A behaviors and beliefs. Support for their view first came from three early treatment studies (Jenni & Wollersheim, 1979; Levenkron et al., 1983; Roskies et al., 1978), which produced more substantial changes in measured Type A variables by using cognitive and behavioral strategies and trying to modify specific components of the Type A behavior pattern than by using various stress management and insight-oriented techniques that did not target specific Type A behaviors. Additional support for M. Friedman and Rosenman's assertion about the kind of treatment needed has come from the three more recent studies, to be described.

*RCPP and USAWC treatment programs.*   The experimental treatment in both the RCPP and the USAWC studies was based on a conceptualization of the Type A behavior pattern as a life-style that involves a chronic struggle to accomplish more and more in less and less time, and often against the opposing efforts of other people and the limitations of time (M. Friedman, 1977). This struggle, which involves chronic feelings of time urgency and chronic and excessive hostility, was seen as the outgrowth of a "faulty" belief system and excessive environmental demands.

The treatment programs used in the RCPP and the USAWC studies were very similar, differing mostly in duration (4.5 years compared to 9 months) and in the absence of cardiologic counseling in the USAWC study.* The treatment was based on an expanded cognitive social learning model of Type A behavior (e.g., Price, 1982; Thoresen, Friedman, Gill, & Ulmer, 1982). It focused on changing the cognitive, behavioral, physiological, and environmental factors associated with two major components of Type A: time urgency and hostility. As part of the treatment, patients learned how

---

*Military officer–students are on a 1-year tour of duty at the United States Army War College, so the experimental Type A treatment program had to be reduced in length to fit into that time frame. Having just completed the 4.5-year Recurrent Coronary Prevention Project, we felt we had a pretty good idea about what treatment components worked best. We therefore designed the intervention for the USAWC around those components.

to make needed changes in their social and physical environments to reduce time pressures, provocations of hostility, and threats to self-esteem. They also learned how to examine and modify their beliefs, their self-image, and their habit of misconstruing a wide range of ordinary stimuli as threats to their egos. They learned to respond to perceived threats with a variety of alternative responses, such as self-instruction and mental and physical relaxation. The ultimate goal of this treatment was to minimize the need for the chronic mobilization of the fight–flight response, which is thought by many (e.g., M. Friedman & Rosenman, 1969; Herd, 1981; Krantz, Glass, Schaeffer, & Davia, 1982; Williams, 1978) to link Type A behavior and coronary heart disease (CHD). Another important part of the treatment was the systematic practice of specific behaviors antithetical to Type A, such as walking slowly, leaving one's watch off, and smiling.

Several different treatment strategies based on the principles of social learning theory (Bandura, 1977) were used to try to help participants accomplish all these changes. Strategies included didactic instruction (lecturing about and assigning readings on Type A behavior), social modeling (providing opportunities for participants to observe the differences in how Type A's and Type B's respond to the same stimuli), and rehearsal of alternative "Type B" responses (trying out new behaviors in the group and noticing the consequences). More thorough descriptions of the treatment program used in these two studies can be found elsewhere (M. Friedman et al., 1982; M. Friedman & Ulmer, 1984; Price, 1982; Price & Friedman, 1986; Thoresen, Friedman, Powell, Gill, & Ulmer, 1985).

*MTAIP treatment program.*    The third major treatment study, the MTAIP, compared three treatment protocols, including cognitive–behavioral stress management training, aerobic exercise, and weight lifting. Only the cognitive–behavioral training achieved significant posttreatment reductions in Type A behavior. This latter treatment was based on the notion that Type A's respond to everyday "hassles" in an automatic, stereotyped, all-or-none fashion without considering alternative response options that might be more appropriate or less stressful. Consequently, the treatment consisted mainly in providing a variety of different coping strategies, such as muscular relaxation, improved communication skills, cognitive relabeling, "stress inoculation," and problem solving. It also attempted to increase participants' awareness of situations that typically trigger stress, so that they could anticipate and plan for these events, use their new skills to cope with them, and evaluate the outcome of this process. A further description of the treatment procedures can be found in the report by Roskies and her colleagues (1986).

**Evaluation of Treatment Effects.**    A third limitation of the early studies that attempted to modify Type A behavior has to do with how treatment effects were evaluated. Only four of the six studies used measures of Type

A behavior to evaluate the effects of treatment (Blumenthal et al., 1980; Jenni & Wollersheim, 1979; Levenkron et al., 1983; Roskies et al., 1978). Moreover, these four studies used only self-report measures of Type A, including the Jenkins Activity Survey (JAS) (Jenkins, Zyzanski, & Rosenman, 1971), the Framingham Type A Scale (FTAS) (Haynes, Feinleib, Levine, Scotch, & Kannel, 1978), and the Bortner Self-Rating Scale of Type A Behavior (Bortner, 1969). They did not use either of the two better validated, direct behavioral measures of Type A: the Structured Interview (SI) (Dembroski, MacDougall, Shields, Petitto, & Lushene, 1978; Rosenman, 1978) or the Videotaped Structured Interview (VSI) (M. Friedman & Powell, 1984). The other two studies (Suinn, 1975; Suinn & Bloom, 1978) did not use any Type A dependent measures at all. Consequently, it is extremely difficult to draw definite conclusions about what Type A behaviors actually changed as a result of these treatments.

All three of the more recent studies evaluated treatment efficacy by using behavioral and physiological measures appropriate to the hypotheses under investigation. For instance, the MTAIP used the SI and the RCPP and USAWC studies used the VSI to assess Type A behavior before and after treatment. The RCPP and USAWC studies also used other measures of Type A behavior. For example, questionnaires were completed by participants and by their spouses and colleagues to obtain supplementary information about the specific nature of the changes in Type A behavior that occurred as a result of treatment. Results from these recent studies demonstrated that Type A behavior can be significantly modified in a large percentage of both coronary patients (M. Friedman et al., 1986) and healthy subjects (Gill et al., 1985; Roskies et al., 1986) and that in coronary patients reductions in Type A behavior are associated with significant reductions in coronary recurrences (M. Friedman et al., 1986).

In addition to demonstrating reductions in Type A behavior, Type A modification programs need to provide evidence of reductions in coronary risk. In the absence of data on coronary morbidity and mortality, changes in physiological variables that are thought to link Type A to CHD could provide preliminary evidence of possible risk reduction. Commendably, all of the early treatment studies included some physiological outcome measures (e.g., serum lipids, heart rate, and blood pressure). Unfortunately, these variables did not show consistent changes in the expected directions.

All three of the recent studies also examined changes in biophysiological variables, including serum cholesterol levels (M. Friedman et al., 1986; Gill et al., 1985), high-density lipoprotein cholesterol measures (Gill et al., 1985), and heart rate and blood pressure reactivity in response to a laboratory stress task (Roskies et al., 1986). The studies showed that, aside from significant reductions in coronary recurrence rates in the RCPP, physiological changes attributable to Type A treatment were rather trivial. The MTAIP also attempted to measure cortisol and plasma epinephrine and norepi-nephrine, but difficulties in obtaining accurate measures made it imprudent to use them to evaluate treatment efficacy (Roskies et al., 1986). Judicious selection of physiological variables and careful attention to the procedures and conditions of assessment are needed in Type A treatment research.

**Durability of Treatment Effects.**   A fourth limitation of studies to date is the absence of follow-up data. Only two of the early treatment studies included follow-up measures of change (Jenni & Wollersheim, 1979; Roskies et al., 1978), and, unfortunately, neither study used validated Type A measures to assess treatment outcome. Thus two questions remain unanswered: Do reductions in Type A behavior continue after Type A treatment ends? What effect does Type A behavior modification have on *long*-term coronary recurrence rates?

## Identification of Treatment Issues

The Type A treatment studies just reviewed have highlighted four important issues that need to be addressed in subsequent Type A intervention research. First, the treatment program should be of sufficient duration to produce lasting changes in this complex and deeply entrenched pattern of behavior. Second, the treatment program should be a direct outgrowth of the investigator's conceptual model of Type A. Third, there is a need for careful selection of the instruments and procedures used to evaluate the effects of treatment. And, fourth, follow-up studies are needed in order to evaluate the long-term effects of the treatment on Type A behavior and associated physiological and psychosocial variables. Some of these treatment issues are considered more fully in the sections that follow. Three other key issues in designing Type A treatment studies will also be examined. First is the need for replicating successful treatment studies. Second is the consideration of what populations to treat to expand our present knowledge about Type A behavior and its effects. And the final consideration is whether treatment outcome can be enhanced by using a more systematic and explicit definition of *Type B* behavior. Suggestions are offered about empirical research that could explore these important treatment issues and test the validity of clinical impressions.

## KINDS OF TREATMENT STUDIES NEEDED

The studies suggested here are meant to answer the following questions: How long do the effects of Type A treatment last? Can the significant reductions in Type A behavior (and coronary recurrence rates) that have already been obtained be replicated in new treatment studies? What is the most effective and efficient way to modify Type A behavior? Are there any alternatives to long-term, large-scale group comparison studies?

## Follow-up of Behavior Change

Although we have evidence that significant reductions in Type A behavior can be achieved, we do not yet know how durable these reductions are over time. Nor do we know whether reduced Type A behavior is associated with *sustained* reductions in coronary rates. Of course, the ultimate goal of research on treating Type A behavior is to discover through empirical means a treatment protocol that can bring about sustained reductions in Type A behavior and associated coronary risk so that this treatment can be included in heart disease prevention programs and coronary rehabilitation programs. If Type A behavior modification takes years to achieve and has only temporary effects on disease endpoints, then its value will be severely limited. Many questions need to be examined in regard to the efficacy and durability of treatment effects. How much reduction in Type A behavior is needed to reduce coronary risk? How long do persons need to remain in treatment to be able to achieve these benefits? Long-term follow-up data on successful treatment studies are needed. Perhaps these studies could be modeled after a current follow-up study of the RCPP conducted by Thoresen and his colleagues, in which all available original participants are being reevaluated 3 years after the termination of treatment.* Variables being assessed include subjects' Type A behavior (as measured by the VSI, self-report questionnaires, and the reports of participants' spouses and colleagues), recurrent infarctions and other coronary indices (e.g., high blood pressure, elevated cholesterol levels, angina), several quality of life variables (e.g., depression, anxiety), and subjects' responses to an arousal task designed to provide insights into how they cope with common everyday hassles. Ideally, in future studies, measures of the immediate and long-term effects of treatment will also include the direct systematic observation of Type A subjects in their home and work settings.

## Replication of Successful Treatments

One canon of science is that experimental findings must be replicable. We need to find out whether the treatment programs that have resulted in significant reductions in Type A behavior and its physical correlates, including CHD, can be replicated in other research centers and with different counselors.

## Comparisons of Different Treatment Approaches

Replications should go beyond simply confirming what we have learned in previous studies. New Type A treatment approaches, based on recent

---

*Recurrent Coronary Prevention Project Update (in progress). Three-year follow-up: January 1986 to January 1988.

research findings about the nature of Type A behavior, need to be compared to Type A treatment programs that have already proven successful in reducing Type A behavior. These comparisons will almost certainly yield important conceptual information about Type A and its risk-conferring qualities, as well as show investigators the best way to modify it. For example, a central issue that has important treatment implications is whether the Type A behavior pattern as a coronary risk factor (1) encompasses an entire life-style, (2) is limited to just two or three isolated psychological or behavioral factors, (3) is simply the outward manifestation of underlying cognitive factors that should be modified, or (4) is nothing more than a physiological predisposition toward higher sympathetic nervous system arousal. In the first case, the whole life-style of patients may need to be modified. This was the approach taken in the RCPP and USAWC studies. In the second case, only certain facets of the behavior pattern—those considered most central or most lethal—would be the objects of treatment. In the third situation, the treatment might focus on modifying the cognitions that promote observable Type A behavior. And in the fourth case, pharmacological intervention might be the treatment of choice. The treatment option based on the conceptualization of Type A as an entire life-style has already been described in a previous section of this chapter. The other three treatment options will now be considered.

**Modifying Only Certain Facets of Type A.** To test the hypothesis that a narrowly focused treatment program is sufficient to alter Type A behavior and its associated coronary risk, several specific treatment approaches could be compared. Four possible approaches will now be considered, including treatments that focus on (1) reducing hostility, (2) increasing relaxation, (3) improving physical exercise, and (4) reducing the psychomotor characteristics of Type A.

*Reducing hostility.* This treatment approach is based on the idea that there may be just one or two components of the Type A behavior pattern that account for the coronary risk associated with Type A. The search for the most important component(s) of Type A behavior has dominated the field for the last 10 years (e.g., H. Friedman, Hall, & Harris, 1985; Glass, 1977; Matthews, Glass, Rosenman, & Bortner, 1977; Musante, MacDougall, Dembroski, & Van Horn, 1983; Scherwitz, Berton, & Leventhal, 1977; Schucker & Jacobs, 1977; Williams et al., 1980). Many studies point to hostility as a leading contender (Barefoot, Dahlstrom, & Williams, 1983; Dembroski, MacDougall, Williams, Haney, & Blumenthal, 1985; Haynes, Feinleib, & Kannel, 1980; MacDougall, Dembroski, Dimsdale, & Hackett, 1985; Matthews et al., 1977; Shekelle, Gale, Ostfeld, & Paul, 1983; Williams, Barefoot, & Shekelle, 1984). In a recent review of this body of research, Matthews and Haynes (1986) concluded that hostility seems to be the most toxic element of the Type A behavior pattern and that future Type A studies should include specific measures of hostility to determine whether this is, indeed, the case. Thus the first approach to compare with the comprehensive life-style modification program used in the RCPP is a treatment program aimed at modifying hostility only. In actual clinical practice, it may be very difficult to focus treatment so narrowly (i.e., on a single component), because on cannot ignore the context in which the target behavior occurs. For instance, Type A hostility seems to occur when persons are exposed to time pressures, when they are in competitive situations, when their self-esteem is threatened, and so on. If the treatment were broadened to include modifying these antecedents of hostility, it might eventually become almost indistinguishable from a "life-style treatment."

*Increasing the relaxation response.* The second treatment approach that could be compared with life-style modification is systematic relaxation training (Bernstein & Borkovec, 1973). There are two basic rationales for relaxation training. The first rationale is that Type A's appear to have great difficulty modulating their chronic hard-driving behavior and being able to relax and may, therefore, need explicit training in these areas. The second rationale is based on the observation that Type A's seem to be constantly mobilized as if their well-being were constantly threatened, resulting in chronic sympathetic nervous system arousal. Progressive muscle relaxation has been shown to reduce factors associated with sympathetic arousal, such as accelerated heart rate and elevated blood pressure (Cottier, Shapiro, & Julius, 1984; Johnston, 1985). Thus it is a theoretically promising treatment for reducing some of the physiological correlates of Type A behavior and perhaps even for reducing Type A behavior itself. If systematic relaxation could produce significant reductions in Type A behavior, it might quickly become the treatment method of choice, because of its simplicity and ease of implementation compared to any other Type A treatment method to date. Despite the theoretical rationale for testing relaxation therapy, however, experimental treatment programs that focus on relaxation training have not shown consistent reductions in Type A behavior (e.g., Jenni & Wollersheim, 1979). Moreover, clinical experience in the RCPP and USAWC studies indicates that in actual practice relaxation training has limited value for Type A's. Both studies discovered that, despite extensive training, incentives, and cajoling, few participants practice systematic relaxation consistently or feel it is of much value to them compared to the other treatment components.

*Increasing physical exercise.* The third treatment approach to compare with a life-style modification program for reducing Type A behavior and its associated coronary risk is to increase physical activity through a systematic exercise program. Physical exercise gains credibility as a possible treatment for Type A's from a previous study by Blumenthal and his colleagues (1980), which showed that exercise reduced heart rate, blood pressure, and high (but not low) scores on the JAS. A further rationale for an exercise treatment program is that Type A's often lack regular heart-healthy exercise regimens and those who do engage in consistent exercise often report that it calms them down. Moreover, a sedentary life-style in itself is considered to be a possible coronary risk factor (Paffenbarger, 1984), so that even if regular exercise doesn't reduce Type A behavior it may still decrease the risk of coronary disease. Despite these rationales, the recent report by Roskies and her associates (1986) showed mixed results with respect to the impact of exercise on Type A behavior and cardiovascular reactivity. Specifically, no reductions in Type A behavior occurred in subjects assigned to an aerobic exercise treatment group, and only small reductions in Type A behavior occurred in subjects assigned to a weight-lifting treatment. Moreover, neither of the exercise treatment groups demonstrated significant reductions in heart rate or in systolic or diastolic blood pressure.

*Modifying behavioral indicators that predict high risk.* The original operational definition of Type A behavior as a coronary risk factor was the Structured Interview used in the Western Collaborative Group Study (Rosenman et al., 1975). As other contributors to this volume have already pointed out, there are now several versions of the original interview. But despite serious methodological problems with the interview, it remains the best predictor of coronary disease of all the instruments currently used in the field of Type A research. Recent research has shown that a small number of behavioral indicators from the SI, including, for example, the number of self-references (Scherwitz, Graham, Grandits, Buehler, & Billings, 1986) and vigorous vocal characteristics (Dembroski & MacDougall, 1983; Scherwitz, Graham, Grandits, & Billings, 1987; Schucker & Jacobs, 1977), account for most of the coronary risk associated with the Type A behavior pattern. These findings suggest an unusual but possible fruitful fourth treatment approach to compare with life-style modification. Perhaps treatment should focus exclusively on reducing or eliminating these psychomotor signs and indicators that are predictive of CHD. This treatment might involve teaching subjects to modulate vocal characteristics, reduce self-references, and so on. This approach has limited appeal to clinical researchers, because it conjures up the image of a patient who has learned how to smile but has not learned how to be happy. Nonetheless, the scientific approach cautions us to suspend judgment until we have subjected the hypothesis to empirical test.

*Problems in modifying only certain facets of Type A behavior.* An important concern about the Type A treatment approaches just described has to do with the possible consequences of attempting to modify only selected aspects of Type A behavior. The concern grows out of a working hypothesis widely shared by researchers in the Type A area that the behavior pattern is a coping strategy for dealing with a variety of possible cognitive stressors and environmental demands (e.g., M. Friedman & Ulmer, 1984; Glass, 1977; Price, 1982; Smith & Anderson, 1986). If the Type A behavior pattern is, indeed, a life strategy, then a treatment program that teaches people how to change their day-to-day tactics without changing their overall life strategy may be an unacceptable approach. For instance, if we teach people how to slow down their pace, but ignore the fact that they continue to commit themselves to an inordinate number of tasks and demands, the effect of treatment may be to leave them without their usual means for meeting their commitments. Such tactical changes could result in their experiencing the very failure that the Type A behavior pattern may be meant to ward off (Price, 1982). Given the general life strategy of Type A's, their specific tactics may be quite appropriate. Thus, unless we help Type A's change their life strategy (i.e., their Type A life-style), we may need to leave their tactics alone.

**Modifying Cognitions Associated with Type A.**    A second major treatment option for modifying the Type A pattern is based on the notion that Type A behavior is simply the outward manifestation of underlying cognitive factors. If, as researchers suppose, there *are* some identifiable cognitive components associated with the Type A behavior pattern, then perhaps treatment should focus on modifying these so-called Type A cognitions. Clinical evidence supports the supposition that certain cognitive–emotional factors underlie Type A behavior and that these factors need to be examined and modified for significant and lasting reductions in Type A behavior to occur. For instance, therapists in the RCPP and the USAWC studies observed that success in modifying Type A behavior was severely hampered without sufficient therapeutic attention to these cognitive–emotional issues. Although subjects could often make specific behavioral changes without any discussion of the cognitive facets of Type A, they seemed to have difficulty maintaining the changes and generalizing them to new situations unless they experienced rather substantial changes in their Type A viewpoint. It is important for these clinical impressions to be subjected to rigorous empirical test, because they have far-reaching implications for the treatment of Type A.

From a clinical perspective, the most important single cognitive factor underlying and promoting Type A behavior seems to be a poor private self-image, encapsulated in the belief that "I am not good enough yet." Although Type A's typically try to project a public image of self-confidence (and often succeed), their private self-image seems to involve diffuse and persistent self-doubt and insecurity (e.g., Houston & Kelly, 1987). This private self-view is often manifested in the daily lives of Type A's as an insecurity about their ability to "do enough" in the salient areas of their lives (e.g., in their occupations). Clinical investigation of the antecedents of this personal sense of insecurity points overwhelmingly to a perceived lack of parental love and acceptance as an important ingredient in most cases. But few data exist at present to support or disconfirm these clinical impressions. Thus empirical research is needed to identify the factors that create self-esteem problems in Type A's. With sufficient knowledge about the antecedents of poor self-esteem in Type A's, we may be able ultimately to intervene early enough in the social learning process to prevent the development of the Type A behavior pattern.

A second and related cognitive component of the Type A pattern seems to be the assumption, or belief, that the *only* way to cope with feelings of insecurity is to "try harder" and "do more." Typically, Type A's appear to be convinced that by trying harder and doing more they will eventually subdue or overcome their self-doubt and attain a more secure sense of well-being. This assumption mobilizes Type A's to engage in a chronic struggle to prove to themselves that their self-doubts are unfounded. Despite achieving outward success, however, Type A's seem unable to use this "objective" evidence to allay fears and insecurities. Self-doubt continues to assert itself and the struggle to prove they are "good enough" continues almost uninterrupted. Eventually, nearly everything in their lives, including physical and emotional health and interpersonal relationships, may become subordinated to this chronic struggle.

Because high levels of achievement are sometimes a by-product of this chronic struggle and because individual achievement is highly regarded and reinforced in our culture, many persons believe that their Type A actions are perfectly normal and even praiseworthy. This cultural influence on Type A beliefs sometimes prevents high-risk Type A's from ever coming face to face with the possibility that their relentless achievement striving may be motivated by their own deficit model of self-worth and by the seemingly erroneous assumption that constant attempts to try harder and do more can and *will* overcome these supposed deficits.

What remains to be demonstrated systematically is the relative importance of addressing these cognitive issues as a means of achieving significant reductions in the Type A behavior pattern and its associated coronary risk. If cognitive changes do turn out to be an efficient focus of treatment, then it will be important to resolve the issue of how to assess the presence of Type A cognitions and how to measure the cognitive changes that may occur as a result of Type A treatment. This assessment issue awaits careful thought and well-designed empirical study.

**Modifying Physiological Factors Associated with Type A.**    A third major treatment option is based on the notion that the psychosocial pattern we call Type A should in itself be considered not a very important coronary risk factor but only a behavioral concomitant of the "real" risk factor, namely, chronically elevated levels of certain catecholamines, such as epinephrine and norepinephrine (Goldband, Katkin, & Morell, 1979; Krantz & Manuck, 1984). This notion suggests a radical departure from current treatment approaches to reducing Type A coronary risk. It suggests the possible efficacy of a strictly pharmacological intervention to reduce the impact of chronically excessive sympathetic arousal on the heart.

Considering the resources in time and qualified professional personnel needed to modify Type A behavior through cognitive–behavioral means, a simple drug regimen such as beta-blocker treatment (Frishman, 1984; Opie, 1983) to reduce the risk associated with coronary-prone behaviors may seem to some investigators to be an attractive alternative. There is some evidence that beta-blockers are effective in reducing recurrence rates in the first year after an infarction (Beta-blocker Heart Attack Trial Research Group, 1982; Norwegian Multicenter Study Group, 1981; Pedersen, 1985). In fact, a recent survey shows that as many as half of all coronary patients in the United States may have beta-blockers prescribed for them at one time or another after suffering an infarction (Koch, 1983). There is also some preliminary evidence that beta-blockers may reduce Type A behavior (Krantz, Durel, et al., 1982; Schmieder, Freidrich, Neus, Rüddel, & von Eiff, 1983).

There are, however, at least two drawbacks to beta-blocker treatment as an alternative to Type A behavior modification. First, patients taking beta-blockers often report various side effects, including fatigue, depression, anxiety, reduced sexual desire, and impaired sexual functioning (Beta-blocker Heart Attack Trial Research Group, 1982; Frishman, 1984; Paykel, Fleminger, & Watson, 1982). Second, there is no research indicating that beta-blocker treatment reduces coronary recurrence rates if initiated after the first year following a heart attack (Frishman, Furberg, & Friedewald, 1984; Turi & Braunwald, 1983). On the other hand, evidence does indicate that coronary recurrence rates can be reduced by up to 50 percent in patients who modify their Type A behavior beginning 6 months to *several years* after suffering an infarction (M. Friedman et al., 1986). Moreover, there are no known physical side effects, such as sexual dysfunction or fatigue, associated with Type A modification programs.

## Patients at Risk

From a clinical standpoint the people who should have highest priority for receiving Type A treatment are those who are most likely to suffer the devastating consequences of the Type A behavior pattern. Heading this list are people who are at risk for a myocardial infarction, including people who have already experienced one or more infarctions and people who have not yet had an infarction but possess multiple coronary risk factors (e.g., cigarette smoking, positive family history of coronary disease, elevated levels of serum cholesterol, and elevated blood pressure).

Modifying Type A behavior in high-risk populations meets two clinical goals. First, it offers maximum therapeutic benefit (i.e., a subsequent infarction may be averted). Second, it provides treatment to persons who feel the need for treatment (i.e., high-risk populations may be strongly motivated to change their Type A behavior). It also helps us meet our research goal of learning more about the exact relationship between Type A behavior and CHD. Because of the relatively high rates of heart attacks in these populations, CHD and other coronary indices are appropriate dependent variables in these treatment studies.

Within the coronary population, there are two subgroups that may benefit more than others from Type A behavior modification, according to post hoc analyses of RCPP data (Powell, Thoresen, & Friedman, 1985). Ironically, the first subgroup is composed of the same patients who are most likely to drop out of a Type A treatment program, namely, Type A individuals who at entry score very high on hostility and very low on social support. It could be that the high level of hostility exhibited by these patients has alienated their families, friends, and colleagues, thereby isolating the patients from their ordinary sources of social support. In this context, the group experiences may offer an opportunity for more meaningful relationships than these patients have experienced for many years (Price & Friedman, 1986). On the other hand, the group experience generally forces these patients to recognize their Type A behavior as a strongly defended coping style, and it confronts them—both didactically and experientially—with the inappropriateness of their behavior. Thus confronted, patients may have to make a decision between (1) dropping out of the treatment group in order to maintain their Type A behavior and (2) staying in the group in order to get needed help in changing their behavior pattern. Obviously, if these patients stand to benefit the most from a Type A behavior modification program, then we would do well to try to find effective ways to keep them in treatment.

The other subgroup that fared best in the RCPP was composed of patients who had low Peel indexes at entry* (Peel, Semple, Wong, Lancaster, & Kahl, 1962). That is, patients with mild or moderate coronary disease who modified their Type A behavior had the lowest recurrence rates. By contrast, patients with high Peel indexes at entry did not achieve lower recurrence rates even if they succeeded in reducing their Type A behavior. Thus it appears that the severity of a heart attack (e.g., the amount of structural damage to the heart) may override the cardiovascular health benefits to be gained from modifying Type A behavior.

According the RCPP results, then, it appears that Type A behavior modification may produce its maximum therapeutic benefits in coronary patients

---

*The Peel Index (Peel et al., 1962) consists of physical indices of the severity of myocardial infarction, including shock, complex arrhythmias, congestive heart failure, cardiomegaly, and the appearance of new Q waves. It is calculated at the time the infarction occurs. A low Peel index (8 or below) is associated with a low risk of recurrent infarction. A high Peel index (9 or over) is associated with a high risk of recurrence.

who are mildly or moderately ill, exhibit a lot of hostility, and have very little social support.

## Patients in Distress

Clinical intervention with large numbers of Type A patients indicates that Type A behavior is often associated with chronic mental agitation, family and other interpersonal problems, and difficulties on the job. Research by Burke and Bradshaw (1981), Jamal (1985), and others (Burke, Weir, & DuWors, 1979; Haynes, Levine, Scotch, Feinleib, & Kannel, 1978; Houston & Kelly, 1987; Keegan, Sinha, Merriman, & Shipley, 1979) corroborates these clinical findings. Thus both coronary and healthy individuals whose Type A behavior is associated with significant subjective distress or significant social or occupational impairment may constitute a second population that could benefit substantially from Type A modification. Treating Type A behavior in such populations has considerable face validity for mental health professionals, because subjective distress and impairment in social or occupational functioning are the two basic criteria of mental and emotional disorders in the United States (American Psychiatric Association, 1980). Moreover, patients in distress may also be more highly motivated to change their behavior pattern than persons who are unaware of any deleterious effects of the pattern. For instance, a person whose spouse is threatening divorce because of the negative impact of his or her Type A behavior on the family, or someone whose job security is threatened because of an impatient and irritable way of interacting with colleagues or clients, or an individual who cannot obtain a good night's rest because of chronic mental turmoil may be an ideal candidate to respond to and benefit from Type A behavior modification. Working with this client population would give us an opportunity to substantiate or refute claims that altering Type A behavior results in a substantial improvement in the quality of life.

The second drawback is that there may be long-term negative consequences from intervening pharmacologically to alter the body's own homeostatic regulatory mechanisms (Bateson, 1972). One can make a case for the desirability of chemically altering physical functioning in the face of imminent catastrophic consequences, such as a fatal infarction. But it is more difficult to make a case for long-term pharmacological intervention to reduce the impact of dangerously high levels of catecholamines, if another option such as Type A behavior modification is available that can eliminate the need for such elevated levels of catecholamines. This line of thinking is based on the notion that elevated hormone levels may be a "normal," or at least an appropriate, response to the chronic stress and strain to which Type A's expose themselves daily because of their hard-driving approach to life. Thus if we reduce the impact of chronically elevated levels of norepinephrine and other substances by pharmacological manipulations without inquiring into the person's circumstances to see what makes these so-called abnormally high values necessary, we may not be solving the most important problems in a patient's life that predispose him (or her) to CHD. Worse, we may be creating a new set of problems, including the unpleasant physical and psychological side effects previously mentioned, as well as disturbances in the body's homeostatic mechanisms. Type A behavior modification, by altering the person's life circumstances and cognitive and behavioral habits in ways that alleviate the need for elevated levels of norepinephrine, may be able to demonstrate reductions in catecholamines and other neurohormones without having to resort to pharmacological treatment. Comparisons of drug treatment, cognitive–behavior modification, and combinations of these two treatments will be needed to answer questions about preferred treatment methodologies.

## Small-Scale Studies

The kinds of studies suggested so far, which would compare different approaches to reducing Type A behavior and its associated coronary risk, imply the need for large-scale group comparisons and long-term follow-ups. In most instances, elaborate and sophisticated medical assessment and extensive economic resources are also needed. Thus many investigators interested in treating Type A behavior may find it difficult to conduct such research.

Quasi-experimental designs of the type described by Campbell and Stanley (1963) could provide an alternative approach for investigators who want to do Type A treatment research but who have very limited resources of time or money or limited access to large numbers of subjects or sophisticated medical assessment. These quasi-experimental designs generally involve smaller numbers of subjects and more modest goals. Because quasi-experimental research is usually exploratory in nature, it is especially useful in the early phases of a research program when hypothesis generation is as important as hypothesis testing. Time series design is an example of a quasi-experimental design that can provide a less ambitious and more intimate approach than large-scale group designs for examining the dynamics of the Type A behavior pattern in individuals subjected to Type A treatment. Briefly, a time series design involves taking several repeated measures of the dependent variables (e.g., Type A behavior or a single component of Type A behavior) before and after each new independent variable (e.g., each new phase of treatment) is introduced.

Naturally, the results of such studies need to be regarded with caution because of the lack of true experimental control. Nonetheless, their value would be substantial if they generate promising hypotheses that could later be tested using more rigorous methodology and if they provide research opportunities for investigators who are otherwise unable to study Type A behavior because more optimal experimental conditions and more elaborate designs are impractical or impossible.

## POPULATIONS TO TREAT

The important question of whom to treat involves both research and clinical issues. The research issues revolve around the question of what we hope to learn. What populations will teach us more about the nature of Type A behavior? About how it is learned? About how it confers coronary risk? About how to modify Type A behavior most effectively and efficiently? About how to reduce the coronary risk associated with it? The clinical issues revolve around the question of whom we can best serve. What populations would benefit the most from the modification of their Type A behavior? What populations would be likely to submit to Type A treatment?

### Young People

The possibility of primary prevention of Type A behavior and CHD suggests a third general population, namely, young people, including adolescents, young adults in college, and recent high school and college graduates who are beginning their adult careers. The available research indicates that Type A behavior is already prevalent in this population (Eagleston et al., in press; Hunter et al., 1982; Matthews, 1978; Matthews & Angulo, 1980; Smith, Gerace, Christakis, & Kafatos, 1985; Spiga, 1986; Thoresen & Pattillo, Chapter 6, this volume). It may be, however, that the behavior pattern is not as firmly entrenched in these groups as in older populations whose Type A behavior has been reinforced for many more years. Researchers might expect, therefore, that the pattern would be easier to change and that effective treatment protocols could include preventive as well as remedial components.

On a cautionary note, it may be that some of the aspects of the Type A pattern that are deleterious in adults may be age appropriate in younger populations. For example, excessive self-centeredness, or self-absorption, seems to characterize adult Type A's (see Scherwitz & Canick, Chapter 7, this volume), often blinding them to the needs of others and to the effects of their actions on others. Yet a certain degree of self-centeredness may be necessary in adolescents and young adults who are trying to establish their sense of identity and independence. Even if certain aspects of Type A behavior are developmentally appropriate at younger ages, however, the opportunity to provide Type A counseling to younger populations seems promising. Certainly, the difficulty in changing the Type A behavior pattern once it becomes a way of life and the devastating nature of its effects on physical, mental, and interpersonal well-being suggest that the earlier it is treated the less difficult and more successful the treatment may be and the more far-reaching its therapeutic effects.

A drawback of treatment studies that attempt to modify Type A behavior in young people is the inability of these studies to provide immediate information about the effects of such modification on coronary disease rates. Because of the typically low rates of CHD in young people (American Heart Association, 1986), very large-scale longitudinal studies will be required to find out whether modifying Type A behavior in this population has the long-term effect of reducing their rates of CHD. Of course, the vast array of biophysiological and psychosocial variables that influence the development of CHD and that could intervene in the years between Type A treatment and clinical CHD may nullify the prophylactic effects of reducing Type A behavior. If, on the other hand, CHD rates at middle age are found to be significantly lower in groups that received Type A treatment as young adults than in control groups that did not receive such treatment, then the power of Type A behavior modification as a prophylaxis against coronary disease would be dramatically demonstrated. Despite possible drawbacks, large-scale longitudinal studies of this nature also provide us with excellent opportunities to learn more about the durability of reductions in Type A behavior and about the ease or difficulty of modifying the behavior pattern early in life.

## Leaders in Society

If the ultimate goal of Type A research is to find ways to reduce the incidence of CHD, then one way may be to discourage the development of Type A behavior. Almost certainly, this would require rather pervasive changes in how Type A behavior is viewed in our society. Currently, a large segment of the population in the United States and elsewhere views the behavior pattern as an essential ingredient in academic and vocational success. To engineer social changes—changes similar in scope to increasing public awareness of the value of physical fitness, dietary discipline, and smoking cessation—perhaps we need to focus our treatment efforts on populations that can have a substantial impact on others, such as leaders of industry and government, teachers, and parents. If successful, such treatment programs might in time have some impact on the socialization process that currently promotes rather than discourages Type A behavior (Price, 1982). If leaders who exhibit Type A behavior discover through personal experience that they can modify their Type A behavior without suffering negative effects on the job, they might become convinced that Type A behavior is more of an anchor than a propeller in job success (Friedman & Ulmer, 1984).

In order to convince the leaders of society that reductions in Type A behavior benefit rather than handicap persons in vocational and personal pursuits, we need to provide convincing empirical evidence to that effect by conducting pre- and posttreatment evaluations of subjects' levels of productivity, leadership effectiveness, and other qualities thought to promote occupational success. A wealth of anecdotal evidence from the RCPP suggests that modifying Type A behavior enhances rather than detracts from vocational success. In the USAWC study, classmate-observers of participants in the Type A treatment program filled out confidential questionnaires that included questions about the possible effects of the Type A program on the leadership qualities of participants. Although significant reductions had occurred in participants' Type A behavior, observers reported believing that the Type A counseling program had not had any adverse effects on the military leadership qualities of participating officers (Gill et al., 1985).

Because of the general fear that reductions in Type A behavior might result in reduced productivity, we need to give much more attention to dependent variables related to job effectiveness in future Type A modification studies.

## What Is the Most Appropriate Context for Treatment?

Related to the question of what population to treat is the issue of what context, or milieu, the treatment should occur in. For instance, what is the relative effectiveness of providing Type A behavior modification to individuals in the one-on-one context typical of most psychotherapy versus a group context? Because all the treatment studies to date have used group formats, no empirical data exist on this issue. Experience in the RCPP and USAWC studies, however, indicates that the power of the group to facilitate change in the Type A behavior pattern is immense. This influence seems to occur mainly through social modeling, group support, and peer pressure. Moreover, there are some features of the Type A pattern that make Type A's particularly resistant to change in a one-on-one situation. These clinically observable features include tendencies to be argumentative, combative, wary, suspicious, defensive, resistant to perceived interpersonal control, and often unusually naive psychologically.

A related issue is whether persons trying to change their Type A behavior can be more effectively treated in intact social groups (e.g., in couples or families) or intact occupational groups (e.g., at the place of business), or whether modification of Type A is enhanced by treating persons outside the context of their daily social and occupational experience. Experimental work is needed to answer these questions. Clinical experience leads the author to believe that Type A treatment may be more effective in intact social or occupational groups, largely because group members who have contact with each other on a regular basis outside the group setting have more opportunities to reinforce each other's progress in modifying Type A behavior. There seem to be only two disadvantages to this way of treating Type A behavior: Participants may feel reluctant to reveal personal information in front of coworkers or family members, and members of intact occupational groups tend to support each other's rationalizations about why Type A behavior is "absolutely required" in their particular, unique milieu. In balance, the clinical experience we have had so far indicates that the advantages of intact groups outweigh the disadvantages.

## EVALUATING TREATMENT

No matter how Type A behavior is conceptualized, what populations are treated, or which specific treatment approaches are used to modify the Type A behavior pattern, the most serious limitations on what can be learned from treatment studies are imposed by the present difficulties in measuring Type A behavior. Some of the problems in Type A assessment stem from conceptual problems about exactly what Type A behavior is (McLellarn, Bornstein, & Carmody, 1986). In other words, what is it we are trying to measure? Other problems may result from insufficient knowledge about psychometrics on the part of researchers who developed the early Type A instruments (O'Looney & Harding, 1985). Careful analyses of the conceptual and methodological problems associated with Type A diagnosis and assessment can be found in several excellent reviews (Byrne, Rosenman, Schiller, & Chesney, 1985; Jenkins, 1978; Matthews, 1982; McLellarn et al., 1986; O'Looney & Harding, 1985; Scherwitz, Chapter 3, this volume).

But assessment problems do not end with difficulties in measuring global Type A. Identifying or developing appropriate tools to measure changes in Type A components, such as hostility and time urgency, is needed, too. Problems in deciding about appropriate physiological measures and difficulties involved in obtaining reliable data on these variables further compound the assessment problem in treatment research. Decisions also need to be made about including standardized psychological instruments in Type A treatment evaluation. These decisions will determine how much we can learn about possible concomitant changes that occur in other psychosocial variables, such as depression or anxiety. They will also influence our ability to understand relationships between Type A behavior and other clinically relevant psychological problems. Assessment issues require researchers' careful attention if future treatment research is to be fruitful.

### Reductions in Global Type A Behavior

If we are seeking information about possible reductions in coronary risk that result from Type A treatment programs, then well-validated measures of Type A behavior *must* be part of the assessment. Within this constraint, we should select instruments that are as sensitive as possible to *changes* in Type A behavior. For example, the SI and the VSI are both validated measures of Type A behavior, yet the VSI with its continuous scoring system (0–114) (Friedman & Powell, 1984) allows researchers to detect more subtle changes in Type A behavior than can be detected using the SI with its broad categorical scoring system of A1, A2, X, and B (Rosenman, 1978). Thus the VSI may be the best instrument available for treatment intervention research.

What about using one of the other two prospectively validated Type A measures, the JAS or the FTAS, to assess global changes in Type A behavior? First, evidence is accumulating in favor of abandoning these two questionnaires as primary measures of Type A because of their poor psychometric qualities, including excessively low reliability coefficients (e.g., O'Looney & Harding, 1985). Second, neither instrument was designed to measure *changes* in Type A behavior. For instance, the JAS includes historical items (e.g., "How was your temper when you were younger?") that would not be expected to change as a result of treatment. Third, the JAS does not actually measure Type A *behavior*, but rather it measures certain Type A attitudes and dispositions (Jenkins, Zyzanski, & Rosenman, 1979). Thus if we want to assess possible changes in subjects' awareness of certain Type A *attitudes*, then the JAS can be included as one of the dependent measures (but not the only measure) in treatment studies. Fourth, as for the FTAS, its brevity prohibits it use as a comprehensive measure of changes in Type A behavior. Such a short scale—it contains only 10 items (Haynes, Levine, Scotch, Feinleib, & Kannel, 1978; Haynes, Feinleib, Levine, Scotch, & Kannel, 1978)—is too insensitive to capture the wide range of possible changes in Type A behavior that might occur as a result of treatment. Therefore, if data on actual reductions in coronary risk are sought, the measures that best assess that risk, namely, the SI or the VSI, should be used. At present, then, the interview method of assessment seems to hold the most promise as a predictor of the coronary risk associated with Type A (Matthews & Haynes, 1986). But the picture remains complicated and confusing, because there are at least two different versions of the interview, including the Structured Interview (SI) (Chesney, Eagleston, & Rosenman, 1980; Rosenman, 1978) and a Videotaped Structured Interview (VSI) (M. Friedman, Thoresen, & Gill, 1981). There are also several different scoring systems for the interviews (e.g., Dembroski & MacDougall, 1983; M. Friedman et al., 1981). A similar problem exists with the JAS: Different versions and different scoring systems are used by different researchers (O'Looney & Harding, 1985).

None of the present Type A measures provides a completely adequate assessment of Type A behavior for purposes of treatment research. Further, because the Type A behavior pattern is assessed in so many different ways, it is often difficult to interpret research findings. For example, one treatment study might measure Type A using the VSI while another might use the FTAS or a version of the JAS, making comparisons across research studies very difficult. The research community studying Type A behavior would welcome progress in this critical area. In the meantime, there is an urgent need to establish more standardized procedures for assessing the effects of Type A treatment programs so that the results of different studies can be compared. Until we reach more general agreement on how to assess the Type A behavior pattern, the use of a battery of selected Type A instruments (including the best-validated instruments) would be a way of improving the comparability of treatment studies.

## Changes in Specific Components of Type A

Knowing which specific aspects of the behavior pattern have changed as a result of treatment would be especially useful in trying to pinpoint what it is about Type A behavior that makes it a coronary risk factor. If, as happened in the RCPP, significant reductions occur in both Type A behavior and rates of infarction, then being able to identify exactly what cognitive, behavioral, or physiological changes occurred would give us new insights into what is pathogenic about Type A. We also need to learn more about how to measure the individual components of the Type A behavior pattern, including hostility, time urgency, competitiveness, low self-esteem, certain Type A beliefs (e.g., the belief suggested by Price, 1982, that one must constantly *prove* his or her worth), and so on. In addition to the standard, validated Type A instruments that are presently in use, new instruments will need to be developed to measure the attributes of Type A that are not currently assessed by existing measures.

A word of caution may be needed. A perusal of the Type A literature over the past decade reveals the fact that a wide array of psychological instruments of questionable validity and reliability have been used to measure a number of Type A constructs that seem to be poorly understood by investigators conducting the studies. This lack of understanding may be the result of not having had any clinical contact with Type A patients, but relying instead only on published descriptions of the Type A behavior pattern. If we hope to see progress in the field of Type A research, it will be essential to use greater care in selecting the methods by which we attempt to measure Type A characteristics. And it will be necessary to achieve a better understanding of the particular Type A construct that is of interest to us. For example, if we wish to draw conclusions about the relationship of self-esteem to Type A behavior, we need to be as clear as possible about the specific nature of the self-esteem problems experienced by Type A's. Conducting clinical trials is one way to gain this more thorough understanding.

As long as Type A research was limited mainly to epidemiological studies, there was less need than there is now for comprehensive measures of the Type A behavior pattern. But now that Type A intervention studies are being conducted, it is useful to know exactly what changes occur as a result of treatment. The interview is inadequate to provide a complete answer to this question. Despite its predictive validity with respect to CHD, it does not seem to be sensitive enough to detect all the psychologically significant changes that occur as a consequence of treatment. Behaviorally anchored measures of the various components of Type A and direct observation of subjects in their natural settings could correct this problem in future treatment studies.

## Physiological Changes

In Type A treatment studies with coronary patients, we need to assess rates of fatal and nonfatal coronary recurrences, as was done in the RCPP. In treatment studies with healthy subjects we should attempt, whenever possible, to conduct sufficiently long-term follow-up studies to be able to compare coronary incidence rates in subjects who reduced their Type A behavior and subjects who did not. Other indicators of coronary disease could also be used, such as angina, and when practical, the degree of coronary atherosclerosis. Measuring reductions in catecholamines and other stress-related hormones may throw light on physiological processes that could link Type A behavior to CHD. One approach would be to monitor neuroendocrine functioning before, during, and after Type A treatment to determine levels of epinephrine and norepinephrine, as well as levels of ACTH, cortisol, and other physiological indicators associated with stress. Theoretically, these measures could help us piece together the puzzle of how Type A behavior leads to CHD. It is usually believed that, until physiological changes resulting from Type A behavior modification are documented, cardiac rehabilitation programs will be unlikely to include Type A behavior modification as part of the standard treatment procedures. The recent Type A modification study by Roskies and her colleagues (1986) reported problems in obtaining valid measures of epinephrine, norepinephrine, and cortisol. If these problems are encountered in other studies, they may prevent us from securing accurate information about these important physiological variables. Ideally, certain standard physiological measures thought to be associated with Type A behavior would be routinely included in treatment studies to provide benchmarks for comparing the results of different studies.

## Psychosocial Variables Other Than Type A

In virtually every Type A treatment study conducted to date, subjects have reported substantial reductions in levels of chronic and excessive mental and emotional distress (e.g., Blumenthal et al., 1980; Gill et al., 1985; Jenni & Wollersheim, 1979; Levenkron et al., 1983; Roskies et al., 1978; Suinn & Bloom, 1978). Some of these data come from well-designed and carefully administered self-report measures and some from inadequately controlled informal evaluations of treatment. These self-reports of reductions in subjective distress need further scientific verification; instruments and methods need to be used that will yield more precise information about exactly what it is that has improved. Considering the negative effects that

Type A behavior seems to have on marriage and family life (e.g., Burke et al., 1979), measures of marital satisfaction and careful assessment of family and other interpersonal relationships would also be useful in informing us about other possible benefits of treatment. The effects of Type A behavior modification on job satisfaction and job effectiveness should also be evaluated. Researchers should probably use a variety of methods of assessment, including direct observation and reports by colleagues and spouses, as well as more traditional self-report measures to document as accurately as possible the impact of Type A treatment on these and other psychosocial variables.

Finally, because the Type A behavior pattern is thought to involve an interaction between the individual and his or her environment, measures should take into account situational factors whenever possible (Smith & Anderson, 1986; Smith & Rhodewalt, in press; Thoresen & Ohman, in press). Unobtrusive measures of subjects' responses in real-life situations need to be recorded. Situational measures are particularly important in view of the common clinical observation that Type A individuals often show extreme situation specificity in certain aspects of their Type A behavior. For example, a person may show impatience in one kind of situation (e.g., waiting to be seated at a restaurant) yet be able to maintain composure in what appear to be similar kinds of situations (e.g., waiting in line at a supermarket or bank). Even more dramatic is the observation that Type A individuals who appear calm and composed in the treatment setting— even when provoked—are often described by their spouses as raging tyrants at home. Hypotheses about situational influences on the Type A behavior pattern need to be explored in order to discover what lies behind these intriguing accounts of situation-specific variations in Type A behavior.

## NEED FOR DEFINING THE TYPE B BEHAVIOR PATTERN

The goal of Type A treatment is to reduce Type A behavior. This goal is operationally defined as lower scores after treatment than before treatment on a validated measure of Type A, such as the SI or the VSI. How does this operational definition of the treatment outcome translate into clinical goals for participants who are trying to modify their Type A behavior pattern? Is it enough for people to know what *not* to do? Or do treatment goals also need to specify the Type B behaviors we expect participants to demonstrate?

The idea of trying to define Type B behavior may strike terror in the hearts of researchers who have seen all the problems in describing *Type A* behavior over the past 25 years, many of which still remain unresolved. But now that more treatment studies are getting underway, there are important reasons for defining Type B. These reasons are based in part on the principles of learning theory and behavior change and in part on the particular nature of the Type A behavior pattern.

## Facilitating the Process of Change

In designing a behavior change program based on learning principles, one of the first steps is to define the goals of the treatment (Bandura, 1969). What behaviors do we expect participants to demonstrate by the end of treatment? Stating the goals in specific behavioral terms gives us the needed perspective for evaluating how well the treatment is achieving the desired outcome. The next step is to design a treatment protocol that makes it possible for patients to progress systematically toward the achievement of the treatment goals. The third step is to ensure that participants have some guidelines for evaluating their progress as they move through the program. Participants' observation of specific changes in their Type A behavior can allay the inevitable concerns they have about their ability to modify their Type A behavior. Without this needed encouragement, the impatience and self-discouraging thoughts that characterize Type A's in the face of uncertainty and ambiguity can undermine their willingness to practice new behaviors and the commitment they need to achieve lasting behavioral change. In the absence of concrete information about their progress, the propensity of Type A's to notice the negative ("How poorly I'm doing!") instead of the positive ("How well I'm doing!") compromises their ability to persist in changing their behavior pattern.

Thus the process of change may be facilitated by explicitly stating the treatment goals, providing step-by-step procedures for attaining those goals, and giving systematic feedback to individuals about their progress.

## Shifting the Focus of Type A's from Negative to Positive

One of the pervasive features of the Type A behavior pattern is a tendency to be motivated largely by negative rather than positive goals. In other words, the avoidance or alleviation of negative consequences seems to be a much more powerful motivator of behavior for Type A's than the achievement of positive consequences.

The excessive use of negative motivation by Type A's became apparent clinically very early in the RCPP treatment program (e.g., L. Thompson, personal communication, Dec. 12, 1978). For example, the chronic and excessive hard-driving behavior of Type A's to meet perfectionistic standards (i.e., to be perfect) seems to be motivated by a desire to avoid or alleviate the anxiety and guilt they feel when they are not perfect. Recall the earlier suggestion in this chapter that the cognitive underpinnings of Type A behavior are the belief that "I'm not good enough yet" coupled with the belief that "I *will* be good enough if I just keep trying harder and doing more." Striving to be okay (i.e., to be perfect, and, therefore, beyond reproach) often translates into working continuously and without adequate relaxation. After all, no one can fault a person for failing to achieve more if the person is already working all the time. Thus hard-driving behavior seems to be, in part, a ploy of Type A's to avoid negative self-appraisal and the negative criticism anticipated from others. Ironically, the attempts of Type A's to avoid or alleviate these negative consequences can eventually result in their exposure to even more serious negative consequences, such as poor health and the deterioration of family relationships.

The excessively competitive behavior of Type A's is another example of a Type A characteristic whose primary goal seems to be the avoidance of negative consequences. For example, when Type A's participate in competitive games, the importance of winning seems to be strongly motivated by a need to avoid feeling or appearing inferior compared to others. For Type A's, the satisfaction of winning is almost never as prominent as the intense dissatisfaction, self-criticism, and hostility that almost always accompanies losing.

The hypervigilance (M. Friedman & Rosenman, 1959) and the wariness, suspiciousness, and cynicism (Williams, 1984) said to characterize the Type A behavior pattern appear to be further examples of negatively motivated habits of Type A's. In these cases the goal seems to be the avoidance of being caught off guard by "bad surprises."

Two other clinical facts provide support for the notion that Type A behavior is a negatively motivated pattern. First, as participants in the RCPP modified their Type A behavior, their attention began to focus more on the pursuit of positive consequences than on the avoidance of negative consequences. Early in treatment their only concern was to avoid heart attacks and death. Yet it was not at all unusual in the later phases of treatment to hear anecdotal reports from participants about how much the Type A modification program was improving their lives. The following quote from a 38-year-old businessman participating in Type A group treatment is representative of these reports:

> Even if treating Type A behavior doesn't prevent coronaries, this program has improved the quality of my life. It's an inner feeling—things are better. The bottom line is: So what if it's not true? I am doing more business, with less stress, and I am a more loving, understanding person. The fact is my life has improved 100 percent. (Fischman, 1987, p. 50)

Second, when participants in the RCPP and USAWC studies began to make headway in modifying their Type A behavior, they also began to notice and mention the conspicuous absence of a systematic view of Type B behavior. In fact, their persistent requests for a better definition of Type B prompted the development of the working model of Type B behavior presented later in this chapter.

If, indeed, Type A is a pattern of behavior that is impelled largely by a desire to avoid or alleviate negative consequences, then we need to take this fact into account in designing and describing the treatment. A Type A treatment program that states the goal of the program in negative terms (i.e., to become less Type A) and highlights the possible negative consequences of failing to achieve this goal (e.g., CHD, death, job failure or stagnation, family disintegration, mental turmoil) is based in the same negative conceptual framework as the behavior pattern it is attempting to modify. Under these circumstances, patients' efforts to modify their Type A behavior may simply be one more example of a negatively motivated project in their lives. Perhaps treatment goals should "accentuate the positive" as a way of modeling the needed change of base in thinking. Thus the goal could be "to become more Type B" instead of "to become less Type A." The positive consequences sought could include achieving and maintaining health and vigor, attaining a more secure sense of professional and personal success, improving family relationships, and experiencing more contentment. These goals, whether explicitly stated or not, were reached by many of the RCPP and USAWC participants who modified their Type A behavior. Indeed, this author's clinical impression is that participants whose goal was to become more Type B were more successful in changing their Type A behavior than those whose goal was to become less Type A.

## Applying the Notion of Counterconditioning

Research on behavior change has shown that reducing or eliminating a *negative* behavior or thought will succeed more readily if a person replaces it with an incompatible *positive* behavior or thought than if a person simply tries to abstain from the negative behavior (Karoly & Kanfer, 1982). A well-known example is systematic desensitization in the treatment of phobias (Wolpe, 1969). This procedure can be viewed as a counterconditioning process, in which the subject replaces a maladaptive response to a stimulus with an adaptive response that is incompatible with the maladaptive one. In the case of reducing phobias, a person is taught to remain relaxed in response to successively threatening presentations of the phobic stimulus. Because it is impossible for a person to be relaxed and fearful at the same time, inducing and maintaining a state of relaxation in the face of a feared object systematically extinguishes the fear response. In the case of reducing Type A behavior, if a person makes a Type B response (e.g., is calm, unhurried, and friendly), it is difficult for him or her to exhibit a Type A response (e.g., be upset, hurried, and hostile) at the same time. Responding with Type B behavior to situations that generally have elicited Type A behavior should result in the eventual extinction of Type A behavior. To accomplish this goal, we need to be able to tell patients what Type B behavior is.

Clinical experience with hundreds of coronary and noncoronary Type A patients has persuaded this author that one of the greatest obstacles patients encounter in changing their Type A behavior is not knowing what to do instead. Being able to identify the "wrong" behaviors is not equivalent to being able to identify and use the "right" ones. Awareness of Type A behavior does seem to be necessary but may not be sufficient to enable patients to exhibit Type B behavior.

## Learning through Social Modeling

Another reason for defining Type B behavior to patients who are trying to modify their Type A behavior is so that they can recognize Type B behavior when they observe it in their day-to-day lives. Social modeling (Bandura, 1977) plays an important role in learning new behaviors. Put differently, when we see what we are supposed to do, it is easier for us to do it than if we have never seen it done. Type A's need to be exposed repeatedly to Type B's in order to learn how to act more like Type B's.

Learning what the specific features of the Type B behavior pattern are and then observing Type B's at work, at home, and in the community are critical tasks for Type A's for two reasons. The first reason is that Type A's tend to ignore stimuli that are extraneous to accomplishing their goals (Matthews & Brunson, 1979). If the goal of treatment is not to be Type A, then Type A's will do their best to accomplish this task. In the process of doing so, they become very astute at noticing Type A's but not Type B's, because noticing Type B's seems extraneous to their goal. The opportunity to learn through social modeling requires that the learner notice the presence of the model.

The second reason Type A treatment programs need to teach Type B behavior is that being able to recognize Type B's gives patients opportunities to observe rather than simply to speculate about the *antecedents* and especially the *consequences* of Type B. A key determinant of whether people will actually exhibit a behavior they have learned through social modeling is the nature of the consequences they observe occurring to the model when he or she exhibits the behavior in question (Bandura, 1977). If the observed consequences are negative, then there is less likelihood that the observer will subsequently exhibit that behavior than if the observed consequences are positive. Directly observing Type B consequences is an important part of Type A modification, because a main obstacle to modifying Type A behavior seems to be the fears of Type A's about the consequences of exhibiting Type B behavior. These fears stem from the Type A belief that Type A behavior is a necessary ingredient of success, even though preliminary research indicates that Type A's and Type B's generally fare equally well in vocational endeavors (e.g., Gill et al., 1985; Jamal, 1985).

The misperception of Type A's that all their success is due to their Type A behavior is a particularly pernicious belief (M. Friedman, 1979). Even if they are completely aware of the deleterious effects of their Type A behavior on their relationships with family and friends, Type A's are unlikely to make the necessary commitment or the difficult behavioral and cognitive changes involved in becoming more Type B if they perceive it to be a career-threatening change. Type A's need to observe that the actual consequences of Type B behavior (e.g., getting things accomplished without undue stress, receiving genial responses from others, deriving positive self-esteem from handling difficult situations and people in a self-controlled manner) are almost always different from the imagined consequences (e.g., not accomplishing anything, feeling out of control, losing face). Observing Type B models, especially at work, can help Type A's chip away at these fears.

## Why Is There No Definition of Type B?

If a definition of Type B behavior would facilitate changes in Type A behavior, why has it not been done before? The answer lies in the scientific history of the Type A behavior pattern. It was discovered by two cardiologists (M. Friedman & Rosenman, 1959) who were treating patients with CHD. The conceptual definition of Type A grew out of a medical model, or disease model, in which Type A behavior was associated with the absence of health. Being Type A was seen as the equivalent of having high blood pressure or being a cigarette smoker. The goal, as far as treating CHD was concerned, was to eliminate factors associated with the disease.

The introduction of social learning theory into the research on Type A behavior has provided an opportunity for researchers to go beyond just getting rid of a pathogenic behavior pattern. Clinical researchers now have the tools for helping patients not only to eliminate the chronic struggle to do more and more in less and less time, but also to replace this life-style with the behaviors and qualities that promote more of a sense of mental and emotional well-being, physical health, and satisfaction in interpersonal relationships.

## Is Type B More Than the Absence of Type A?

Perhaps the primary research issue related to defining and studying Type B behavior is whether there actually is an identifiable Type B behavior pattern, or, alternatively, whether Type B behavior is simply the absence of Type A behaviors (e.g., Rosenman et al., 1966). One way to compare these two alternative models is to compare two treatment programs that are identical except that one would focus on increasing Type B behavior while the other would use the more traditional approach of reducing Type A behavior. Such a study would not confirm the existence of a Type B behavior pattern. But if treatment effectiveness were enhanced when the Type B model was explicitly used, it would support the notion that the Type B concept is a useful one for clinical intervention. Another way to explore the Type B concept would be to develop a Type B structured interview. If high Type B scores were associated with low rates of CHD (while other risk factors were controlled for), then the utility of the Type B concept would again be demonstrated.

## TABLE 12.1. THE TYPE B BEHAVIOR PATTERN (A WORKING DEFINITION)

### What does Type B _look_ like?

| | |
|---|---|
| Posture: | Relaxed—not "on your mark, get set . . ." |
| Gestures: | Easy—not jerky, forced, or fast<br>Natural—not tense<br>Few to moderate—not distractingly excessive |
| Face: | Relaxed—not tense<br>Friendly—not hostile<br>Mildly to moderately expressive—not excessively animated and no nervous tics |
| Movement: | Gentle and easy—not forced or abrupt<br>Limbs at rest—no repetitive "nervous" movements |
| Overall impression: | At ease—not struggling or discontented |

### What does Type B _sound_ like?

| | |
|---|---|
| Voice: | Easy to listen to—not sharp, excessively emphatic, dysrhythmic, or rapid |
| Speech: | Other-directed—not egocentric |
| Manner: | Patient—doesn't interrupt, talk over, or speech-hurry |

### What does Type B _feel_ like? What are the internal indicators?

| | |
|---|---|
| Mental indicators: | Being at peace with oneself—not excessively self-demanding or critical |
| | A general sense of harmony with the people, events, and circumstances of one's surroundings—not a sense of opposition, wariness, readiness for battle, nor fear, apprehension, dread |
| | Awareness of what is good about a situation—instead of a preoccupation with what is wrong with it |
| | Generally more trusting than wary |
| | Self-encouraging thoughts about being able to handle one's business and personal affairs—not self-discouraging thoughts about one's possible inadequacies |
| Physiological indicators: | Muscles are relaxed—not tense and tight |
| | Breathing is diaphragmatic and effortless—not shallow/upper-chest, or forced or irregular |
| | Naturally energetic—neither "hyper" nor exhausted |

### What is Type B like to _live with_ or _work with_?

| | |
|---|---|
| Mood: | Pleasant mood is pretty dependable—not subject to frequent bouts of hostility, impatience, guilt, remorse, anxiety, depression |

**TABLE 12.1.** (*Continued*)

| | |
|---|---|
| Attention: | Interested in others—not too self-absorbed or easily distracted |
| Attitude: | An accepting attitude about trivial mistakes and others' different ways of doing things; a problem-solving attitude toward big mistakes and major disasters—not contemptuous of imperfection in self or others, nor paralyzed by big problems |
| Reaction to unexpected: | Flexible; handles the unexpected with some equanimity; takes a long-range enough perspective on the present to avoid being overwhelmed by what is happening at the moment |
| Effort: | Matches effort to the task: the amount of effort used is based on how hard the task is and how important it is—everything doesn't get an "all-out effort" |
| Work satisfaction: | Associates a sense of enjoyment and fulfillment with work—not just with the achievement of work goals but also with the process by which the goals are achieved |
| Interactions with others: | A good team member; able to lead and able to let others lead—not chronically dominating, controlling, critical, or judgmental |

## A Working Model of the Type B Behavior Pattern

A working model of Type B behavior is outlined in Table 12.1 for the consideration of researchers who are interested in beginning to define and study the converse of Type A behavior. This working model of Type B is based on three things: (1) a composite picture of Type A "treatment successes" formed by clinical observation, observation of VSI psychomotor responses, participants' self-reports, and reports by participants' spouses and colleagues; (2) behavioral and cognitive factors that seem to be the opposite of what is readily observable in unmodified Type A's; and (3) behaviors and attitudes that appear to keep the fight–flight response from being elicited on a chronic basis. The main purpose of offering a working conceptual definition of Type B is to provide a point of departure for specifying more precisely and more comprehensively the behaviors, cognitive factors, physiological factors, and interpersonal characteristics we expect people to demonstrate at the end of a Type A treatment program. Explicitly defining Type B may help us gear our interventions to achieve these treatment goals and to evaluate more comprehensively whether these changes have occurred.

Finally, it is hoped that empirical research on Type B behavior may also add conceptual clarity to our present, far-from-complete picture of what the Type A behavior pattern really is.

## REFERENCES

American Heart Association (1986). *1987 heart facts*. Dallas: Author.

American Psychiatric Association (1980). *Diagnostic and statistical manual of mental disorders* (3rd ed.). Washington, DC: Author.

Bandura, A. (1969). *Principles of behavior modification*. New York: Holt, Rinehart, & Winston.

Bandura, A. (1977). *Social learning theory*. Englewood Cliffs, NJ: Prentice-Hall.

Barefoot, J. L., Dahlstrom, W. G., & Williams, R. B. (1983). Hostility, CHD incidence, and total mortality: A 25-year follow-up study of 255 physicians. *Psychosomatic Medicine, 45*, 59–63.

Bateson, G. (1972). *Steps to an ecology of mind*. New York: Ballantine.

Bernstein, D. A., & Borkovec, T. D. (1973). *Progressive relaxation training: A manual for the helping professions*. Champaign, IL: Research Press.

Beta-blocker Heart Attack Trial Research Group (1982). A randomized trial of propranolol in patients with acute myocardial infarction: I. Mortality results. *Journal of the American Medical Association, 247*, 1707–1714.

Blumenthal, J. A., Williams, R. S., Williams, R. B., & Wallace, A. G. (1980). Effects of exercise on Type A (coronary-prone) behavior pattern. *Psychosomatic Medicine, 42*, 289–296.

Bortner, R. W. (1969). A short rating scale as a potential measure of Pattern A behavior. *Journal of Chronic Diseases, 22*, 87–91.

Burke, R. J., & Bradshaw, P. (1981). Occupational and life stress and the family. *Small Group Behavior, 12*, 329–375.

Burke, R. J., Weir, T., & DuWors, R. E. (1979). Type A behavior of administrators and wives' reports of marital satisfaction and well-being. *Journal of Applied Psychology, 67*, 57–65.

Byrne, D. G., Rosenman, R. H., Schiller, E., & Chesney, M. A. (1985). Consistency and variation among instruments purporting to measure the Type A behavior pattern. *Psychosomatic Medicine, 47*, 242–261.

Campbell, D. T., & Stanley, J. C. (1963). *Experimental and quasi-experimental designs for research*. Chicago: Rand McNally.

Chesney, M. A., Eagleston, J. R., & Rosenman, R. H. (1980). The Type A Structured Interview: A behavioral assessment in the rough. *Journal of Behavioral Assessment, 2*, 255–272.

Cottier, C., Shapiro, K., & Julius, S. (1984). Treatment of mild hypertension with progressive muscle relaxation: Predictive value of indexes of sympathetic tone. *Archives of Internal Medicine, 144*, 1954–1958.

Dembroski, T. M., & MacDougall, J. M. (1983). Behavioral and psychophysiological perspectives on coronary-prone behavior. In T. M. Dembroski, T. H., Schmidt, & G. Blumchen (Eds.), *Biobehavioral bases of coronary heart disease*. New York: Karger.

Dembroski, T. M., MacDougall, J. M., Shields, J. L., Petitto, J., & Lushene, R. (1978). Components of the Type A coronary-prone behavior pattern and cardiovascular responses to psychomotor performance challenge. *Journal of Behavioral Medicine, 1*, 159–176.

Dembroski, T. M., MacDougall, J. M., Williams, R. B., Haney, T. L., & Blumenthal, J. R. (1985). Components of Type A, hostility, and anger-in: Relationship to angiographic findings. *Psychosomatic Medicine, 47*, 219–233.

Eagleston, J. R., Kirmil-Gray, K., Thoresen, C. E., Wiedenfeld, S. A., Bracke, P., Heft, L., & Arnow, B. (in press). Physical correlates of Type A behavior in children and adolescents. *Journal of Behavioral Medicine.*

Fischman, J. (1987). Type A on trial. *Psychology Today*, February, pp. 42–50.

Friedman, H. S., Hall, J. A., & Harris, M. J. (1985).Type A behavior, nonverbal expressive style, and health. *Journal of Personality and Social Psychology, 48*, 1299–1315.

Friedman, M. (1977). Type A behavior pattern: Some of its pathophysiological components. *Bulletin of the New York Academy of Medicine, 53*, 593–604.

Friedman, M. (1979). The modification of Type A behavior in post-infarction patients. *American Heart Journal, 97*, 551–560.

Friedman, M., & Powell, L. H. (1984). The diagnoses and quantitative assessment of Type A behavior: Introduction and description of the Videotaped Structured Interview. *Integrative Psychiatry, 2*, 123–129.

Friedman, M., & Rosenman, R. H. (1959). Association of specific overt behavior pattern with blood and cardiovascular findings. *Journal of the American Medical Association, 169*, 1286–1296.

Friedman, M., & Rosenman, R. H. (1969). The possible general causes of coronary artery disease. In M. Friedman, *Pathogenesis of coronary artery disease.* New York: McGraw-Hill.

Friedman, M., & Rosenman, R. H. (1974). *Type A behavior and your heart.* Englewood Cliffs, NJ: Knopf.

Friedman, M., Thoresen, C. E., & Gill, J. J. (1981). Type A behavior, its possible role, detection and alteration in patients with ischemic heart disease. In J. W. Hurst (Ed.), *The heart update V.* New York: McGraw-Hill.

Friedman, M., Thoresen, C. E., Gill, J. J., Ulmer, D., Powell, L. H., Price, V. A., Brown, B., Thompson, L., Rabin, D. D., Breall, W. S., Bourg, E., Levy, R., & Dixon, T. (1986). Alteration of Type A behavior and its effect on cardiac recurrences in post myocardial infarction patients: Summary results of the Recurrent Coronary Prevention Project. *American Heart Journal, 112*, 653–665.

Friedman, M., Thoresen, C. E., Gill, J. J., Ulmer, D., Powell, L., Thompson, L., Price, V. A., Elek, S. R., Rabin, D. R., Piaget, G., Dixon, T. R., Bourg, E., Levy, R. A., & Tasto, D. L. (1982). Feasibility of altering Type A behavior pattern in post-myocardial infarction patients. *Circulation, 66*, 83–92.

Friedman, M., & Ulmer, D. (1984). *Treating Type A and your heart.* Englewood Cliffs, NJ: Knopf.

Frishman, W. H. (1984). *Clinical pharmacology of the beta-adrenoceptor blocking drugs* (2nd ed.). Norwalk, CT: Appleton-Century-Crofts.

Frishman, W. H., Furberg, C. D., & Friedewald, W. T. (1984). B-adrenergic blockade for survivors of acute myocardial infarction. *New England Journal of Medicine, 310*, 830–837.

Gill, J. J., Price, V. A., Friedman, M., Thoresen, C. E., Powell, L. H., Ulmer, D., Brown, B., & Drews, F. R. (1985). Reduction in Type A behavior in healthy middle-aged American military officers. *American Heart Journal, 110*, 503–514.

Glass, D. C. (1977). *Behavior patterns, stress, and coronary disease.* Hillsdale, NJ: Erlbaum.

Goldband, S., Katkin, E. S., & Morell, M. A. (1979). Personality and cardiovascular disorder. Steps toward demystification. In C. Spielberger & I. Sarason (Eds.), *Stress and anxiety* (Vol. 6). Washington, DC: Hemisphere.

Haynes, S. G., Feinleib, M., & Kannel, W. B. (1980). The relationship of psychosocial factors to coronary heart disease in the Framingham Study: III. Eight-year incidence of coronary heart disease. *American Journal of Epidemiology, 111*, 37–58.

Haynes, S. G., Feinleib, M., Levine, S., Scotch, N., & Kannel, W. B. (1978). The relationship of psychosocial factors to coronary heart disease in the Framingham Study: II. Prevalence of coronary heart disease. *American Journal of Epidemiology, 107*, 384–402.

Haynes, S., Levine, S., Scotch, N., Feinleib, M., & Kannel, W. B. (1978). The relationship of psychosocial factors to coronary heart disease in the Framingham Study: I. Methods and risk factors. *American Journal of Epidemiology*, *107*, 362–383.

Herd, J. A. (1981). Behavioral factors in the physiological mechanisms of cardiovascular disease. In S. M. Weiss, J. A. Herd, & B. H. Fox (Eds.), *Perspectives on behavioral medicine*. New York: Academic.

Houston, B. K., & Kelly, K. E. (1987). Type A behavior in housewives: Relation to work, marital adjustment, stress, tension, health, fear of failure, and self-esteem. *Journal of Psychosomatic Research*, *31*, 55–61.

Hunter, S., Wolf, T., Sklov, M. C., Webber, L. S., Watson, R. M., & Berenson, G. S. (1982). Type A coronary-prone behavior pattern and cardiovascular risk factor variables in children and adolescents: The Bogalusa Heart Study. *Journal of Chronic Diseases*, *35*, 613–621.

Jamal, M. (1985). Type A behavior and job performance: Some suggestive findings. *Journal of Human Stress*, *11*, 60–68.

Jenkins, C. D. (1978). A comparative review of the interview and questionnaire methods in the assessment of the coronary-prone behavior pattern. In T. M. Dembroski, S. M. Weiss, J. L. Shields, S. G. Haynes, & M. Feinleib (Eds.), *Coronary-prone behavior*. New York: Springer-Verlag.

Jenkins, C. D., Zyzanski, S. J., & Rosenman, R. H. (1971). Progress toward validation of a computer-scored test for the Type A coronary-prone behavior pattern. *Psychosomatic Medicine*, *33*, 193–202.

Jenkins, C. D., Zyzanski, S. J., & Rosenman, R. H. (1979). *Jenkins Activity Survey*. New York: Psychological Corporation.

Jenni, M. A., & Wollersheim, J. P. (1979). Cognitive therapy, stress management training, and the Type A behavior pattern. *Cognitive Therapy & Research*, *3*, 61–73.

Johnston, D. W. (1985). Invited review: Psychological interventions in cardiovascular disease. *Journal of Psychosomatic Research*, *5*, 447–456.

Karoly, P., & Kanfer, F. H. (Eds.). (1982). *Self-management and behavior change: From theory to practice*. New York: Pergamon.

Keegan, D. L., Sinha, B. N., Merriman, J. E., & Shipley, C. (1979). Type A behavior pattern: Relationship to coronary heart disease, personality, and life adjustment. *Canadian Journal of Psychiatry*, *24*, 724–730.

Koch, H. (1983). Drugs most frequently used in office practice, a summary of findings: National ambulatory medical care survey, 1981. *Advancedata*, *89*, 1–11.

Krantz, D. S., & Durel, L. A. (1983). Psychobiological substrates of the Type A behavior pattern. *Health Psychology*, *2*, 393–411.

Krantz, D., Durel, L. A., Davia, J. E., Shaffer, R. T., Arabian, J. M., Dembroski, T. M., & MacDougall, J. M. (1982). Propranolol medication among coronary patients: Relationship to Type A behavior and cardiovascular response. *Journal of Human Stress*, *8*(3), 4–12.

Krantz, D. S., Glass, D. C., Schaeffer, M. A., & Davia, J. E. (1982). Behavior patterns and coronary disease: A critical evaluation. In T. J. Cacioppo & R. E. Petty (Eds.), *Perspectives on cardiovascular physiology*. New York: Guilford.

Krantz, D. S., & Manuck, S. B. (1984). Acute psychophysiologic reactivity and risk of cardiovascular disease: A review and methodological critique. *Psychological Bulletin*, *96*, 435–464.

Levenkron, J. C., Cohen, J. D., Mueller, H. S., & Fisher, E. B., Jr. (1983). Modifying the Type A coronary prone behavior pattern. *Journal of Consulting & Clinical Psychology*, *51*, 192–204.

MacDougall, J. M., Dembroski, T. M., Dimsdale, J. E., & Hackett, T. P. (1985). Components of Type A, hostility, and anger-in: Further relationships to angiographic findings. *Health Psychology*, *4*, 137–152.

Matthews, K. A. (1978). Assessment and developmental antecedents of the Pattern A behavior in children. In T. M. Dembroski, S. M. Weiss, J. L. Shields, S. G. Haynes, & M. Feinleib (Eds.), *Coronary-prone behavior*. New York: Springer-Verlag.

Matthews, K. A. (1982). Psychological perspectives on the Type A behavior pattern. *Psychological Bulletin, 91,* 293–323.

Matthews, K., & Angulo, J. (1980). Measurement of the Type A behavior pattern in children: Assessment of children's competitiveness, impatience–anger, and aggression. *Child Development, 51,* 466–475.

Matthews, K. A., & Brunson, B. I. (1979). Allocation of attention and the Type A coronary-prone behavior pattern. *Journal of Personality & Social Psychology, 37,* 2081–2090.

Matthews, K. A., Glass, D. C., Rosenman, R. H., & Bortner, R. W. (1977). Competitive drive, pattern A, and coronary heart disease: A further analysis of some data from the Western Collaborative Group Study. *Journal of Chronic Diseases, 30,* 489–498.

Matthews, K. A., & Haynes, S. G. (1986). Type A behavior pattern and coronary disease risk: Update and critical evaluation. *American Journal of Epidemiology, 123,* 923–960.

McLellarn, R. W., Bornstein, P. H., & Carmody, T. P. (1986). A methodological critique of the Structured-Interview assessment of Type A behavior. *Journal of Cardiopulmonary Rehabilitation, 6,* 21–25.

Musante, L., MacDougall, J. M., Dembroski, T. M., & Van Horn, A. E. (1983). Component analysis of the Type A coronary-prone behavior pattern in male and female college students. *Journal of Personality & Social Psychology, 45,* 1104–1117.

Norwegian Multicenter Study Group. (1981). Timolol-induced reduction in mortality and reinfarction in patients surviving acute myocardial infarction. *New England Journal of Medicine, 304,* 801–807.

O'Looney, B. A., & Harding, C. M. (1985). A psychometric investigation of two measures of Type A behaviour in a British sample. *Journal of Chronic Diseases, 38,* 841–848.

Opie, L. H. (1983). Basis for cardiovascular therapy with beta-blocking agents. *American Journal of Cardiology, 52,* 2D–9D.

Paffenbarger, R. S., Jr., & Hyde, R. T. (1984). Exercise and the prevention of coronary heart disease. In A. Leon (Ed.), Exercise and health (special issue). *Preventive Medicine, 13,* 3–22.

Paykel, E. S., Fleminger, R., & Watson, J. P. (1982). Psychiatric side effects of antihypertensive drugs other than reserpine. *Journal of Clinical Psychopharmacology, 2,* 14–39.

Pedersen, T. D. (1985). Six-year follow-up of the Norwegian Multicenter Study on timolol after acute myocardial infarction. *New England Journal of Medicine, 313,* 1055–1058.

Peel, A., Semple, T., Wong, I., Lancaster, W. M., & Kahl, J. L. G. (1962). A coronary prognostic index for grading the severity of infarction. *British Heart Journal, 24,* 745–760.

Powell, L. H., Thoresen, C. E., & Friedman, M. (1985). Modification of the Type A behavior pattern after myocardial infarction. In H. Hofmann (Ed.), *Primary and secondary prevention of coronary heart disease.* Berlin-Heidelberg: Springer-Verlag.

Price, V. A. (1982). *Type A behavior pattern: A model for research and practice.* New York: Academic.

Price, V. A., & Friedman, M. (1986). Modifying Type A behavior and reducing coronary recurrence rates. *Proceedings of the 15th European Conference on Psychosomatic Research* (pp. 178–183). London: John Libbey.

Rosenman, R. H. (1978). The interview method of assessment of the coronary-prone behavior pattern. In T. M. Dembroski, S. M. Weiss, J. L. Shields, S. G. Haynes, & M. Feinleib (Eds.), *Coronary-prone behavior*. New York: Springer-Verlag.

Rosenman, R. H., Brand, R. J., Jenkins, C. D., Friedman, M., Straus, R., & Wurm, M. (1975). Coronary heart disease in the Western Collaborative Group Study: Final follow-up experience of 8½ years. *Journal of the American Medical Association, 233,* 872–877.

Rosenman, R. H., Friedman, M., Straus, R., Wurm, M., Jenkins, C. D., Messinger, H. B.,

Kositchek, R., Hahn, W., & Werthessen, N. T. (1966). Coronary heart disease in the Western Collaborative Group Study. *Journal of the American Medical Association, 195,* 86–92.

Roskies, E. (1979). Considerations in developing a treatment program for the coronary-prone (Type A) behavior pattern. In P. Davidson (Ed.), *Behavioral medicine: Changing health life styles.* New York: Brunner/Mazel.

Roskies, E., Kearney, H., Spevack, M., Surkis, A., Cohen, C., & Gilman, S. (1979). Generalizability and durability of treatment effects in an intervention program for coronary-prone (Type A) managers. *Journal of Behavioral Medicine, 2,* 195–207.

Roskies, E., Seraganian, P., Oseasohn, R., Hanley, J. A., Collu, R., Martin, N., & Smilga, C. (1986). The Montreal Type A Intervention Project: Major findings. *Health Psychology, 5,* 45–69.

Roskies, E., Spevack, M., Surkis, A., Cohen, C., & Gilman, S. (1978). Changing the coronary-prone (Type A) behavior pattern in a non-clinical population. *Journal of Behavioral Medicine, 1,* 201–216.

Scherwitz, L., Berton, I., & Leventhal, H. (1977). Type A assessment and interaction in the behavior pattern interview. *Psychosomatic Medicine, 39,* 229–240.

Scherwitz, L., Graham, L. E., Grandits, G., & Billings, J. (1987). Speech characteristics and behavior type assessment in the MRFIT structured interview. *Journal of Behavioral Medicine, 10,* 173–195.

Scherwitz, L., Graham, L. E., Grandits, K. G., Buehler, J., & Billings, J. (1986). Self-involvement and coronary heart disease incidence in the Multiple Risk Factor Intervention Trial. *Psychosomatic Medicine, 48,* 187–199.

Schmieder, R., Friedrich, G., Neus, H., Rüddel, H., & von Eiff, A. W. (1983). The influence of beta-blockers on cardiovascular reactivity and Type A behavior pattern in hypertensives. *Psychosomatic Medicine, 45,* 417–423.

Schucker, B., & Jacobs, E. R., Jr. (1977). Assessment of behavioral risk for coronary disease by voice characteristics. *Psychosomatic Medicine, 39,* 219–228.

Shekelle, R. B., Gale, M., Ostfeld, A. M., & Paul, O. (1983). Hostility, risk of CHD, and mortality. *Psychosomatic Medicine, 45,* 109–114.

Smith, J. C., Gerace, T. A., Christakis, G., & Kafatos, A. (1985). Cross-cultural validity of the Miami Structured Interview—1 for Type A in children: The American-Hellenic Heart Study. *Journal of Chronic Diseases, 38,* 793–799.

Smith, T. W., & Anderson, N. B. (1986). Models of personality and disease: An interactional approach to Type A behavior and cardiovascular risk. *Journal of Personality & Social Psychology, 50,* 1166–1173.

Smith, T. W., & Rhodewalt, F. (in press). On states, traits, and processes: A transactional alternative to the individual difference assumptions in Type A behavior and physiological reactivity. *Journal of Research in Personality.*

Spiga, R. (1986). Social interaction and cardiovascular response of boys exhibiting the coronary-prone behavior pattern. *Journal of Pediatric Psychology, 11,* 59–69.

Suinn, R. M. (1975). The cardiac stress management program for Type A patients. *Cardiac Rehabilitation, 5,* 13–15.

Suinn, R. M., & Bloom, L. J. (1978). Anxiety management program for pattern A behavior. *Journal of Behavioral Medicine, 1,* 25–35.

Suinn, R. M. (1980). Pattern A behaviors and heart disease: Intervention approaches. In J. M. Ferguson & C. B. Taylor (Eds.), *Comprehensive handbook of behavioral medicine: Volume I. Systems intervention.* Jamaica, NY: SP Medical and Scientific Books.

Thoresen, C. E., Friedman, M., Gill, J. J., & Ulmer, D. K. (1982). The Recurrent Coronary Prevention Project. Some preliminary findings. *Acta Medica Scandinavia, 660* (Suppl.), 172–192.

Thoresen, C. E., Friedman, M., Powell, L. H., Gill, J. J., & Ulmer, D. (1985). Altering the Type A behavior pattern in postinfarction patients. *Journal of Cardiopulmonary Rehabilitation, 5*, 258–266.

Thoresen, C. E., & Ohman, A. (in press). The Type A behavior pattern: A person-environment interaction perspective. In D. Magnusson & A. Ohman (Eds.), *Psychopathology: An interaction perspective*. New York: Academic.

Thoresen, C. E., Telch, M. J., & Eagleston, J. R. (1981). Approaches to altering the Type A behavior pattern. *Psychosomatics, 22*, 472–479.

Turi, Z. G., & Braunwald, E. (1983). The use of b-blockers after myocardial infarction. *Journal of the American Medical Association, 249*, 2512–2516.

Williams, R. B., Jr. (1978). Psychophysiological processes, the coronary-prone behavior pattern, and coronary heart disease. In T. M. Dembroski, S. M. Weiss, J. L. Shields, S. G. Haynes, & M. Feinleib (Eds.), *Coronary-prone behavior*. New York: Springer-Verlag.

Williams, R. B., Jr. (1984). An untrusting heart. *The Sciences, 5*(7), 31–36.

Williams, R. B., Barefoot, J. C., & Shekelle, R. B. (1984). The health consequences of hostility. In M. A. Chesney, S. E. Goldston, & R. H. Rosenman (Eds.), *Anger, hostility, and behavioral medicine*. New York: Hemisphere/McGraw-Hill.

Williams, R. B., Jr., Haney, T. L., Lee, K. L., Kong, Y. H., Blumenthal, J. A., & Whalen, R. E. (1980). Type A behavior, hostility, and coronary atherosclerosis. *Psychosomatic Medicine, 42*, 539–549.

Wolpe, J. (1969). *The practice of behavior therapy*. New York: Pergamon.

# 13

## The Type A Behavior Pattern: Summary, Conclusions, and Implications

DIANE F. O'ROURKE, B. KENT HOUSTON,

JANEL K. HARRIS, AND C. R. SNYDER

It is evident from the previous chapters in this volume that the formulation of the Type A behavior pattern has had a revolutionary impact on the conceptualization of the etiology of heart disease. It has arguably done as much as any other system of thought to make interdisciplinary research between the social and medical sciences a reality. However, it is just as evident from the information presented that at the present time the area is in a quandary. In contrast to the promising results obtained in early population-based studies such as the Western Collaborative Group Study (WCGS), the results of research completed after 1980 have been unclear and generally disappointing (see Haynes & Matthews, Chapter 4, this volume). These failures have generated some very hard questions about the status of the Type A behavior pattern; and questions typically posed when an area such as this is just beginning now need to be answered anew.

Heading the list of important questions are: What exactly is the Type A behavior pattern? Can this construct be reliably identified in given populations? What are the pathogenic elements of the construct? However, a more hard-nosed and central issue must also be addressed: Has the Type A construct outlived its usefulness? Is Type A dead? In Chapter 2, Rosenman, Swan, and Carmelli contend that it is not, while Williams and Barefoot, in Chapter 9, come to the opposite conclusion.

The purpose underlying this volume was to provide the opportunity to review and rethink this area in order to formulate provisional answers to these very difficult questions. The present chapter broadly reviews the major issues brought out by the authors of the chapters in this volume and highlights some of the most intriguing of the current trends and future directions in this ever-changing area.

## WHAT IS THE TYPE A BEHAVIOR PATTERN?

### Original Conceptualization

As is by now folklore in the field, the original conceptualization of the Type A behavior pattern (TABP) stemmed from the observation of two cardiologists, Drs. Friedman and Rosenman, that their patients (particularly the younger and middle-aged ones) seemed to share similar attributes and behaviors. The association of behavioral and psychological characteristics with heart disease was not a new one (see Chapter 9 by Williams & Barefoot), but Drs. Friedman and Rosenman pioneered the attempt to define the construct well enough that it could be assessed and empirically tested. The major result of their efforts was a large-scale epidemiological study, the WCGS, which prospectively tested the association of the TABP with development of coronary heart disease (CHD) in a population of more than 3000 white, middle-class males. The outcome of this study was more than promising: Subjects identified as having the Type A behavior pattern proved to be almost twice as likely (even after adjustment for more traditional risk factors) to develop clinical signs of CHD as subjects who were assessed as not evidencing these behaviors. These results provided the cornerstone for the scientific credibility of the TABP field of research.

What did Drs. Friedman and Rosenman mean by the *Type A behavior pattern*? As described in Chapter 2 by Rosenman and colleagues, the mix of behaviors and psychological characteristics noted in these patients was conceptualized as representing a specific action-emotion complex that can be observed in individuals who are "in a chronic struggle to achieve poorly defined goals or to obtain an excessive number of things from their environment and to be in habitual conflict with others and with time" (p. 8). More concretely, TABP can be described as a set of observable behaviors (e.g., accelerated pace, rapid and emphatic speech stylistics, involvement in many activities), observable emotional responses (e.g., irritation, hostility, anger), and inferred behavioral dispositions (e.g., competitiveness, ambitiousness).

The Type A behavior pattern was not conceptualized as a stable trait. Rather, Type A behaviors were conceptualized as occurring *only* in response to certain environmental stimuli. Nor was the TABP meant to imply psychopathology. The pattern was clearly described as distinct from stress-related characteristics such as chronic anxiety, worry, or neuroticism.

Obviously, in order to evaluate the association of this construct with CHD, the success or lack of success in measuring the construct must be judged. In doing this, three questions arise. First, how well do existing measures of TABP fit with the original conceptualization of the Type A construct? Second, how well do these measures predict CHD? And, third, given the recent failures to find TABP–CHD associations, is it still appropriate to measure TABP as it was originally conceptualized?

## Measurement of the Type A Behavior Pattern

**Structured Interview.** As is evident from Chapter 2 by Rosenman and colleagues and Chapter 4 by Haynes and Matthews, the general consensus at this time is that the Structured Interview (SI) is the best (at least for males) of the various TABP measurement tools available today. It was the first assessment procedure developed and was initially constructed specifically for use in the WCGS. It is unique in its emphasis on creating a context that is intended to elicit Type A behaviors from susceptible individuals. Structurally, the SI consists of a number of questions selected to obtain information about the presence of TABP characteristics. However, the wording of the questions and the manner in which the interview is conducted are intended to be somewhat challenging, to rush the interviewee to some extent, and to evoke memories of challenging or provocative situations. Speech stylistics noted by auditors of the interviews are weighted more than the content of respondents' answers to the questions in making the A–B classifications.

Given the above emphasis, it is obvious that the manner in which the interview is conducted is integral to the assessment process. Unfortunately, recent evidence suggests that this manner may have changed subtly over time. More important, Scherwitz has proposed that this change in the style of administering the SI may have promoted the recent failure of the MRFIT study to find an association between TABP and CHD (see Chapter 3).

Scherwitz and colleagues compared the style of administering the SI used in the recent MRFIT study with that employed in the earlier WCGS. This comparison revealed that the MRFIT interviewers asked questions more rapidly following interviewees' responses and interrupted the interviewees more frequently, particularly in a manner that was inconsiderate of their train of thought. Scherwitz has suggested that this interruptive style tends to disengage individuals from the interview process. Furthermore, because of the hypothesized importance of the environment in eliciting TABP behaviors, he contends that engagement with the interview is necessary to provide the context needed to elicit valid Type A behaviors from interviewees. In this view, the manner in which SI interviews were conducted in the MRFIT study did not result in valid A–B classifications, and this may be one reason why an association between TABP and CHD was not found in this study.

Data collected by Houston and colleagues (see Chapter 10 by Houston) support the contention that the style in which the SI is administered affects the findings associated with A–B status. In a study in which reactivity to a laboratory stressor was used as an outcome measure, diastolic blood pressure reactivity was found to be negatively related to Type A ratings made from interviews conducted in the more rapid "disengaging" style, while it was positively related to Type A ratings made from interviews conducted in a style modeled after that originally used in the WCGS.

These data suggest that the style in which the SI interview is conducted may be crucial to ensure that the Type A ratings that are obtained are maximally predictive of relevant cardiovascular endpoints. It does appear that to obtain Type A ratings that are predictive the interview must successfully engage individuals in the interview process.

**Self-Report Measures.**    In hopes of assessing the TABP in a more objective, cost-effective, and generally accessible manner than is possible with the SI, a number of self-report measures of TABP have been developed. By far, the most widely used self-report measure is the Jenkins Activity Survey (JAS). It was constructed specifically to mimic the SI, and items were retained based on their ability to discriminate SI-determined Type A's and Type B's. Unfortunately, even in the original validation study, the JAS was not found to predict CHD after adjustment for other risk factors (Matthews & Haynes, 1986).

The Framingham Type A Scale (FTAS) was developed from data collected for a large prospective study of heart disease, the Framingham Heart Study. The only frequently used self-report scale not validated against the SI, the FTAS consists of 10 items that were extracted from a 300-item life history questionnaire. Items were initially selected if they were judged to relate to the Type A construct and were retained on the basis of item and factor-analytic techniques (see Chapter 5 by Eaker & Castelli).

Finally, another measure that has been used in several European epidemiological studies is the Bortner Rating Scale. This measure consists of 14 adjective rating scales selected because of their applicability to the Type A construct.

**Summary.**    While the SI certainly seems to have proven vulnerable to a problem of unstandardized drift in the style of administration, the use of self-report measures in this area has been subject to even more damaging limitations. Besides the fact that self-reports are always influenced by the biases of the respondent, the absence of any method to evaluate observed behaviors is a major problem for all self-report measures given the importance of observed behaviors to the TABP conceptualization. Moreover, there is no mechanism within the administration of a self-report measure to provide the stimulus necessary to evoke the Type A behaviors.

Furthermore, as data on the various measures have accumulated, the evidence indicates that the different self-report inventories seem to assess different aspects of the TABP construct and show only modest correlations among themselves (cf. Chapter 2 by Rosenman et al. and Chapter 4 by Haynes & Matthews). The SI relates most closely to TABP as it was originally conceptualized because it measures observable behaviors. For males, it has been found to be the most sensitive in measuring general psychophysiological reactivity to events that are frustrating, difficult, or moderately competitive. Not surprisingly, it has also proven to be the most sensitive at measuring verbal characteristics such as rapid, loud, and explosive speech. The JAS is intermediate in its assessment of the original TABP concept as it taps self-reports of many of the Type A characteristics. The strength of the JAS has been in identifying achievement-oriented individuals. However, the JAS has proven to be a poor measure of the Type A characteristics of competitive drive, impatience, and potential for hostility. It also has the problem that any self-report measure will have in that it misses the observable behaviors of the TABP. The FTAS appears to have the poorest conceptual fit. First, it misses the emotional responses that are associated with the TABP. Also, it measures dissatisfaction and discomfort with a competitive orientation and with job pressures, a job and life strain factor that was not part of the original conceptual definition of the TABP.

Thus while the advantages of self-report over behavioral interviewing are readily apparent in terms of objectivity and efficiency, these inventories have not been effective in serving as an alternative to the SI. They have proven to be inadequate measures for assessing the Type A behavior pattern as it was originally conceptualized. Finally, the empirical evidence that these measures predict CHD is more equivocal for the JAS and less plentiful for the FTAS than that for the SI (see Chapter 4 by Haynes & Matthews). Although the FTAS predicted total CHD and myocardial infarction in males in the Framingham Heart Study, the relationship of this measure to the TABP is unclear.

A critical question about assessment concerns its validity across diverse populations. It has been suggested that the TABP measures available today are only appropriate for use with Caucasian, middle-class (i.e., white-collar) males. The absence of positive findings in populations such as women suggests that if coronary-prone behaviors do exist in these populations they may be manifested differently, and therefore require different assessment techniques. Thoresen and Pattillo, in Chapter 6, report an example indicative of this problem. In a study of Type A children, these authors found that the mothers of Type A children did not appear more Type A than the mothers of Type B children during assessment using the SI. However, when these women were observed during laboratory sessions in which their children were being evaluated, they did evidence significantly more Type A behaviors than did the mothers of Type B children. This suggests that the SI, as it has been administered with men, may not provide the context necessary to elicit the Type A behavior from certain types of women. Thus the context that engages Type A behavior in individuals who are predisposed to exhibiting the TABP may vary depending on gender, occupational status, and other important factors.

## WHAT IS THE ASSOCIATION OF TYPE A TO CHD?

Chapter 4 by Haynes and Matthews and Chapter 5 by Eaker and Castelli review in detail the research that has evaluated the relationship of TABP measures to various CHD outcomes. On first reading, the data produced by these studies seem confusing. However, as nicely outlined in Chapter 4, there are several important patterns to this mix of positive and negative findings. First, as was noted in the introduction to this chapter, there seems to be an important time factor to this mix. The promise of earlier research has faded in the face of the disappointing results produced by studies completed since 1978.

The type of research design employed and the population characteristics of the sample studied also seem to have been consistently associated with whether or not the TABP–CHD relation has been found. Most of the research done in this area that has used some form of CHD as an outcome can be classified into one of three types: large-scale prospective population-based studies (e.g., WCGS, the Framingham Heart Study, Belgian Heart Disease Prevention Trial, Honolulu Heart Study), prospective studies of persons designated as "high risk" (e.g., the MRFIT study), and cross-sectional angiography studies.

Population-based prospective studies that have used symptom-free males have generally provided the strongest support for the TABP as an independent risk factor for CHD. In fact, the only failure to find an association between TABP and CHD was in the Honolulu Heart Study (see Haynes & Matthews, Chapter 4, for a discussion of the possible reasons for this failure). Conversely, the results from prospective studies of individuals at high risk for CHD have failed consistently to support the idea that TABP is a risk factor either for recurrent events or for first-time CHD events in men with high levels of traditional risk factors. Results of cross-sectional studies evaluating the link between TABP and coronary artery disease (CAD) have been just as inconsistent. Additionally, the studies evaluating the association of TABP with CHD in women have consistently failed to find an association between TABP and CHD endpoints such as myocardial infarction or atherosclerosis.

The fact that these studies often used different measures of TABP, employed different subject populations, and were sometimes completed decades and continents apart enormously complicates the process of understanding the meaning of the inconsistencies. Is it that the association between TABP and CHD is actually very weak, or are there other factors that may account for the unusual patterning of positive and null findings in this area? Two prominent explanatory themes for the latter possibility have appeared throughout many of the chapters in this volume. The following sections review the major points involved in each.

## Methodological Considerations

The first theme suggests that one reason for the inconsistencies is the numerous methodological problems (see Chapter 4 by Haynes & Matthews and Chapter 9 by Williams & Barefoot) that have plagued the more recent research. Preeminent among these methodological problems has been the difficulty in obtaining accurate measurement of the construct. First, the low intercorrelations between the various self-report measures and the SI highlight concern that the various assessment instruments are actually measuring different phenomena. Several authors (e.g., Matthews & Haynes, 1986) contend that the JAS is not a valid measure of coronary-prone behavior. Thus the results from studies in which this instrument was employed are suspect. The problem of a possible shift over time in the style of administering the SI (see Chapter 3 by Scherwitz) suggests that recent studies that have used the SI may have also inaccurately assessed A–B status. Finally, as noted previously, it has been strongly suggested that there are no valid measures of TABP for any population other than Caucasian, middle-class males. The failures to find the CHD–TABP association in women and men of Japanese descent may be due to inappropriate assessment.

The growing concern that the truly pathogenic element of the TABP may be buried within the global Type A pattern also leads to questions about the appropriateness of current methods of assessment. For instance, Williams and Barefoot present strong evidence in Chapter 9 that it may be the "hostility complex" within the TABP that is the pathogenic factor. If the critical aspect of the TABP is actually only one element of the entire TABP, research in the field should be reoriented toward evaluating this possibility, and new assessment techniques would need to be developed. The search for the pathogenic element(s) within the complex of Type A behaviors makes the continued use of current assessment methods questionable (see Chapter 8 by Chesney, Hecker, & Black, Chapter 9 by Williams & Barefoot).

Most of the coronary angiography studies have been completed since 1980. As a group, these studies have suffered from several methodological problems that have reduced their statistical power to detect an association between TABP and CAD to unacceptable levels. The studies generally have been characterized by inadequate sample sizes, and in those studies using the SI, there has been a consistent overrepresentation of Type A's. The predominance of Type A's in these angiographic samples suggests that a selection factor may have been operating, and this is illustrative of the type of subtle interactional complication that can plague research in this area. For example, given the hypothesized association of the behavior pattern with CHD, physicians may take the complaints of suspected Type A patients more seriously and refer them more often for an angiographic procedure than they do their Type B patients. Also, it is possible that Type A's may be more aggressive than Type B's in obtaining care for their symptoms. Thus the very presence of the behavior pattern and its correlates may bias study populations in a manner that makes it more statistically difficult to detect the TABP–CAD relation.

Another, and perhaps more important, problem with coronary angiography studies has to do with their logic. If investigators are going to try to evaluate the relation between CAD and a risk factor, whether psychosocial or traditional, they should either study a random sample of subjects or compare subjects who are and are not suspected of having CAD. As nicely articulated in an article by Pickering (1986), studying only subjects who are suspected of having CAD, for example, angiographic patients, in an attempt to investigate the relation between CAD and a risk factor is methodologically unsound. The only study that may have been close to having employed a suitable subject sample was an autopsy study conducted on individuals who had died for reasons independent of CHD (Friedman, Rosenman, Straus, Wurm, & Kositchek, 1968). And, in this study, Type A's were found to have greater coronary occlusion than Type B's.

Other methodological problems concerning study sample characteristics have also been noted. In Chapter 9, Williams and Barefoot contend that one reason for negative findings in the angiographic studies may be that the study samples have comprised primarily older individuals who by the time of the study have already proven themselves to be "survivors." Thus Type A's for whom the pattern is a risk factor have already been naturally selected out of the study because of earlier mortality. Secondly, it may be that in studies using volunteers (such as the MRFIT project) the Type A's who are willing to commit time and energy to be studied comprise a distinct, nonrepresentative subpopulation of Type A's. Also, in studies of high-risk groups, the effects of disease status on behavior are unknown, while in the angiography studies, completing the TABP assessment just before the procedure (when subjects would be expected to be more tense and apprehensive) could conceivably bias the assessment results.

A final methodological consideration concerns identifying the population for which TABP may and may not be a risk factor. TABP may simply not be a risk factor for females. To date, the only prospective study that has included a large sample of females is the Framingham Heart Study. As detailed in Chapter 5 by Eaker and Castelli, the data indicate that Type A behavior, as defined by the FTAS, does not have the predictive relationship with CHD for females that is found in males. It is important to recognize that this failure could mean either that TABP is not a risk factor for women, or that the overt form of the behaviors and/or the characteristic environment that elicits the behaviors may be different in women than in men.

Is the prognostic value of the TABP limited to white-collar Caucasian males? The TABP as a prognostic risk factor was originally conceptualized and validated on a sample of Caucasian men employed in white-collar occupations. The Framingham Heart Study found that the prognostic value of Type A status was limited to white-collar males, and the failure to find associations of TABP with CHD for different populations such as women and white-collar men of Japanese descent certainly argues that the answer to the above question may be yes. Although it is promising that significant effects have been found for both factory workers and civil servants in the French-Belgian Cooperative Heart Study (see Chapter 4 by Haynes & Matthews), it may be that at this time, the TABP is best viewed only as a risk factor for Caucasian, white-collar males.

## Societal Changes Over Time

Moving away from methodology as an explanation, a second, intriguing, explanatory theme for the shift in the success of research in this area following the late seventies was proposed by Haynes and Matthews in Chapter 4. They suggest that one reason for the absence of positive findings in the later studies may be that changes in society have actually altered the manifestation and impact of TABP behaviors. Although the original conceptualization clearly emphasized the contextual nature of the risk associated with TABP, the unstated assumption during the 25 or so years of research that have followed its formulation is that the characteristics of both the pattern and the eliciting environment have remained stable over time. Yet the incidence of CHD is dropping. Just as widespread media attention to the health effects of smoking has drastically altered the incidence of smoking during the past 10 years, it is reasonable to assume that the same kind of attention to the danger of the "Type A personality" may have altered the behavior of individuals, as well as the behavior of organizations that had provided the environment necessary for the elicitation of these behaviors. The lone failure of a population-based prospective study was the Honolulu Heart Study, a failure that involved a sample from a population with a distinctly different cultural milieu and significantly lower incidence rates for both CHD and TABP than their Caucasian United States or European counterparts. Haynes and Matthews speculate that it may be that as changes in our society discourage many of the previously highly esteemed TABP behaviors (such as aggressive competitiveness), the prevalence and risk of Type A behaviors may decline. Thus both the nature of the beast and its habitat may be changing.

## BIOBEHAVIORAL MECHANISMS: THE LINK BETWEEN TABP AND CHD

Given the chapters of Houston (10), Williams and Barefoot (9), and Contrada, Krantz, and Hill (11), it is clear that considerable attention has been given to evaluation of the physiological mechanisms in persons assessed as being Type A that may either directly promote CHD or serve as markers of pathogenic processes. Although the exact etiology of CAD is unknown, the most widely accepted theory is that CAD results from injury to the inner walls of the arteries, the endothelium. Coronary heart disease is thought by most cardiologists to result from complications of CAD. The reasoning of researchers in this area has been that, if the presence of the Type A behaviors does increase risk for developing CHD, it should be possible to demonstrate an association between Type A and the biobehavioral mechanisms that may contribute to processes related to endothelial injury (see Chapter 9 by Williams & Barefoot).

The physiological mechanisms by which TABP is assumed to mediate the development of CAD are the activities of the sympathetic adrenal–medullary and the pituitary adrenal–cortical systems. The connection between these systems, TABP, and CHD is associational. It is known that psychological and behavioral factors can influence the activity of these systems, while excessive activity in these same systems has been implicated in CAD (see Krantz & Manuck, 1984, Chapter 9 by Williams & Barefoot for more detailed explanations). Both acute and chronic excesses have been suggested as possible avenues for the coronary pathophysiology associated with the TABP. The following sections review research on four specific biobehavioral mechanisms thought to be associated with, or markers for, the pathophysiology associated with the TABP. These mechanisms are excessive catecholamine and cardiovascular reactivity, testosterone hyper-responsivity, chronic corticoid excess, and deficient parasympathetic antagonism of sympathetic nervous system effects.

To date, the lion's share of attention has been devoted to evaluating acute changes in response to environmental stressors; that is, whether or not Type A's are characterized by excessive cardiovascular and catecholamine reactivity to stressful or challenging events (i.e., those events that have the characteristics necessary to elicit the Type A behaviors). Most investigators have evaluated cardiovascular hyperreactivity (e.g., heart rate, blood pressure) while there are also a number of studies that have looked at catecholamine differences (namely, norepinephrine, epinephrine). Other measures such as cortisol and testosterone responsivity have been investigated much less frequently. The research in this area is fully reviewed in Chapter 10 by Houston, so the following will only focus on the most salient issues.

To answer the question of whether or not Type A's are characterized by excessive physiological reactivity to their environment, it has also proven necessary to determine the nature of the environmental events that would be expected to elicit excessive reactivity from Type A's. Perusal of Chapter 10 by Houston makes it immediately clear that, as in the research linking TABP to CHD endpoints, evaluation of these questions requires that a number of factors be considered simultaneously. Different measures of TABP, different subject groups, different laboratory conditions, and different tasks have all influenced the results that have been obtained.

In general, for males working on solitary tasks, SI-defined Type A behavior has been associated with greater cardiovascular and/or catecholamine reactivity to the tasks. And in men performing tasks in a social context, SI-defined Type A behavior has been consistently associated with greater catecholamine and/or cardiovascular reactivity. The environmental stressors that most frequently produced hyperreactivity in Type A's working in the presence of others were tasks that were of moderate difficulty and involved competition, harassment, or incentive for winning.

Studies that have defined Type A behavior via the JAS have found that the optimal task and situational characteristics needed to elicit hyperresponsivity from Type A's differ slightly from those found to elicit this hyperresponsivity from SI-defined Type A's. Cardiovascular reactivity has generally been found to be higher in JAS-defined Type A, versus B, males when performing solitary tasks involving moderate probability of failure, moderate incentive, and moderate speed requirements. However, in a social context, a situation that has consistently produced differences between SI-defined A's and B's, JAS-defined Type A and B men exhibit no significant differences in reactivity. Houston speculated that this may be due to the inability of the JAS adequately to assess the TABP anger and hostility upon which reactivity in a social context may depend.

Very few studies have examined the association of reactivity with FTAS-defined Type A, and, for those studies that have, the results have been equivocal. Like the SI and JAS, the FTAS appears to measure different dimensions within the Type A pattern.

There is also evidence of A–B differences in the responsivity of testosterone. The link between excessive testosterone and CAD is circumstantial. However, increases in testosterone are associated with decreased HDL cholesterol levels (the "good" cholesterol), while exogenously administered testosterone has produced increased atheroma in rats. SI-defined Type A's have been found to respond to sensory intake tasks with greater plasma testosterone levels than are found in Type B's. A further refinement of this relationship found that Type B subjects with low Cook-Medley Hostility

(Ho) scores evidenced the smallest testosterone increases, while Type A's with high Ho scores exhibited the largest increases. Type A men have also been found to excrete excess testosterone during daytime working hours, as compared to Type B men (see Chapter 9 by Williams & Barefoot).

Chronic corticosteroid excess and deficient parasympathetic antagonism of sympathetic effects have also been proposed as mediators of the association between Type A and CHD. Corticosteroid excess is implicated in CHD development as glucocorticoids have functions that could be atherogenic (e.g., increasing serum lipids and the number of dead or injured arterial endothelial cells). Again, Chapter 9 by Williams and Barefoot details the work linking Type A to both of these biobehavioral mechanisms. Suffice it to say that this research has shown that Type A men, as compared to Type B, show increased cortisol response to laboratory tasks. Evidence of a different sort suggests that Type A's may also have a less robust parasympathetic antagonism of sympathetic effects than is found in Type B's. For example, Type A's, as compared to Type B's, show a more prolonged decrease in EKG T-wave amplitude in response to infusions of isoproterenol (a beta-adrenergic agonist). Although these results are promising, there are only a few studies that have evaluated these last two mechanisms.

In bleak contrast to the findings that relate catecholamine and cardiovascular reactivity to Type A behavior in males, there is little evidence that such a relation exists in Type A females defined by either the SI or the JAS. Few of the studies that have investigated reactivity in females have found A–B differences in reactivity. Again, it may be that one reason for these failures is that the context needed to elicit Type A behavior from females is different from that for males (perhaps due to sex-role expectations or the fact that TABP in females is not being accurately assessed). However, the generality of the failures certainly points to the possibility that TABP just may not be a useful predictor of either reactivity or CHD in women.

Researchers have also studied the relationships between reactivity and SI-defined components of Type A behavior. A summary of these findings can be found in Chapter 10 by Houston. In brief, this research indicates that cardiovascular reactivity is not related to SI components of latency, rate of response, voice emphasis, or loudness of speech. An association tends to be found between reactivity and potential for hostility, and this is the one component that has also been found to predict CHD (see Chapter 8 by Chesney et al., Chapter 10 by Houston, Chapter 2 by Rosenman et al.). However, while some studies report strong, positive associations between reactivity and the potential for hostility, other studies have found a significant negative relation with this factor. Thus overall, the findings from this body of literature are disappointing.

In conclusion, the bulk of the evidence supports the contention that, under certain conditions, there are differences between Type A and Type B males in their physiological reactivity to laboratory stressors. When SI-defined Type A males are exposed to conditions that annoy or harass them, or motivate them to accomplish something in a short time, they exhibit cardiovascular and plasma catecholamine responses that are significantly greater than those of Type B men. Possible reasons for the failure of other studies to find reactivity differences between Type A's and Type B's are the presence of uncontrolled variables (e.g., beta-blockers, physical conditioning), the use of self-report measures that do not adequately assess some critical components of the Type A pattern (e.g., potential for hostility), and the use of various types of laboratory stressors that do not provide the stimuli necessary to elicit the Type A behaviors.

## HOW DO TYPE A BEHAVIORS DEVELOP?

### The Nature-Versus-Nurture Question

If the assumption is made that TABP is associated in some fashion with an increased risk for CHD, the question of how these behaviors develop becomes important for those interested in prevention. As with questions about the etiology of almost any syndrome, researchers in this area have been interested in evaluating the possible contributions of genetics and biology versus those of environment. However, as is the case with most attempts to untangle the enmeshed contributions of these two factors, the relative role of each in the development of Type A behaviors will probably remain subject to debate for some time.

**Nature.** Although the predominant notion is that Type A behaviors are responsible for exaggerated cardiovascular and neuroendocrine reactivity to stress, there are investigators who propose that the excessive arousal noted in Type A individuals may well be the cause, rather than the consequence, of Type A behaviors. This view and the research stemming from it are described by Contrada and colleagues in Chapter 11. The precursor to the idea that Type A behaviors may have a biological basis is the early James and Lange theory of emotion that posited that emotions reflect the perception of physiological status; that is, certain visceral, skeletal, and muscular responses promote certain emotional states (cf., Fehr & Stern, 1970). Although this theory, and the more cognitively oriented reformulation of Schacter and Singer (1962), have both been controversial, there is no question that physiological arousal can affect emotions. Thus it may be that some of the emotional and behavioral characteristics of TABP comprise a response to the biological substrata of excessive autonomic arousal.

The approach of researchers interested in testing this notion has been to evaluate the effects on Type A behaviors of administering pharmacological agents capable of either blocking or enhancing sympathetic nervous system activity. The reasoning is that, if the Type A behaviors are a consequence of sympathetic nervous system (SNS) hyperreactivity, then suppression of this hyperreactivity through pharmacological means should decrease the intensity of these behaviors, while pharmacological enhancement of SNS activity should increase the intensity of the Type A behaviors.

The results produced by this line of research have been mixed. In coronary and hypertensive patients, both correlational and experimental studies have found that beta-blockers decrease SI-rated speech stylistics and potential for hostility as well as Type A scores that are assessed by self-report. Conversely, one study in which nonpatient subjects (normotensives) were used found no evidence that administration of beta-blockers moderated Type A behaviors.

Moreover, although the reports of reduced Type A behavior in coronary patients in association with beta-blocking medications are promising, the confidence that can be placed in these results is undermined by several methodological problems. The omission of placebo conditions as well as the failure to distinguish among the various classes of beta-blocking medications are two critical limitations to this research.

As detailed by Contrada and colleagues in Chapter 11, a study by Krantz and colleagues that did include the necessary controls obtained perplexing results. The effects of a beta-adrenergic agonist (isoproterenol), a beta-blocker (propranolol), and a placebo were compared. The expected physiological effects of these drugs were obtained: Cardiovascular reactivity increased following administration of the beta agonist and decreased following administration of the beta-blocker. However, *both* drugs were associated with decreases in the rated components of the Type A behavior pattern!

Data have also been obtained that indicate that there are important differences between beta-blockers that freely penetrate the blood–brain barrier (i.e., propranolol) versus those that do not (i.e., atenolol) in the impact that they have on Type A behaviors. One study that compared the two found that only the beta-blocker that freely penetrated the blood–brain barrier (propranolol) decreased overall ratings of Type A behavior. This suggests that central nervous system mechanisms may be important in mediating the behavioral effects. This finding provides little support for the notion that it may be excessive peripheral somatic feedback that fuels the overt Type A behaviors.

Thus evidence associating a reduction in autonomic arousal with an attenuation of Type A behaviors in coronary and hypertensive patients is at this time unconvincing. Further study is needed on this topic.

A second approach to evaluating the notion that biology may provide a constitutional predisposition for expression of the Type A behaviors has been to evaluate whether or not there is a genetic link to TABP. Thoresen and Pattillo outline this work in Chapter 6. To date, the data on the heritability of SI-defined Type A suggest that global Type A is not genetically determined, although some of its components such as speech stylistics and potential for hostility may be. Type A ratings between parents and their offspring tend to show similarities, and the association between fathers and sons shows the strongest correspondence. However, the degree to which these similarities reflect genetic or environmental influences remains unclear.

A–B differences linked to gender or ethnicity have also been explored (see Chapter 6 by Thoresen & Pattillo). Gender and ethnic differences in global and component measures of Type A have been reported, with boys being rated more Type A than girls, and White children rating themselves more Type A than Black children. These findings, however, have been very inconsistent.

**Nurture.**    Even if global Type A and/or its components are ultimately found to have a genetic or biological contribution, environmental events such as parent–child interactions would still have an effect on behaviors. Nurture is important, even in the event that it only influences the substrate provided by nature.

Studies that have examined the different patterns of parent (or caregiver) and child interactions for Type A and Type B children generally provide evidence suggesting that the interpersonal environment in which these two types of children grow up is likely to be significantly different. For example, both parents and caregivers tend to interact differently with Type A children than they do with non-A children. Parents of Type A children have been found to be more active and less discriminating in giving praise and criticism during their children's performance of challenging tasks than are the parents of Type B children. Also, during their child's performance of challenging tasks, fathers of Type A children were found to model more Type A behaviors while the mothers pushed the child to perform better more frequently than was observed with the parents of low Type A children. In turn, Type A children were more often found to describe their parents as more punishing or disapproving than were Type B children.

Thus the evidence associating environmental factors and A–B status is stronger than that accumulated for the biological association. A review of the careful, intriguing work undertaken by Thoresen and colleagues suggests that this research offers promise of yielding important information concerning how this behavior pattern may develop.

## Recent Conceptualizations of the TABP

Following a review of the research that has focused on Type A in children, Thoresen and Pattillo propose that the original conceptualization of the Type A behaviors needs to be expanded to include theories relevant to the development of this pattern. How does one become a person prone to exhibit Type A behaviors? These authors contend that several theories concerning the origins of insecurity are relevant to the study of Type A behavior. They contend that the anger and hostility that characterize the Type A pattern may actually stem from the quality of parent–child relationships. These authors suggest that some of the evidence produced by research on attachment theory yields potentially relevant data concerning precursors to the Type A behavior pattern. For instance, the quality of early mother–child attachment has been found to be highly predictive of the quality of social relationships the child experiences as an adult. There is also evidence that children who are described as insecurely attached–avoidant have been found to develop an anger-oriented appraisal and coping style that has many similarities to the Type A behavior pattern described in adults. Thoresen and Pattillo detail this interesting idea, and it is clear that parent–child interactions offer, if studied appropriately, a wealth of information about some of the behavioral mechanisms important to the development of Type A behaviors.

In Chapter 6, Thoresen and Pattillo propose numerous theoretical ideas that should be more systematically incorporated into research on the development of Type A behaviors. For instance, they recommend the study of narcissism and its resemblance to the Type A behaviors, the study of social–cognitive processes in understanding how Type A's construct their everyday reality, the study of coping theory and its relevance to the ways in which Type A's cope, and the study of how Type A's assign personal meaning to life events.

Another conceptualization that is remarkedly akin to the thinking espoused by Thoresen and Pattillo is the conceptualization of the origin of the Type A behaviors that is promoted by Scherwitz and Canick in Chapter 7. These authors contend that the critical factor in the Type A complex is actually an inadequately defined sense of self. This idea evolved from the empirical finding that one particular aspect of behavior during the SI, verbalized self-references, was associated with behavioral, autonomic, and emotional reactivity, as well as with overall Type A ratings and CHD. The rationale for this reasoning is detailed in their chapter. Basically, these authors suggest that a flaw in self-identity renders Type A individuals excessively vulnerable to perceiving threat in the environment. In this scheme, the competitive, aggressive, and hurried behaviors that have comprised the overt manifestations of the TABP are viewed as defensive responses to the perceived threats of the environment.

## TREATMENT OF TYPE A BEHAVIOR

At this time, the Type A behavior pattern occupies the unique position of being the first psychosocial risk factor for which there is evidence suggesting that modification of it may be associated with a reduction in clinical disease. Given the problems with measurement, conceptualization, and obtaining appropriate study samples that have been reviewed throughout this volume, the evidence concerning the impact of modification of the Type A behaviors on future disease is remarkable. The issues that emerge from the attempts to construct and evaluate treatment and the results that have been obtained from these efforts are reviewed in Chapter 12 by Price. The following simply summarizes her most salient points.

There are two interrelated questions that have been addressed in this area: Can Type A behaviors be changed via treatment? and, more important, If Type A behaviors are changed, will this change be associated with a reduction in either the incidence or the recurrence of CHD? There are currently three well-designed studies that address these questions: the Recurrent Coronary Prevention Project (RCPP); the Montreal Type A Intervention Project (MTAIP); and the United States Army War College Study (USAWC).

Although there are numerous small-scale studies of Type A modification, the confidence placed in the results of these studies is generally limited by various conceptual or methodological problems evident in their designs. In contrast, the RCPP, and MTAIP, and the USAWC have provided rather convincing evidence that Type A behaviors can be altered. And one of these, the RCPP, suggests that reduction in manifest Type A behavior is associated with reduced risk for recurring coronary disease. Each of these studies used a structured interview method of assessing Type A behavior (either the SI or the Videotaped Structured Interview; see Chapter 12 by Price) and also collected data on the physiological variables believed to mediate the Type A–CHD relation.

The treatment approaches varied somewhat across studies. In both the RCPP, a 4.5-year comprehensive treatment program designed to reduce Type A behavior in postcoronary patients, and the USAWC, a 9-month study of healthy Type A military officers, treatment components were theoretically linked to the Type A construct and were designed to have a direct impact on Type A behaviors such as hostility, competitiveness, and time urgency. The programs included instruction, modeling, and reinforcement for making behavioral (and cognitive) changes that were regarded as being in the Type B direction. Results of these studies indicated that overt Type A behaviors were modified in a large percentage of the subjects, while the data from the RCPP indicated that in the coronary patients, these reductions were also associated with significant reductions in coronary recurrences.

In contrast to the RCPP and USAWC, the MTAIP adopted a treatment approach designed to enhance general coping abilities rather than to modify specific aspects of the Type A behavior pattern. Program components included relaxation training, communication training, cognitive restructuring, stress inoculation, and problem solving. Participants also planned, self-monitored, practiced, and evaluated their newly learned coping strategies. The results of this study revealed that healthy Type A managers who received coping skills training showed significant decreases in Type A behavior, as compared to their peers who participated in either an aerobic training or a weight-lifting program. It is interesting to note that finding that improving general coping skills actually reduced manifested Type A behaviors is compatible with the notion that the Type A behaviors may be an assortment of rather maladaptive, defensive coping behaviors.

Although each of the three Type A behavior treatment programs just described produced changes in overt Type A behaviors, none produced changes in the physiological variables believed to mediate the relation between Type A and CHD. This anomaly suggests that the biobehavioral mechanisms whereby Type A behavior increases risk for incidence or recurrence of CHD may be inadequately measured by traditional procedures for physiological assessment.

Clarification of the biobehavioral mechanisms that mediate reduced risk for recurring CHD is just one of several issues raised by this area of research. Price argues that a much more important goal for those interested in treatment is the need to define Type B behavior, and she details a conceptual and working model for the definition of Type B behavior in Chapter 12. Price points to the need for more sensitive and more direct behaviorally anchored measures of Type A. Another issue of concern highlighted by Price is the need for greater emphasis on altering the components of Type A that are found to be toxic. Finally, she suggests that persons interested in the modification of TABP should pay greater attention to the individual's work and family milieu and the interaction of these with other personality characteristics that may influence coronary proneness such as anger expression (also see Chapter 4 by Haynes & Matthews).

## BEYOND TYPE A

Given the multiplicity and the complexity of these problems, what steps are needed to respond adequately to the contradictory findings within the field? Certainly, the bulk of the evidence weighs in favor of the hypothesized relationship of TABP with manifestations of CHD. The data do not suggest that the usefulness of the construct is over. However, both the contradictions in the field and the thoughtful reasons that have been promoted to explain these contradictions suggest that the original conceptualization of the Type A behavior pattern and the methodology in this field are currently too immature to address the multitude of factors that are encompassed by this construct.

There are scattered references in each of the chapters in this volume to potential methodological refinements that should be incorporated into future research. For instance, Haynes and Matthews suggest that obtaining estimates over time of the prevalence of Type A behavior as well as data regarding the prevalence of TABP in populations other than Caucasian males would help. If this were done, the makeup of future study samples could then be more closely matched to the characteristics of the population of interest. The statistical power of such studies would then be strengthened.

Thoresen and Pattillo argue that appropriate assessment *requires* a multimethod, multimodal approach. And they suggest that naturalistic observations should be included among the various measures designed to tap the perceptual–cognitive, behavioral, and physiologic features of the Type A pattern. They also contend that carefully documented clinical case studies that employ naturalistic observation techniques could be used as a means of discovering the possible antecedents and consequences of Type A behavior and of tracking its development over time. In this manner, the development of these behaviors could be studied in the context in which they occur.

Another potential methodological improvement has been suggested by Houston in Chapter 10. Houston contends that it may be very important to identify the natural interrelationships between the various Type A characteristics. He proposes that one way to do this in the future may be through cluster analysis. Cluster-analytic techniques could be employed to identify different groups of individuals who share the same patterns or interrelations of Type A characteristics. Houston details one study in which he and his colleagues applied cluster analyses to identify empirically derived subgroups within the global Type A pattern. They found that, for both men and women, assignment to the empirically derived subgroups improved the prediction of cardiovascular reactivity over what was obtained when they were assigned to the groups according to the traditional A–B classification scheme. Thus another alternative available to future investigators that has not been used in previous research would be to employ empirically defined subgroups of Type A subjects.

Despite the numerous methodological flaws that have been uncovered and the various remedies that have been promoted to correct these, the strongest pressure in the field seems to be toward fashioning basic changes in the conceptualization of the Type A construct. There appears to be a simultaneous push within this area in two ostensibly diverse directions. One direction emphasizes isolating and breaking out the pathogenic elements from the total matrix of TABP behaviors (microanalysis), while a second direction emphasizes the importance of exploring the contribution of the environment in both defining and eliciting the TABP (macroanalysis). Both views are similar in the emphasis that, in order for the ideas encapsulated in the original notion of Type A to continue to contribute to our knowledge of the association of psychosocial factors to CHD, investigators must flexibly respond to the questions raised by the ambiguities of the more recent research.

### Microanalysis

As is clear from the previous chapters, the original emphasis on one global pattern has yielded ground to a second perspective in which the components of the overall pattern have been investigated separately in the hopes of finding the "toxic" elements. For the most part, the recent component emphasis is not theory driven, but has evolved in response to empirical findings that some aspects of SI-derived measures of TABP have proven to be more predictive of CHD than the global measure. The work by Chesney and colleagues that is described in this volume exemplifies very systematic and careful research of this kind.

The component of Type A that has been found to be the most consistent and strongest predictor of CHD is the potential for hostility. Several other characteristics or components have also been found to predict CHD. Specifically, studies have found relations between CHD and measures of self-involvement, competitiveness, speech stylistics, and self-reports of anger. Unfortunately, there have been some inconsistencies in the evidence concerning the predictiveness of these various components and/or how these components are measured. Once again, the problems of measurement (e.g., differences between studies in delineating and operationalizing what is to be measured; problems of reliability, etc.) may be some of the reasons for the discrepancies that have been found.

If one considers the findings for these characteristics in terms of conceptual categories, the search for the pathogenic elements within the TABP has produced some results that do have some consistency. As is obvious from reading Chapter 2 by Rosenman and colleagues and Chapter 9 by Williams and Barefoot, individual investigators differentiate research that has evaluated the potential for hostility regarded as reflecting TABP hostility (see Chapter 2 by Rosenman et al.) from the research on the Cook-Medley Ho scale (see Chapter 9 by Williams and Barefoot). However, both lines of research are complementary: Scores on both measures have been found to predict the extent of CAD, and scores for potential for hostility and the Ho scale show modest intercorrelations. The Type A hostility as measured by a component scoring system for the SI is defined behaviorally as a hostile style of interacting with the interviewer and a predisposition to respond to numerous situations with various manifestations of anger, while Ho as measured by the Cook-Medley scale is conceptualized more as an attributional tendency toward cynicism and a generalized distrust of others. Despite this, both constructs seem to share a common conceptual theme, although the supraordinate construct that encompasses them both has yet to be defined.

Williams and Barefoot contend that the Cook-Medley Ho scale taps into a coronary-prone "hostility complex" that represents a distillation of the "toxic" element contained within the Type A behavior pattern. Even though the Ho scale may not measure hostility that traditionally has been related to the TABP, the constellation of anger-related attributes and behaviors reflected in the hostility complex has been demonstrated to have important consequences for CHD. Thus investigation of the contribution of hostility and related attributes to CHD represents an area of substantial current interest and a major direction for future research regarding coronary-prone behaviors.

## Macroanalysis

Turning next to the macroanalysis of Type A, there is growing interest in identifying environmental factors and/or other personality dimensions that may influence the predictiveness of Type A. One reason for the inconsistent findings on the association between Type A and either CAD or CHD may be that important moderators of the TABP–CHD relationship have not been considered in the typical research design.

For example, variations in both vocational and interpersonal environments have been associated with modifications of the TABP–CHD relation. A greater incidence of CHD has been found for FTAS-defined Type A males than for Type B males in white-collar jobs, but this A–B association with CHD has not been found for males in blue-collar occupations (see Chapter 4 by Haynes & Matthews). With regard to interpersonal environment, relatively greater CHD has been found for SI-defined Type A men married to women who were more dominant, exhibited a greater activity level, and had 13 or more years of schooling (Carmelli, Swan, & Rosenman, 1985). Similarly, relatively greater CHD was found for FTAS-defined Type A men who were married to women who were Type B, had 13 or more years of schooling, and worked outside the home (Eaker, Haynes, & Feinleib, 1983). The latter association was more prominent for blue-collar than white-collar men. With regard to other personality characteristics, Haynes (in Matthews & Haynes, 1986) reports finding relatively greater incidence of CHD for FTAS-defined Type A white-collar males who inhibit their anger (i.e., do not show their anger outwardly).

It appears, then, that certain environmental circumstances as well as personality characteristics may confer a greater risk of CHD for Type A's and thus provide a larger context in which to view the operation of coronary-prone behaviors. This makes sense because psychosocial variables operate not in isolation, but rather in the framework of environmental factors and other psychosocial variables.

The findings concerning the environmental factors that interact with Type A strengthen the original emphasis in the formulation of Type A (see Chapter 2 by Rosenman et al.) that the milieu plays an important role in eliciting the TABP. These results reinforce the recommendation of Haynes and Matthews to broaden the scope of the typical research inquiry. Specific research is needed to delineate how the factors that are found in the work environment (e.g., job demands, job control, competition with others), in the family environment (e.g., marital conflict, social support), and in other aspects of personality (e.g., anger expression, trust of others) may interact with Type A to confer greater risk.

Given all of the above, it is clear that there will not be one right answer to the question of how to ensure the continuation of the ground-breaking work started by Rosenman and Friedman. Even if the microanalytic dissection of the TABP was successful in identifying the important risk-related components of the TABP, the data that have been collected indicate that the context in which these risk factors operate is of great importance. Thus the way for the future seems to be one that synthesizes the microanalytic approach with the macroanalytic view.

In conclusion, Type A is at a crossroads. Progress in this area will continue only if keen and inventive solutions to the problems that have been enumerated throughout this volume are devised. There is no question that measurement is a momentous problem. Self-report methods have not proven to be a viable alternative to individualized interviews for measurement of the entire Type A complex. The best assessment device available, the SI, seems to be effective only with Caucasian middle-class males. Conceptualization is also in flux. Although there does seem to be a general consensus about the behaviors originally portrayed by Friedman and Rosenman as pivotal to the Type A construct, the more important question seems now to be what aspect or component of the original construct should be measured. Once answered, the question then needs to be reanswered for women and populations other than Caucasian males. It is now obvious that researchers can no longer ignore the other half of the risk equation originally developed by Friedman and Rosenman. The influence of the environment must be incorporated into the designs of future research so that impact of the person–situation interactions on the TABP–CHD relation can be assessed. Consideration needs to be given to how the job, family, and perhaps other environments interact with coronary-prone characteristics in increasing risk for CHD.

The list of problems is long, yet the possibilities seem exciting. Despite all of the obstacles just named, the data continue to suggest that, for males, there is an association between something captured within the Type A construct and manifestations of CHD. It is hoped that the issues that have been addressed in this volume will serve as useful guides to investigators interested in continuing to define and refine what is meant by "coronary-prone behaviors."

## REFERENCES

Carmelli, D., Swan, G. E., & Rosenman, R. H. (1985). The relationship between wives' social and psychologic status and their husbands' coronary heart disease: A case-control family study from the Western Collaborative Group Study. *American Journal of Epidemiology, 122,* 90–100.

Eaker, E. D., Haynes, S. G., & Feinleib, M. (1983). Spouse behavior and coronary heart disease in men: Prospective results from the Framingham Heart Study II. Modifications of risk in Type A husbands according to the social and psychological status of their wives. *American Journal of Epidemiology, 118,* 23–41.

Fehr, F. S., & Stern, J. A. (1970). Peripheral physiological variables and emotion: The James-Lange theory revisited. *Psychological Bulletin, 74,* 411–424.

Friedman, M., Rosenman, R. H., Straus, R., Wurm, M., & Kositchek, R. (1968). The relationship of behavior pattern A to the state of the coronary vasculature: A study of 51 autopsied subjects. *American Journal of Medicine, 44,* 525–538.

Krantz, D. S., & Manuck, S. B. (1984). Acute psychophysiologic reactivity and risk of cardiovascular disease: A review and methodologic critique. *Psychological Bulletin, 96,* 435–465.

Matthews, K. A., & Haynes, S. G. (1986). Type A behavior pattern and coronary risk: Update and critical evaluation. *American Journal of Epidemiology, 123,* 923–960.

Pickering, T. G. (1985). Should studies of patients undergoing coronary angiography be used to evaluate the role of behavioral risk factors for coronary heart disease? *Journal of Behavioral Medicine, 8,* 203–213.

Schacter, S., & Singer, J. (1962). Cognitive, social and physiologic determinants of emotional state. *Psychological Review, 69,* 379–399.

# Author Index

# Subject Index